Cardiovascular
Physiology

OTHER BOOKS IN THE SERIES

Endocrine Physiology
by Susan P. Porterfield, PhD

Gastrointestinal Physiology, 5th edition
by Leonard R. Johnson, PhD

Renal Physiology, 2nd edition
by Bruce M. Koeppen, MD, PhD, and Bruce A. Stanton, PhD

Cardiovascular Physiology

Seventh Edition

Robert M. Berne, MD, DSc (Hon)

Professor of Physiology, Emeritus
Department of Physiology
University of Virginia School of Medicine
Charlottesville, Virginia

Matthew N. Levy, MD

Chief of Investigative Medicine
Mount Sinai Medical Center;
Professor Emeritus of Physiology and Biomedical
Engineering
Case Western Reserve University
Cleveland, Ohio

 Mosby

St. Louis Baltimore Boston Carlsbad Chicago Naples New York Philadelphia Portland
London Madrid Mexico City Singapore Sydney Tokyo Toronto Wiesbaden

Vice President and Publisher: Anne S. Patterson
Editor: Emma D. Underdown
Developmental Editor: Christy Wells
Project Manager: Linda Clarke
Associate Production Editor: Deborah Ann Cicirello
Series Design: Elizabeth Fett
Manufacturing Manager: William A. Winneberger, Jr.
Cover Art: GW Graphics

SEVENTH EDITION

Copyright © 1997 by Mosby–Year Book, Inc.

Previous editions copyrighted 1967, 1972, 1977, 1981, 1986, 1992

Printed in the United States of America
Composition by Top Graphics
Printing/binding by R.R. Donnelley & Sons Co.

Mosby–Year Book, Inc.
11830 Westline Industrial Drive
St. Louis, Missouri 63146

Library of Congress Cataloging-in-Publication Data
Berne, Robert M., 1918-
    Cardiovascular physiology / Robert M. Berne, Matthew N. Levy.—
7th ed.
        p.   cm.
    Includes bibliographical references and index.
    ISBN 0-8151-0901-6
    1. Cardiovascular system—Physiology.   I. Levy, Matthew N., 1922-
II. Title.
    [DNLM: 1. Cardiovascular System—physiology.   WG 102 B525c 1997]
QP102.B47   1997
612.1—dc20
DNLM/DLC
for Library of Congress   96-28899
                                                                    CIP

97 98 99 00 01 / 9 8 7 6 5 4 3 2 1

To our Grandchildren
Alex, Ari, Christopher, Daniel, Kyle, Madelyn,
Maggie, Molly, Nicolas, Sarah, Todd, and Tracy

Preface

This book is designed primarily for medical and graduate students. Therefore, we have emphasized general concepts and have minimized extraneous, isolated facts. Furthermore, we carefully selected the references at the end of each chapter. Review articles were preferred over scientific papers, and the scientific articles we included were chosen for their depth, clarity, and timeliness; for their appropriateness for the beginning student; and for their bibliographies.

Throughout the book we have incorporated the most recent information and have indicated which subjects are still controversial. Emphasis is placed on control mechanisms. To present a clear view of the various regulatory mechanisms, the component parts of the system are first discussed individually. Then, to show how the entire cardiovascular system operates in an intact subject, the last chapter describes how various individual components are coordinated to allow the body to respond to two important stresses—exercise and hemorrhage.

Normal physiology serves as a frame of reference that students of medicine must comprehend before they can understand the derangements caused by disease or toxic agents. Pathophysiology is considered very selectively in this text. Many examples of abnormal function have been added in this edition to illustrate and clarify normal physiologic processes. These clinical examples are scattered throughout the text and are emphasized by color boxes.

The book has been updated and revised extensively. Several old figures have been deleted and many new figures have been added to facilitate comprehension of the textual material. Throughout the book, italics are used to emphasize important facts and concepts, and boldface type is used for new terms and definitions. Each chapter includes a summary to highlight key points. To help in review, self-study problems are provided at the end of each chapter. Appendix A contains the answers to these problems, and Appendix B includes a multiple choice review examination with answers.

We wish to thank our readers for their constructive comments in the past, and we hope that they will continue to provide the input necessary for us to improve future editions. We also wish to thank the numerous investigators and publishers who have granted us permission to use illustrations from their publications. In most cases these illustrations have been altered somewhat to increase their didactic utility. In some cases unpublished data from our own investigations have been presented.

Robert M. Berne
Matthew N. Levy

vii

Contents

1 The Circuitry, 1

SUMMARY, 4
KEY WORDS AND CONCEPTS, 6
SELF-STUDY PROBLEMS, 6

2 Electrical Activity of the Heart, 7

TRANSMEMBRANE POTENTIALS, 7
  Principal Types of Cardiac Action
    Potentials, 9
  Ionic Basis of the Resting Potential, 9
  Ionic Basis of the Fast Response, 12
  Ionic Basis of the Slow Response, 22
CONDUCTION IN CARDIAC FIBERS, 22
  Conduction of the Fast Response, 23
  Conduction of the Slow Response, 24
CARDIAC EXCITABILITY, 24
  Fast Response, 25
  Slow Response, 25
  Effects of Cycle Length, 26
NATURAL EXCITATION OF THE HEART, 26
  Sinoatrial Node, 27
  Ionic Basis of Automaticity, 29
  Overdrive Suppression, 30
  Atrial Conduction, 31
  Atrioventricular Conduction, 32
  Ventricular Conduction, 36
REENTRY, 38
TRIGGERED ACTIVITY, 39
  Early Afterdepolarizations, 39
  Delayed Afterdepolarizations, 40
ELECTROCARDIOGRAPHY, 41
  Scalar Electrocardiography, 41
ARRHYTHMIAS, 44
  Altered Sinoatrial Rhythms, 44
  Atrioventricular Transmission
    Blocks, 45
  Premature Depolarizations, 45
  Ectopic Tachycardias, 46
  Fibrillation, 47
SUMMARY, 49
KEY WORDS AND CONCEPTS, 51
SELF-STUDY PROBLEMS, 52

3 The Cardiac Pump, 55

STRUCTURE OF THE HEART IN RELATION TO
    FUNCTION, 55
  Myocardial Cell, 55
  Excitation-Contraction Coupling, 61
  Myocardial Contractile Machinery and
    Contractility, 63
  Indices of Contractility, 66
  Cardiac Chambers, 66
  Cardiac Valves, 68
  The Pericardium, 71
  Heart Sounds, 71
CARDIAC CYCLE, 73
  Ventricular Systole, 73
  Ventricular Diastole, 74
MEASUREMENT OF CARDIAC OUTPUT, 76
  Fick Principle, 76
  Indicator Dilution Techniques, 78
SUMMARY, 79
KEY WORDS AND CONCEPTS, 79
SELF-STUDY PROBLEMS, 80

4   Regulation of the Heartbeat, 83

NERVOUS CONTROL OF HEART RATE, 83
   Parasympathetic Pathways, 84
   Sympathetic Pathways, 86
   Control by Higher Centers, 87
   Baroreceptor Reflex, 88
   Bainbridge Reflex and Atrial Receptors, 89
   Respiratory Cardiac Arrhythmia, 90
   Chemoreceptor Reflex, 92
   Ventricular Receptor Reflexes, 94
INTRINSIC REGULATION OF MYOCARDIAL
   PERFORMANCE, 95
   Frank-Starling Mechanism, 96
   Rate-Induced Regulation, 99
EXTRINSIC REGULATION OF MYOCARDIAL
   PERFORMANCE, 102
   Nervous Control, 102
   Chemical Control, 106
SUMMARY, 110
KEY WORDS AND CONCEPTS, 110
SELF-STUDY PROBLEMS, 111

5   Hemodynamics, 113

VELOCITY OF THE BLOODSTREAM, 113
RELATIONSHIP BETWEEN VELOCITY AND
   PRESSURE, 114
RELATIONSHIP BETWEEN PRESSURE AND FLOW, 116
RESISTANCE TO FLOW, 120
   Resistances in Series and in Parallel, 121
LAMINAR AND TURBULENT FLOW, 124
SHEAR STRESS ON THE VESSEL WALL, 126
RHEOLOGIC PROPERTIES OF BLOOD, 126
SUMMARY, 131
KEY WORDS AND CONCEPTS, 132
SELF-STUDY PROBLEMS, 132

6   The Arterial System, 135

HYDRAULIC FILTER, 135
ARTERIAL ELASTICITY, 137
DETERMINANTS OF ARTERIAL BLOOD
   PRESSURE, 140
   Mean Arterial Pressure, 141
   Pulse Pressure, 144
PERIPHERAL ARTERIAL PRESSURE CURVES, 147
BLOOD PRESSURE MEASUREMENT IN HUMANS, 149
SUMMARY, 150

KEY WORDS AND CONCEPTS, 151
SELF-STUDY PROBLEMS, 151

**7   The Microcirculation and
     Lymphatics, 153**

VASOACTIVE ROLE OF ENDOTHELIUM, 157
PASSIVE ROLE OF ENDOTHELIUM, 158
   Transcapillary Exchange, 158
LYMPHATICS, 167
SUMMARY, 168
KEY WORDS AND CONCEPTS, 168
SELF-STUDY PROBLEMS, 169

**8   The Peripheral Circulation and Its
     Control, 171**

VASCULAR SMOOTH MUSCLE, 171
INTRINSIC OR LOCAL CONTROL OF PERIPHERAL
   BLOOD FLOW, 175
   Autoregulation and Myogenic Regulation, 175
   Endothelium-Mediated Regulation, 177
   Metabolic Regulation, 177
EXTRINSIC CONTROL OF PERIPHERAL BLOOD
   FLOW, 180
   Neural Sympathetic Vasoconstriction, 180
   Sympathetic Constrictor Influence on
      Resistance and Capacitance Vessels, 181
   Parasympathetic Neural Influence, 182
   Humoral Factors, 182
   Vascular Reflexes, 183
BALANCE BETWEEN EXTRINSIC AND INTRINSIC
   FACTORS IN REGULATION OF PERIPHERAL
   BLOOD FLOW, 190
SUMMARY, 192
KEY WORDS AND CONCEPTS, 192
SELF-STUDY PROBLEMS, 193

**9   Control of Cardiac Output: Coupling
     of Heart and Blood Vessels, 195**

VASCULAR FUNCTION CURVE, 195
   Venous Pressure Dependence on Cardiac
      Output, 200
   Blood Volume, 201
   Venomotor Tone, 202
   Blood Reservoirs, 202

Peripheral Resistance, 203
INTERRELATIONSHIPS BETWEEN CARDIAC OUTPUT
   AND VENOUS RETURN, 204
COUPLING BETWEEN HEART AND
   VASCULATURE, 204
   Myocardial Contractility, 205
   Blood Volume, 207
   Peripheral Resistance, 208
FUNCTION OF THE RIGHT VENTRICLE, 208
ROLE OF HEART RATE, 211
ANCILLARY FACTORS THAT AFFECT THE VENOUS
   SYSTEM AND CARDIAC OUTPUT, 213
   Gravity, 214
   Muscular Activity and Venous Valves, 216
   Respiratory Activity, 217
   Artificial Respiration, 219
SUMMARY, 219
KEY WORDS AND CONCEPTS, 220
SELF-STUDY PROBLEMS, 220

10   Coronary Circulation, 223

FUNCTIONAL ANATOMY OF CORONARY
   VESSELS, 223
FACTORS THAT INFLUENCE CORONARY BLOOD
   FLOW, 225
   Physical Factors, 225
   Neural and Neurohumoral Factors, 227
   Metabolic Factors, 228
EFFECTS OF DIMINISHED CORONARY BLOOD
   FLOW, 230
CORONARY COLLATERAL CIRCULATION AND
   VASODILATORS, 231
CARDIAC OXYGEN CONSUMPTION AND WORK, 233
CARDIAC EFFICIENCY, 234
SUBSTRATE UTILIZATION, 235
SUMMARY, 236
KEY WORDS AND CONCEPTS, 236
SELF-STUDY PROBLEMS, 237

11   Special Circulations, 239

CUTANEOUS CIRCULATION, 239
   Regulation of Skin Blood Flow, 239
   Skin Color: Relationship to Skin Blood
      Volume, Oxyhemoglobin, and Blood
      Flow, 242
SKELETAL MUSCLE CIRCULATION, 242
   Regulation of Skeletal Muscle Blood Flow, 243

CEREBRAL CIRCULATION, 244
   Estimation of Cerebral Blood Flow, 245
   Regulation of Cerebral Blood Flow, 246
PULMONARY CIRCULATION, 248
   Functional Anatomy, 248
   Pulmonary Hemodynamics, 250
   Regulation of the Pulmonary Circulation, 252
RENAL CIRCULATION, 253
   Anatomy, 253
   Renal Hemodynamics, 253
   Regulation of the Renal Circulation, 255
SPLANCHNIC CIRCULATION, 257
   Intestinal Circulation, 258
   Hepatic Circulation, 259
FETAL CIRCULATION, 261
   Circulatory Changes That Occur at Birth, 263
SUMMARY, 264
KEY WORDS AND CONCEPTS, 266
SELF-STUDY PROBLEMS, 266

**12   Interplay of Central and Peripheral
       Factors in the Control of the
       Circulation, 269**

EXERCISE, 269
   Mild to Moderate Exercise, 270
   Severe Exercise, 273
   Postexercise Recovery, 274
   Limits of Exercise Performance, 274
   Physical Training and Conditioning, 275
HEMORRHAGE, 276
   Course of Arterial Blood Pressure
      Changes, 276
   Compensatory Mechanisms, 276
   Decompensatory Mechanisms, 280
   Interactions of Positive and Negative
      Feedback Mechanisms, 282
SUMMARY, 283
KEY WORDS AND CONCEPTS, 283
SELF-STUDY PROBLEMS, 284

**APPENDIX A   Answers to Self-Study
             Problems, 287**

APPENDIX B   Review Examination, 299

The Circuitry

The circulatory, endocrine, and nervous systems constitute the principal coordinating and integrating systems of the body. Whereas the nervous system is primarily concerned with communications and the endocrine glands with regulation of certain body functions, the circulatory system serves to transport and distribute essential substances to the tissues and to remove by-products of metabolism. The circulatory system also shares in such homeostatic mechanisms as regulation of body temperature, humoral communication throughout the body, and adjustments of oxygen and nutrient supply in different physiologic states.

The cardiovascular system that accomplishes these chores is made up of a pump, a series of distributing and collecting tubes, and an extensive system of thin vessels that permit rapid exchange between the tissues and the vascular channels. The primary purpose of this text is to discuss the function of the components of the vascular system and the control mechanisms (with their checks and balances) that are responsible for alteration of blood distribution necessary to meet the changing requirements of different tissues in response to a wide spectrum of physiologic and pathologic conditions.

Before considering the function of the parts of the circulatory system in detail, it is useful to consider it as a whole in a purely descriptive sense. The heart consists of two pumps in series: one to propel blood through the lungs for exchange of oxygen and carbon dioxide (the **pulmonary circulation**) and the other to propel blood to all other tissues of the body (the **systemic circulation**). Unidirectional flow through the heart is achieved by the appropriate arrangement of effective flap valves. Although the cardiac output is intermittent, continuous flow to the periphery occurs by distension of the aorta and its branches during ventricular contraction **(systole)** and elastic recoil of the walls of the large arteries with forward propulsion of the blood during ventricular relaxation **(diastole).** Blood moves rapidly through the aorta and its arterial branches. The branches become narrower and their walls become thinner and change histologically toward the periphery. From a predominantly elastic structure, the aorta, the peripheral arteries become more muscular until at the arterioles the muscular layer predominates (Figure 1-1).

1

Figure 1-1 ■ Internal diameter, wall thickness, and relative amounts of the principal components of the vessel walls of the various blood vessels that compose the circulatory system. Cross sections of the vessels are not drawn to scale because of the huge range from aorta and venae cavae to capillary. (Redrawn from Burton AC: *Physiol Rev* 34:619, 1954.)

In the large arteries, frictional resistance is relatively small and pressures are only slightly less than in the aorta. However, the small arteries offer moderate resistance to blood flow and this resistance reaches a maximal level in the arterioles, sometimes referred to as the stopcocks of the vascular system. Hence *the pressure drop is significant in the small arteries and is greatest across the arterioles* (Figure 1-2). Adjustment in the degree of contraction of the circular muscle of these small vessels permits regulation of tissue blood flow and aids in the control of arterial blood pressure.

In addition to a sharp reduction in pressure across the arterioles, there is also a change from pulsatile to steady flow as pressure continues to decline from the arterial to the venous end of the capillaries (Figure 1-3). *The **pulsatile arterial blood flow**, caused by the intermittency of cardiac ejection, is damped at the capillary level by the combination of distensibility of the large arteries and frictional resistance in the arterioles.*

In a patient with hyperthyroidism **(Graves disease),** the basal metabolism is elevated and is often associated with arteriolar vasodilation. This reduction in arteriolar resistance diminishes the dampening effect on the pulsatile arterial pressure and is manifest as pulsatile flow in the capillaries, as observed in the finger nailbed of patients with this ailment.

Many capillaries arise from each arteriole so that the total cross-sectional area of the capillary bed is very large, despite the fact that the cross-sectional area of each capillary is less than that of each arteriole. As a result, blood flow velocity becomes quite slow in the capillaries, analogous to the decrease in velocity of flow (Figure 1-3) seen at the wide regions of a river. Because the capillaries consist of short tubes whose walls are only one cell thick and because flow velocity is low, conditions in the capillaries are ideal for the ex-

Figure 1-2 ■ **Pressure drop across the vascular system in the hamster cheek pouch.** *AP*, **Mean arterial pressure;** *VP*, **venous pressure.** (Redrawn from Davis MJ et al: *Am J Physiol* 250:H291, 1986.)

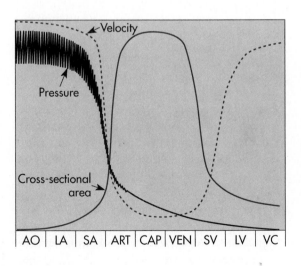

Figure 1-3 ■ **Phasic pressure, velocity of flow, and cross-sectional area of the systemic circulation.** *The important features are the inverse relationship between velocity and cross-sectional area, the major pressure drop across the small arteries and arterioles, and the maximal cross-sectional area and minimal flow rate in the capillaries.* *AO*, Aorta; *LA*, large arteries; *SA*, small arteries; *ART*, arterioles; *CAP*, capillaries; *VEN*, venules; *SV*, small veins; *LV*, large veins; *VC*, venae cavae.

change of diffusible substances between blood and tissue.

On its return to the heart from the capillaries, blood passes through venules and then through veins of increasing size with a progressive decrease in pressure until the blood reaches the right atrium (Figure 1-2). As the heart is approached, the number of veins decreases, the thickness and composition of the vein walls change (Figure 1-1), the total cross-sectional area of the venous channels diminishes, and the **velocity of blood flow** increases (Figure 1-3). Note that the velocity of blood flow and the cross-sectional area at each level of the vasculature are essentially mirror images (Figure 1-3).

Data from a 20-kg dog (Table 1-1) indicate that between the aorta and the capillaries the number of vessels increases about 3 billion fold, and the total cross-sectional area increases about 500-fold. The volume of blood in the systemic vascular system is greatest in the veins and venules (67%). It is only 5% of the total blood volume in the capillaries and 11% in the aorta, arteries, and arterioles. In contrast, blood volume in the pulmonary vascular bed is about equally divided among the arterial, capillary, and venous vessels. The cross-sectional area of the venae cavae is larger than that of the aorta. Therefore, the velocity of flow is slower in the venae cavae than that in the aorta (Figure 1-3).

Blood entering the right ventricle via the right atrium is pumped through the pulmonary arterial system at a mean pressure about one seventh that in the systemic arteries. The blood then passes through the lung capillaries, where carbon dioxide is released and oxygen taken up. The oxygen-rich blood returns via the pulmonary veins to the left atrium and ventricle to complete the cycle. Thus, in the normal intact circulation, the total volume of blood is constant, and an increase in the volume of blood in one area must be accompanied by a decrease in an-

other. However, the distribution of the circulating blood to the different regions of the body is determined by the output of the left ventricle and by the contractile state of the arterioles (resistance vessels) of these regions. The circulatory system is composed of conduits arranged in series and in parallel (Figure 1-4).

■ SUMMARY

1. The greatest resistance to blood flow, and hence the greatest pressure drop, in the arterial system occurs at the level of the small arteries and the arterioles.

TABLE 1 - 1

Vascular dimensions in a 20-kg dog

Vessels	No.	Total cross-sectional area (cm^2)	Total blood volume (%)
Systemic			
Aorta	1	2.8	
Arteries	40-110,000	40	11
Arterioles	2.8×10^6	55	
Capillaries	2.7×10^9	1357	5
Venules	1×10^7	785	
Veins	660,000-110	631	67
Venae cavae	2	3.1	
Pulmonary			
Arteries and arterioles	$1-1.5 \times 10^6$	137	3
Capillaries	2.7×10^9	1357	4
Venules and veins	2×10^6 -4	210	5
Heart			
Atria	2		5
Ventricles	2		

Data from Milnor WR: *Hemodynamics,* Baltimore, 1982, Williams & Wilkins.

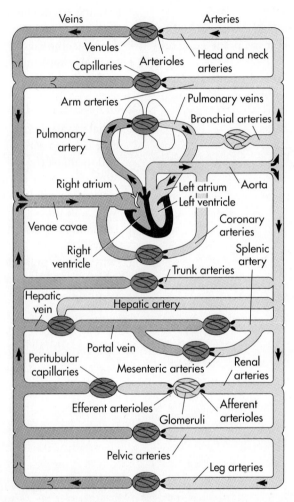

Veins

Arteries

Figure 1-4 ■ Schematic diagram of the parallel and series arrangement of the vessels composing the circulatory system. The capillary beds are represented by thin lines connecting the arteries (on the right) with the veins (on the left). The crescent-shaped thickenings proximal to the capillary beds represent the arterioles (resistance vessels). (Redrawn from Green HD: In Glasser O, editor: *Medical physics*, vol 1, Chicago, 1944, Mosby–Year Book.)

2. Pulsatile pressure is progressively damped by the elasticity of the arteriolar walls and the functional resistance of the arterioles, so that capillary blood flow is essentially nonpulsatile.
3. Velocity of blood flow is inversely related to the cross-sectional area at any point along the vascular system.
4. Most of the blood in the systemic vascular bed is located in the venous side of the circulation.

■ KEY WORDS AND CONCEPTS

- Pulmonary circulation
- Systemic circulation
- Systole
- Diastole
- Vascular resistance
- Capacity of capillaries
- Resistance at arterioles
- Velocity of blood flow
- Vascular cross-sectional area
- Intravascular pressure profile
- Vascular blood volume
- Pulsatile arterial blood flow
- Damped pulsations
- Venous compliance
- Arterial compliance
- Graves disease

■ SELF-STUDY PROBLEMS

1. What physical characteristics of arterioles enable them to maintain arterial blood pressure and to adjust the distribution of blood flow?
2. Why does most of the blood in the systemic circulation reside in the veins and venules?
3. Where in the systemic circulation is velocity of blood flow fastest and where is it slowest? Why?
4. Why is flow pulsatile in the systemic arterial system but nonpulsatile in the capillaries and venous systems?

Electrical Activity of the Heart

The experiments on "animal electricity" conducted by Galvani and Volta two centuries ago led to the discovery that electrical phenomena were involved in the spontaneous contractions of the heart. In 1855 Kölliker and Müller observed that when they placed the nerve of an innervated skeletal muscle preparation in contact with the surface of a frog's heart, the muscle twitched with each cardiac contraction.

The electrical events that normally take place in the heart initiate its contraction. Disorders in electrical activity can induce serious and sometimes lethal rhythm disturbances.

■ TRANSMEMBRANE POTENTIALS

The electrical behavior of single cardiac muscle cells has been investigated by inserting microelectrodes into the interior of the cell. The potential changes recorded from a typical ventricular muscle fiber are illustrated in Figure 2-1, *A*. When two electrodes are placed in an electrolyte solution near a strip of quiescent cardiac muscle, no potential difference (point *a*) is measurable between the two electrodes. At point *b* one of the electrodes, a microelectrode, was inserted into the interior of a cardiac muscle fiber. Immediately the galvanometer recorded a po-

tential difference (V_m) across the cell membrane; the potential of the interior of the cell was about 90 mV lower than that of the surrounding medium. Such electronegativity of the interior of the resting cell with respect to the exterior is also characteristic of skeletal and smooth muscle, of nerve, and indeed of most cells within the body.

At point *c* the ventricular cell was excited by an electrical stimulator. Very rapidly the cell membrane became depolarized; actually, the potential difference was reversed (positive overshoot), so that the potential of the interior of the cell exceeded that of the exterior by about 20 mV. The rapid upstroke of the **action potential** is designated phase 0. Immediately after the upstroke, there was a brief period of partial repolarization (phase 1), followed by a **plateau** (phase 2) that persisted for about 0.1 to 0.2 s. The potential then became progressively more negative (phase 3), until the resting state of polarization was again attained (at point *e*). **Repolarization** (phase 3) is a much slower process than is **depolarization** (phase 0). The interval from the end of repolarization until the beginning of the next action potential is designated phase 4.

The relationships between the electrical

events and the actual mechanical contraction are shown in Figure 2-2. Rapid depolarization (phase 0) precedes force development, and completion of repolarization coincides approximately with peak force. The duration of contraction parallels the duration of the action potential. Also, as the frequency of cardiac contraction is increased, the durations of the action potential and the mechanical contraction decrease as explained below (Figure 2-20).

Figure 2-1 ■ **Changes in transmembrane potential recorded from a fast-response (A) and slow-response (B) cardiac fiber in isolated cardiac tissue immersed in an electrolyte solution. A, At time *a* the microelectrode was in the solution surrounding the cardiac fiber. At time *b* the microelectrode entered the fiber. At time *c* an action potential was initiated in the impaled fiber. Time *c* to *d* represents the effective refractory period *(ERP)*; time *d* to *e* represents the relative refractory period *(RRP)*. B, An action potential recorded from a slow-response cardiac fiber. Note that compared with the fast-response fiber, the resting potential of the slow fiber is less negative, the upstroke (phase *0*) of the action potential is less steep, the amplitude of the action potential is smaller, phase *1* is absent, and the RRP extends well into phase *4*, after the fiber has fully repolarized.**

Figure 2-2 ■ **Time relationships between the mechanical force developed by a thin strip of ventricular muscle and the changes in transmembrane potential.** (Redrawn from Kavaler F, Fisher VJ, Stuckey JH: *Bull NY Acad Med* 41:592, 1965.)

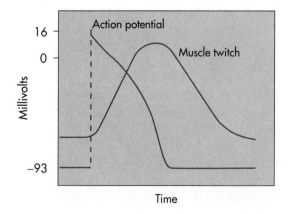

Principal Types of Cardiac Action Potentials

Two main types of action potentials are observed in the heart, as shown in Figure 2-1. One type, the **fast response,** occurs in the normal atrial and ventricular myocytes and in the specialized conducting fibers **(Purkinje fibers).** The other type of action potential, the **slow response,** is found in the **sinoatrial (SA) node,** the natural pacemaker region of the heart, and in the **atrioventricular (AV) node,** the specialized tissue that conducts the cardiac impulse from atria to ventricles.

As shown in Figure 2-1, not only is the **resting membrane potential** (phase 4) of the fast response considerably more negative than that of the slow response, but also the slope of the

Fast responses may change to slow responses under certain pathologic conditions. For example, in patients with coronary artery disease, when a region of cardiac muscle is deprived of its normal blood supply, the K^+ concentration in the interstitial fluid that surrounds the affected muscle cells rises because K^+ is lost from the inadequately perfused **(ischemic)** cells. The action potentials in some of these cells may then be converted from fast to slow responses. An experimental conversion from a fast to a slow response is illustrated in Figure 2-3.

Figure 2-3 ■ **Effect of tetrodotoxin on the action potential recorded in a calf Purkinje fiber perfused with a solution containing epinephrine and 10.8 mM K^+. The concentration of tetrodotoxin was 0 M in A, 3×10^{-8} M in B, 3×10^{-7} M in C, and 3×10^{-6} M in D and E; E was recorded later than D.** (Redrawn from Carmeliet E, Vereecke J: *Pflugers Arch* 313:300, 1969.)

upstroke (phase 0), the amplitude of the action potential, and the extent of the overshoot of the fast response are greater than those of the slow response. The amplitude of the action potential and the steepness of the upstroke are important determinants of propagation velocity. Hence, in cardiac tissue characterized by the slow response, conduction velocity is much slower and conduction is more likely to be blocked than in tissues that display the fast response. Slow conduction and a tendency toward block increase the likelihood of certain rhythm disturbances.

Ionic Basis of the Resting Potential

The various phases of the cardiac action potential are associated with changes in the permeability of the cell membrane, mainly to sodium, potassium, and calcium ions. Changes in cell membrane permeability alter the rate of ion passage across the membrane. The permeability of the membrane to a given ion defines the net quantity of the ion that will diffuse across each unit area of the membrane per unit concentration difference across the membrane. Changes in permeability are accomplished by the opening and closing of **ion channels** that are specific for the individual ions.

Just as with all other cells in the body, the concentration of potassium ions inside a cardiac muscle cell, $[K^+]_i$, greatly exceeds the concentration outside the cell, $[K^+]_o$, as shown in Figure 2-4. The reverse concentration gradient exists for Na ions and for free Ca ions (not bound to protein). Estimates of the extracellular and intracellular concentrations of Na^+, K^+, and Ca^{++}, and of the equilibrium potentials (defined below) for these ions, are compiled in Table 2-1.

The resting cell membrane is relatively permeable to K^+ but much less so to Na^+ and Ca^{++}. Hence, K^+ tends to diffuse from the inside to the outside of the cell, in the direction of the concentration gradient, as shown on the right side of the cell in Figure 2-4.

$$\text{Electrostatic:} \qquad\qquad \text{Chemical:}$$
$$E_K \qquad\qquad -61.5 \log ([K^+]_i/[K^+]_o)$$

Figure 2-4 ■ The balance of chemical and electrostatic forces acting on a resting cardiac cell membrane, based on a 30:1 ratio of the intracellular to extracellular K⁺ concentrations, and the existence of a nondiffusible anion (A⁻) inside but not outside the cell.

T A B L E   2 - 1

Intracellular and extracellular ion concentrations and equilibrium potentials in cardiac muscle cells

Ion	Extracellular concentrations (mM)	Intracellular concentrations (mM)*	Equilibrium potential (mV)
Na⁺	145	10	70
K⁺	4	135	−94
Ca⁺⁺	2	10^{-4}	132

Modified from Ten Eick RE, Baumgarten CM, Singer DH: *Prog Cardiovasc Dis* 24:157, 1981.
*The intracellular concentrations are estimates of the free concentrations in the cytoplasm.

Any flux of K⁺ that occurs during phase 4 takes place through certain specific **K⁺ channels.** Several types of K⁺ channels exist in cardiac cell membranes. Some of these channels are controlled (i.e., opened and closed) by the transmembrane potential, whereas others are controlled by some chemical signal (e.g., a neurotransmitter). The specific K⁺ channel through

which K⁺ passes during phase 4 is a voltage regulated channel that conducts the K⁺ current, called i_{K1}, which is an **inwardly rectifying K⁺ current,** as explained below (Figure 2-5). Many of the anions (labeled A⁻) inside the cell, such as the proteins, are not free to diffuse out with the K⁺ (Figure 2-4). Therefore, as the K⁺ diffuses out of the cell and leaves the A⁻ behind, the deficiency of cations causes the interior of the cell to become electronegative.

Therefore, two opposing forces are involved in the movement of K⁺ across the cell membrane. A chemical force, based on the concentration gradient, results in the net outward diffusion of K⁺. The counterforce is an electrostatic one; the positively charged K ions are attracted to the interior of the cell by the negative potential that exists there, as shown on the left side of the cell in Figure 2-4. If the system came into equilibrium, the chemical and electrostatic forces would be equal.

This equilibrium is expressed by the **Nernst equation** for potassium:

$$E_K = -61.5 \log ([K^+]_i/[K^+]_o) \qquad (1)$$

The right-hand term represents chemical potential difference at the body temperature of 37° C. The left-hand term, E_K, represents the electrostatic potential difference that would exist across the cell membrane if K⁺ were the only diffusible ion. E_K is called the **potassium equilibrium potential.**

An experimental disturbance in the equilibrium between electrostatic and chemical forces imposed by **voltage clamping** would cause K⁺ to move through the K⁺ channels. If the transmembrane potential (V_m) were clamped at a level negative to E_K, the electrostatic forces would exceed the diffusional forces, and K⁺ would be attracted into the cell (i.e., the K⁺ current would be **inward**). Conversely, if V_m were clamped at a level positive to E_K, the diffusional forces would exceed the electrostatic forces, and

Figure 2-5 ■ **The K⁺ currents recorded from a rabbit ventricular myocyte when the potential was changed from a holding potential of −80 mV to various test potentials. Positive values along the vertical axis represent outward currents; negative values represent inward currents. The V$_m$ coordinate of the point of intersection** *(open circle)* **of the curve with the X axis is the reversal potential; it denotes the Nernst equilibrium potential** *(E$_K$)* **at which the chemical and electrostatic forces are equal.** (Redrawn from Giles WR, Imaizumi Y: *J Physiol [Lond]* 405:123, 1988.)

K⁺ would leave the cell (i.e., the K⁺ current would be **outward**).

When the measured concentrations of [K⁺]$_i$ and [K⁺]$_o$ for mammalian myocardial cells are substituted into the Nernst equation, the calculated value of E$_K$ equals about −94 mV (Table 2-1). This value is close to, but slightly more negative than, the resting potential actually measured in myocardial cells. Therefore, the electrostatic force is slightly weaker than the chemical (diffusional) force, and K⁺ tends to leave the resting cell.

The balance of forces acting on the Na ions is entirely different from that acting on the K ions in resting cardiac cells. The intracellular Na⁺ concentration, [Na⁺]$_i$, is much lower than the extracellular concentration, [Na⁺]$_o$. At 37° C, the

sodium equilibrium potential, E$_{Na}$, expressed by the Nernst equation is:

$$-61.5 \log ([Na^+]_i / [Na^+]_o) \qquad (2)$$

For cardiac cells, E$_{Na}$ is about 40 to 70 mV (Table 2-1). At equilibrium, therefore, a transmembrane potential of +40 to +70 mV would be necessary to counterbalance the chemical potential for Na⁺. However, the actual polarization of the resting cell membrane is just the opposite. The resting membrane potential of myocardial fibers is about −90 mV. Hence, both chemical and electrostatic forces act to pull extracellular Na⁺ into the cell. The influx of Na⁺ through the cell membrane is small, however, because the permeability of the resting membrane to Na⁺ is very low. Nevertheless, it is mainly this small inward current of positively charged Na ions that causes the potential on the inside of the resting cell membrane to be slightly less negative than the value predicted by the Nernst equation for K⁺.

The steady inward leak of Na⁺ would gradually depolarize the resting cell membrane were it not for the metabolic pump that continuously extrudes Na⁺ from the cell interior and pumps in K⁺. The metabolic pump involves the enzyme, **Na⁺, K⁺-ATPase,** which is located in the cell membrane itself. Because the pump must move Na⁺ against both a chemical and an electrostatic gradient, operation of the pump requires the expenditure of metabolic energy. Increases in [Na⁺]$_i$ or in [K⁺]$_o$ accelerate the activity of the pump. The quantity of Na⁺ extruded by the pump exceeds the quantity of K⁺ transferred into the cell by a 3:2 ratio. Therefore, the pump itself tends to create a potential difference across the cell membrane, and thus it is termed an **electrogenic pump.** If the pump is partially inhibited, as by **digitalis,** the resting membrane potential becomes less negative than normal.

The dependence of the transmembrane potential, V$_m$, on the intracellular and extracellular concentrations of K⁺ and Na⁺ and on the conductances (g_K and g_{Na}) of these ions is described by the **chord conductance equation:**

$$V_m = \frac{g_K}{g_K + g_{Na}} E_K + \frac{g_{Na}}{g_K + g_{Na}} E_{Na} \quad (3)$$

For a given ion (X), the conductance (g_x) is defined as the ratio of the current (i_x) carried by that ion to the difference between the V_m and the Nernst equilibrium potential (E_x) for that ion; that is,

$$g_x = \frac{i_x}{V_m - E_x} \quad (4)$$

The chord conductance equation reveals that the relative, not the absolute, conductances to Na^+ and K^+ determine the resting potential. In the resting cardiac cell, g_K is about 100 times greater than g_{Na}. Therefore, the chord conductance equation reduces essentially to the Nernst equation for K^+.

When the ratio $[K^+]_i/[K^+]_o$ is decreased experimentally by raising $[K^+]_o$, the measured value of V_m (Figure 2-6) approximates that predicted by the Nernst equation for K^+. For extracellular K^+ concentrations of about 5 mM and above, the measured values correspond closely with the predicted values. The measured levels are slightly less than those predicted by the Nernst equation because of the small but finite value of g_{Na}. For values of $[K^+]_o$ below about 5 mM, g_K decreases as $[K^+]_o$ is diminished. As g_K decreases, the effect of the Na^+ gradient on the transmembrane potential becomes more important, as predicted by equation 3. This change in g_K accounts for the greater deviation of the measured V_m from that predicted by the Nernst equation for K^+ at low levels of $[K^+]_o$ (Figure 2-6). Also, in accordance with equation 3, changes in $[Na^+]_o$ scarcely affect the resting V_m (Figure 2-7), because of the low value of g_{Na}.

Ionic Basis of the Fast Response

Genesis of the Upstroke Any process that abruptly changes the resting membrane poten-

Figure 2-6 ■ **The transmembrane potential *(V_m)* of a cardiac muscle fiber varies inversely with the potassium concentration of the external medium *(curved line)*. The straight line represents the change in transmembrane potential predicted by the Nernst equation for E_K.** (Redrawn from Page E: *Circulation* 26:582, 1962. By permission of the American Heart Association, Inc.)

tial to a critical value (called the **threshold**) will result in a propagated action potential. The characteristics of fast-response action potentials are shown in Figure 2-1, *A*. The rapid depolarization (phase 0) is related almost exclusively to the inrush of Na^+ by virtue of a sudden increase in g_{Na}. The **amplitude** of the action potential (the potential change during phase 0) varies linearly with the logarithm of $[Na^+]_o$, as shown in Figure 2-7. When $[Na^+]_o$ is reduced from its normal value of about 140 mM to about 20 mM, the cell is no longer excitable.

The physical and chemical forces responsible for these transmembrane movements of Na^+ are explained in Figure 2-8. When the resting membrane potential, V_m, is suddenly changed to the threshold level of about -65 mV, the properties of the cell membrane change dramatically. Specific **fast channels** for Na^+ exist in the membrane. These channels can be blocked specifically by the puffer fish toxin **tetrodotoxin.** Also, many of the drugs used to treat certain cardiac arrhythmias act principally on these fast Na^+ channels.

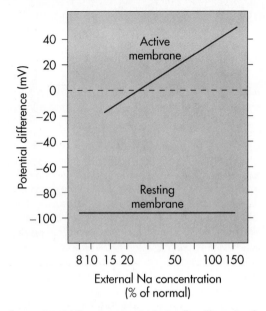

Figure 2-7 ■ **The concentration of sodium in the external medium is a critical determinant of the amplitude of the action potential in cardiac muscle** *(upper line)* **but has relatively little influence on the resting potential** *(lower line).* (Redrawn from Weidmann S: *Elektrophysiologie der Herzmuskelfaser,* Bern, 1956, Verlag Hans Huber.)

Na$^+$ moves through these channels in a manner that suggests that the flux is controlled by two types of "gates" in each channel. One of these gates, the **m gate,** tends to open the channel as V$_m$ becomes less negative and is therefore called an **activation gate.** The other, the **h gate,** tends to close the channel as V$_m$ becomes less negative and hence is called an **inactivation gate.** The m and h designations were originally employed by Hodgkin and Huxley in their mathematical model of conduction in nerve fibers.

With the cell at rest, V$_m$ is about − 90 mV. At this level, the m gates are closed and the h gates are wide open, as shown in Figure 2-8, *A.* The concentration of Na$^+$ is much greater outside than inside the cell, and the interior of the cell is electrically negative with respect to the exterior.

Hence, both chemical and electrostatic forces are oriented to draw Na$^+$ into the cell.

The electrostatic force in Figure 2-8, *A* is a potential difference of 90 mV, and it is represented by the white arrow. The chemical force, based on the difference in Na$^+$ concentration between the outside and inside of the cell, is represented by the black arrow. For a Na$^+$ concentration difference of about 130 mM, a potential difference of 60 mV (inside more positive than the outside) would be necessary to counterbalance the chemical, or diffusional, force, according to the Nernst equation for Na$^+$ (equation 2). Therefore, we may represent the net chemical force favoring the inward movement of Na$^+$ in Figure 2-8 (black arrows) as being equivalent to a potential of 60 mV. With the cell at rest the total electrochemical force favoring the inward movement of Na$^+$ is 150 mV (panel A). The m gates are closed, however, and the conductance of the resting cell membrane to Na$^+$ is very low. Hence, virtually no Na$^+$ moves into the cell; that is, the **inward Na$^+$ current** is negligible.

Any process that makes V$_m$ less negative tends to open the m gates and thereby "activates" the fast Na$^+$ channels. The activation of the fast channels is therefore called a **voltage-dependent** phenomenon. The precise potential at which the m gates swing open varies somewhat from one Na$^+$ channel to another in the cell membrane. As V$_m$ becomes less negative, the m gates open and Na$^+$ enters the cell (Figure 2-8, *B*) by virtue of the chemical and electrostatic forces.

The entry of positively charged Na$^+$ into the interior of the cell neutralizes some of the negative charges inside the cell and thereby diminishes further the transmembrane potential, V$_m$. The resultant reduction in V$_m$ in turn opens more m gates and thereby augments the inward Na$^+$ current. This is called a **regenerative process.** As V$_m$ approaches about − 65 mV, the remaining m gates rapidly swing open in the fast Na$^+$ channels until virtually all of the m gates are open (Figure 2-8, *B*).

$V_m = -90$ mV

$V_m = -65$ mV

$V_m = 0$ mV

A, During phase 4, the chemical (60 mV) and electrostatic (90 mV) forces favor influx of Na⁺ from the extracellular space. Influx is negligible, however, because the activation (**m**) gates are closed.

B, If V_m is brought to about −65 V, the **m** gates begin to swing open, and Na⁺ begins to enter the cell. This reduces the negative charge inside the cell, and thereby opens still more Na⁺ channels, which accelerates the influx of Na⁺. The change in V_m also initiates the closure of inactivation (**h**) gates, which operate more slowly than the **m** gates.

C, The rapid influx of Na⁺ rapidly decreases the negativity of V_m. As V_m approaches 0, the electrostatic force attracting Na⁺ into the cell is neutralized. Na⁺ continues to enter the cell, however, because of the substantial concentration gradient, and V_m begins to become positive.

$V_m = +20$ mV

$V_m = +30$ mV

D, When V_m is positive by about 20 mV, Na⁺ continues to enter the cell, because the diffusional forces (60 mV) exceed the opposing electrostatic forces (20 mV). The influx of Na⁺ is slow, however, because the net driving force is small, and many of the inactivation gates have already closed.

E, When V_m reaches about 30 mV, the **h** gates have now all closed, and Na⁺ influx ceases. The **h** gates remain closed until the first half of repolarization, and thus the cell is absolutely refractory during this entire period. During the second half of repolarization, the **m** and **h** gates approach the state represented by panel A, and thus the cell is relatively refractory.

Figure 2-8 ■ The gating of a sodium channel in a cardiac cell membrane during phase 4 (A) and during various stages of the action potential upstroke (B to E). The positions of the m and h gates in the fast Na⁺ channels are shown at the various levels of V_m. The electrostatic forces are represented by the white arrows and the chemical (diffusional) forces by the black arrows.

The rapid opening of the m gates in the fast Na⁺ channels is responsible for the large and abrupt increase in Na⁺ conductance, g_{Na}, coincident with phase 0 of the action potential (Figure 2-9). The rapid influx of Na⁺ accounts for the steep upstroke of V_m during phase 0. The maximal rate of change of V_m varies from 100 to 200 V/s in myocardial cells and from 500 to 1000 V/s in Purkinje fibers. Although the quantity of Na⁺ that enters the cell during one action potential alters V_m by over 100 mV, that quantity of Na⁺ is too small to change the intracellular Na⁺ concentration measurably. The chemical force remains virtually constant, and only the electrostatic force changes throughout the action potential. Hence, the lengths of the black arrows in Figure 2-8 remain constant at 60 mV, whereas the white arrows change in magnitude and direction.

As Na⁺ rushes into the cardiac cell during phase 0, the negative charges inside the cell are neutralized, and V_m becomes less negative. When V_m becomes zero (Figure 2-8, C), an electrostatic force no longer pulls Na⁺ into the cell. As long as the fast Na⁺ channels are open, however, Na⁺ continues to enter the cell because of the large concentration gradient. This continuation of the inward Na⁺ current causes the inside of the cell to become positively charged (Figure 2-8, D). This reversal of the membrane polarity is the so-called **overshoot** of the cardiac action potential. Such a reversal of the electrostatic gradient would, of course, tend to repel the entry of Na⁺ (Figure 2-8, D). However, as long as the inwardly directed chemical forces exceed these outwardly directed electrostatic forces, the net flux of Na⁺ will still be inward, although the rate of influx will be diminished.

The inward Na⁺ current finally ceases when the h (inactivation) gates close (Figure 2-8, E). The activity of the h gates is governed by the value of V_m just as is that of the m gates. The opening of the m gates occurs very rapidly (in about 0.1 to 0.2 ms), whereas the closure of the h gates is slower, requiring 1 ms or more. Phase 0 is finally terminated when the h gates have closed and have thereby **inactivated** the fast Na⁺ channels. The closure of the h gates so soon after the opening of the m gates accounts for the quick return of g_{Na} to near its resting value (Figure 2-9).

The h gates then remain closed until the cell has partially repolarized during phase 3 (at about time d in Figure 2-1, A). From time c to time d, the cell is in its **effective refractory period** and will not respond to further excitation. This mechanism prevents a sustained, tetanic contraction of cardiac muscle. Tetanus would, of course, preclude the normal intermittent pumping action of the heart.

Figure 2-9 ■ Changes in the conductances of Na⁺ (g_{Na}), Ca⁺⁺ (g_{Ca}), and K⁺ (g_K) during the various phases of the action potential of a fast-response cardiac cell. The conductance diagram shows directional changes only.

About midway through phase 3 (time d in Figure 2-1, A), the m and h gates in some of the fast Na⁺ channels have resumed the states shown in Figure 2-8, A. Such channels are said to have **recovered from inactivation.** The cell can begin to respond (but weakly at first) to further excitation (Figure 2-10). Throughout the remainder of phase 3, the cell completes its recovery from inactivation. By time e in Figure 2-1, A, the h gates have reopened and the m gates have reclosed in the remaining fast Na⁺ channels (Figure 2-8, A).

Statistical Characteristics of the "Gate" Concept The **patch-clamping technique** has made it possible to measure ionic currents through single membrane channels. The individual channels open and close repeatedly in a quasirandom sequence. This process is illustrated in Figure 2-11, which shows the current flow through single Na⁺ channels in a myocardial cell. To the left of the arrow, the membrane potential was clamped at −85 mV. At the arrow, the potential was suddenly changed to −45 mV, at which value it was held for the remainder of the record.

Figure 2-11 indicates that immediately after the membrane potential was made less negative, one Na⁺ channel opened three times in sequence. It remained open for about 2 or 3 ms each time and was closed for about 4 or 5 ms between openings. In the open state, it allowed 1.5 pA of current to pass. During the first and second openings of this channel, a second channel also opened, but for periods of only 1 ms. During the brief times that both channels were open simultaneously, the total current was 3 pA. After the first channel closed for the third time, both

Figure 2-10 ■ The changes in action potential amplitude and slope of the upstroke as action potentials are initiated at different stages of the relative refractory period of the preceding excitation. (Redrawn from Rosen MR, Wit AL, Hoffman BF: *Am Heart J* 88:380, 1974.)

channels remained closed for the rest of the recording, even though the membrane was held constant at -45 mV.

The overall change in **ionic conductance** of the entire cell membrane at any given time reflects the number of channels that are open at that time. Because the individual channels open and close in an irregular pattern, the overall membrane conductance represents the statistical probability of the open or closed state of the individual channels. The temporal characteristics of the activation process then represent the time course of the increasing probability that the specific channels will be open, rather than the kinetic characteristics of the activation gates in the individual channels. Similarly, the temporal characteristics of inactivation reflect the time course of the decreasing probability that the channels will be open and not the kinetic characteristics of the inactivation gates in the individual channels.

Genesis of Early Repolarization In many cardiac cells that have a prominent plateau, phase 1 constitutes an early, brief period of limited repolarization between the end of the upstroke and the beginning of the plateau. Phase 1 reflects the activation of a **transient outward current,** i_{to}, mostly carried by K^+. Activation of these K^+ channels during phase 1 leads to a brief

Figure 2-11 ■ The current flow (in picoamperes) through two individual Na^+ channels in a cultured cardiac cell, recorded by the patch-clamping technique. The membrane potential had been held at -85 mV but was suddenly changed to -45 mV at the arrow and held at this potential for the remainder of the record. One channel opened three times for about 3 ms each time, which allowed about 1.5 pA of current to flow through the membrane. During the first and second openings, a second channel opened for about 1 ms each time, permitting an additional 1.5 pA of current to flow. (Redrawn from Cachelin AB, DePeyer JE, Kokubun S, Reuter H: *J Physiol* 340:389, 1983.)

efflux of K⁺ from the cell because the interior of the cell is positively charged and because the internal K⁺ concentration greatly exceeds the external concentration (Figure 2-12). This brief efflux of positively charged ions brings about the brief, limited repolarization (phase 1).

Phase 1 is prominent in Purkinje fibers (Figure 2-3) and in epicardial fibers from the ventricular myocardium (Figure 2-13); it is much less developed in endocardial fibers. When the basic cycle length at which the epicardial fibers are stimulated is increased from 300 to 2000 ms,

phase 1 becomes more pronounced and the action potential duration is increased substantially. The same increase in basic cycle length has no effect on the early portion of the plateau in endocardial fibers, and it has a smaller effect on the action potential duration than it does in epicardial fibers (Figure 2-13).

Genesis of the Plateau During the plateau (phase 2) of the action potential, Ca⁺⁺ enters the cell through calcium channels that activate and inactivate much more slowly than do the fast Na⁺ channels. During the flat portion of phase 2 (Fig-

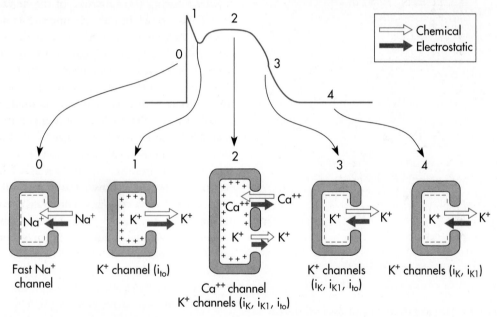

Figure 2-12 ■ The principal ionic currents and channels that generate the action potential in a cardiac cell.

Phase 0. The chemical and electrostatic forces both favor the entry of Na⁺ into the cell through fast Na⁺ channels to generate the upstroke.

Phase 1. The chemical and electrostatic forces both favor the efflux of K⁺ through i_{to} channels to generate early, partial repolarization.

Phase 2. During the plateau, the net influx of Ca⁺⁺ through Ca⁺⁺ channels is balanced by the efflux of K⁺ through i_K, i_{K1}, and i_{to} channels; these channels are defined on pages 16 to 22.

Phase 3. The chemical forces that favor the efflux of K⁺ through i_K, i_{K1}, and i_{to} channels predominate over the electrostatic forces that favor the influx of K⁺ through these same channels.

Phase 4. The chemical forces that favor the efflux of K⁺ through i_K and i_{k1} channels exceed very slightly the electrostatic forces that favor the influx of K⁺ through these same channels.

Figure 2-13 ■ **Action potentials recorded from canine epicardial and endocardial strips driven at basic cycle lengths of 300 and 2000 ms.** (From Litovsky SH, Antzelevitch C: *J Am Coll Cardiol* 14:1053, 1989.)

Figure 2-14 ■ **Effects of isoproterenol on the Ca^{++} currents conducted by T-type *(upper panel)* and L-type *(lower panel)* Ca^{++} channels in canine atrial myocytes. *Upper panel,* Potential changed from −80 to −20 mV; *lower panel,* potential changed from −30 to +30 mV.** (Redrawn from Bean BP: *J Gen Physiol* 86:1, 1985.)

ure 2-12), this influx of positive charge (carried by Ca^{++}) is balanced by the efflux of an equal amount of positive charge (carried by K^{+}). The K^{+} exits through various specific K^{+} channels.

Ca^{++} Conductance During the Plateau The Ca^{++} channels are voltage-regulated channels that are activated as V$_{m}$ becomes progressively less negative during the upstroke of the action potential. Two types of Ca^{++} channels (**L-type** and **T-type**) have been identified in cardiac tissues. Some of their important characteristics are illustrated in Figure 2-14, which displays the Ca^{++} currents generated by voltage-clamping an isolated atrial myocyte. Note that when V$_{m}$ is suddenly increased to +30 mV from a holding potential of −30 mV (lower panel), an inward Ca^{++} current (denoted by a downward deflection) is activated. Note also that after the inward current reaches its maximal value (in the downward direction), it returns toward zero very gradually (i.e., the channel inactivates very slowly). Thus, the current that passes through these channels is **long lasting,** and they have therefore been designated L-type channels. They are the predominant type of Ca^{++} channels in the heart and are activated during the action potential upstroke when V$_{m}$ reaches about −10 mV. The L-type channels are blocked by the so-called **Ca^{++} channel antagonists,** such as verapamil, nifedipine, and diltiazem.

The T-type (transient) Ca^{++} channels are much less abundant in the heart. They are activated at more negative potentials (about −70 mV) than are the L-type channels. Note in Figure 2-14 (upper panel) that when V$_{m}$ is suddenly increased to −20 mV from a holding potential of −80 mV, a Ca^{++} current is activated and then is inactivated very quickly.

Opening of the Ca^{++} channels is reflected by an increase in Ca^{++} conductance (g_{Ca}), which begins immediately after the upstroke of the action potential (Figure 2-9). Because the intracellular Ca^{++} concentration is much less than the extracellular concentration (Table 2-1), when the Ca^{++} channels open, Ca^{++} enters the cell throughout the plateau. The Ca^{++} that enters the myocardial cell during the plateau is involved in **excitation-contraction coupling,** as described in Chapter 3.

Various factors may influence g_{Ca}. An increase in g_{Ca} by **catecholamines,** such as **isoproterenol** and **norepinephrine,** is probably the principal mechanism by which catecholamines enhance cardiac muscle contractility. Catecholamines interact with **β-adrenergic receptors** located in the cardiac cell membranes. This interaction stimulates the membrane bound enzyme, **adenylyl cyclase,** which raises the intracellular concentration of **cyclic AMP.** This change enhances the activation of the L-type Ca^{++} channels in the cell membrane (Figure 2-14, lower panel) and thus augments the influx of Ca^{++} into the cells from the interstitial fluid. However, catecholamines do not affect the Ca^{++} current through the T-type channels (upper panel).

K^+ Conductance During the Plateau During the plateau of the action potential, the concentration gradient for K^+ between the inside and outside of the cell is virtually the same as it is during phase 4, but the V_m is positive. Therefore, the chemical and electrostatic forces greatly favor the efflux of K^+ from the cell during the plateau (Figure 2-12). If g_K were the same during the plateau as it is during phase 4, the efflux of K^+ during phase 2 would greatly exceed the influx of Ca^{++}, and a sustained plateau could not be achieved. However, as V_m approaches and attains positive values near the end of phase 0, g_K suddenly decreases (Figure 2-9).

The changes in g_K during the different phases of the action potential may be appreciated by examining the current-voltage relationship for the

The Ca^{++} channel antagonists decrease g_{Ca}. By reducing the amount of Ca^{++} that enters the myocardial cells during phase 2, these drugs diminish the strength of the cardiac contraction (Figure 2-15). Despite this direct depressant effect of the Ca^{++} channel antagonists on the contractile strength of the heart, these agents are used widely in the treatment of **congestive heart failure,** a common clinical condition in which the heart is not able to generate enough blood flow to meet the needs of the tissues. These drugs also diminish the contraction of the vascular smooth muscle, and thereby induce generalized vasodilation. This reduces the counterforce **(afterload)** that opposes the propulsion of blood from the ventricles into the arterial system, as explained in Chapters 3 and 4. Hence, vasodilator drugs, such as the Ca^{++} channel antagonists, are often referred to as **afterload reducing drugs.** This ability to diminish the counterforce enables the heart to provide a more adequate cardiac output, despite the direct depressant effect that these drugs exert on myocardial fibers.

i_{K1} channels (the channels that mainly determine g_K during phase 4). An example of this relationship in an isolated ventricular myocyte is shown in Figure 2-5. Note that the current-voltage curve intersects the voltage axis at a V_m of -70 mV. The absence of ionic current flow at the intersection indicates that the electrostatic forces must have been equal to the chemical (diffusional) forces (Figure 2-4) at this potential. Thus, in this isolated ventricular cell, the Nernst equilibrium potential (E_K) for K^+ was -70 mV; in a myocyte in the intact ventricle, E_K normally is about -95 mV.

When the membrane potential was clamped at levels negative to -70 mV in this isolated cell (Figure 2-5), the electrostatic forces exceeded the chemical forces and an inward K^+ current was induced (as denoted by the negative values of K^+

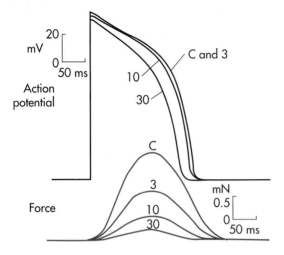

Figure 2-15 ■ **The effects of diltiazem, a Ca^{++} channel blocking drug, on the action potentials (in millivolts) and isometric contractile forces (in millinewtons) recorded from an isolated papillary muscle of a guinea pig. The tracings were recorded under control conditions *(C)* and in the presence of diltiazem, in concentrations of 3, 10, and 30 μmol/L.** (Redrawn with permission from Hirth C, Borchard U, Hafner D: *J Mol Cell Cardiol* 15:799, 1983.)

current over this range of voltages). Note also that for V_m more negative than -70 mV, the curve has a steep slope. Thus, when V_m equals or is negative to E_K, a small change in V_m induces a substantial change in K$^+$ current; that is, g_K is large. During phase 4, the V_m of a myocardial cell is slightly less negative than E_K (Figure 2-6).

When the transmembrane potential of this isolated myocyte was clamped at levels less negative than -70 mV (Figure 2-5), the chemical forces exceeded the electrostatic forces. Therefore, the net K$^+$ currents were outward (as denoted by the positive values along the corresponding section of the Y axis).

Thus, during phase 4 of the cardiac cycle, the **driving force** for K$^+$ (the difference between V_m and E_K) favored the efflux of K$^+$, mainly through

the i_{K1} channels. Note that for V_m values positive to -70 mV, the curve is relatively flat; this is especially pronounced for values of V_m positive to -40 mV. Thus, a given change in voltage causes only a small change in ionic current (i.e., g_K is small). Thus g_K *is small for outwardly directed K$^+$ currents but substantial for inwardly directed K$^+$ currents;* i.e., the i_{K1} current is **inwardly rectified.** This rectification is most marked over the plateau (phase 2) range of transmembrane potentials (Figure 2-5). *This characteristic prevents excessive loss of K$^+$ during the prolonged plateau, during which the electrostatic and chemical forces both favor the efflux of K$^+$.*

The **delayed rectifier K$^+$ channels,** which conduct the i_K current, are also activated at voltages that prevail toward the end of phase 0. However, activation proceeds very slowly, over several hundreds of milliseconds. Hence, activation of these channels tends to increase g_K very slowly and slightly during phase 2. Thus, these channels play only a minor role during phase 2, but they do contribute to repolarization (phase 3), as described below. The action potential plateau persists as long as the efflux of charge carried by certain cations (mainly K$^+$) is balanced by the influx of charge carried by other cations (mainly Ca^{++}). The effects of altering this balance are demonstrated by administration of a calcium channel antagonist. Figure 2-15 shows that with increasing concentrations of diltiazem, the voltage of the plateau becomes less positive, and the duration of the plateau diminishes. Similarly, administration of certain K$^+$ channel antagonists prolongs the action potential substantially.

Genesis of Final Repolarization The process of final repolarization (phase 3) starts at the end of phase 2, when the efflux of K$^+$ from the cardiac cell begins to exceed the influx of Ca^{++}. At least three outward K$^+$ currents (i_{to}, i_K, and i_{K1}) bring about the rapid repolarization (phase 3) of the cardiac cell (Figure 2-12).

The transient outward current (i_{to}) not only accounts for the brief, partial repolarization (phase 1), as previously described, but it also helps determine the duration of the plateau; hence, it also helps initiate repolarization. For example, the transient outward current is much more pronounced in atrial than in ventricular myocytes. In atrial cells, therefore, the outward K+ current exceeds the inward Ca++ current early in the plateau, whereas the outward and inward currents remain equal for a much longer time in ventricular myocytes. Hence, the plateau of the action potential is much less pronounced in atrial than in ventricular myocytes (Figure 2-16).

The **delayed rectifier K+ current** (i_K) is activated near the end of phase 0, but activation is very slow. Hence, the outward i_K current tends to increase throughout the plateau. Concurrently, the Ca++ channels are inactivated after the beginning of the plateau, and therefore the inward Ca current decreases. As the efflux of K+ begins to exceed the influx of Ca++, V_m becomes progressively less positive, and repolarization is initiated.

The **inwardly rectified K+ current** (i_{K1}) contributes substantially to repolarization. As the net efflux of cations causes V_m to become more negative during phase 3, the conductance of the channels that carry the i_{K1} current progressively increases. This is reflected by the hump that is evident in the flat portion of the current-voltage curve at V_m values between -20 and -70 mV in Figure 2-5. Thus, as V_m passes through this range of values less negative than E_K, the outward K+ current increases and thereby accelerates repolarization.

Restoration of Ionic Concentrations The excess Na+ that had entered the cell rapidly during phase 0 and more slowly throughout the action potential is removed from the cell by the action of the enzyme Na+,K+-ATPase. This enzyme ejects Na+ in exchange for the K+ that had exited mainly during phases 2 and 3.

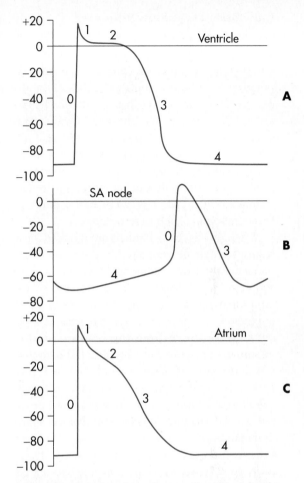

Figure 2-16 ■ **Typical action potentials (in millivolts) recorded from cells in the ventricle (A), SA node (B), and atrium (C). Sweep velocity in B is one half that in A or C.** (From Hoffman BF, Cranefield PF: *Electrophysiology of the heart,* New York, 1960, McGraw-Hill.)

Similarly, most of the excess Ca++ that had entered the cell during phase 2 is eliminated by an Na+/Ca++ exchanger, which exchanges 3 Na+ for 1 Ca++. However, a small fraction of the Ca++ is eliminated by an ATP-driven Ca++ pump (see p 63).

Ionic Basis of the Slow Response

Fast-response action potentials (Figure 2-1, *A*) may be considered to consist of four principal components: an upstroke (phase 0), an early repolarization (phase 1), a plateau (phase 2), and a period of repolarization (phase 3). In the slow response (Figure 2-1, *B*), phase 0 is much less steep, phase 1 is absent, phase 2 is brief and not flat, and phase 3 is not separated very distinctly from phase 2. In the fast response, the upstroke is produced by the influx of Na^+ through the fast channels. These channels can be blocked by certain compounds, such as tetrodotoxin.

When the fast Na^+ channels are blocked, slow responses may be generated in the same fibers under appropriate conditions. The Purkinje fiber action potentials shown in Figure 2-3 clearly exhibit the two response types. In the control tracing (panel *A*), a prominent notch (phase 1) separates the upstroke from the plateau. Action potential *A* in Figure 2-3 is a typical fast-response action potential. In action potentials *B* to *E*, progressively larger quantities of tetrodotoxin were added to the bathing solution to gradually block the fast Na^+ channels. It is evident that the sharp upstroke becomes progressively less prominent in action potentials *B* to *D,* and it disappears entirely in *E*. Thus, the tetrodotoxin had a pronounced effect on the steep upstroke, and only a negligible influence on the plateau. With elimination of the steep upstroke (panel *E*), the action potential resembles a typical slow response.

Certain cells in the heart, notably those in the SA and AV nodes, are normally slow-response fibers. In such fibers, depolarization is achieved by the inward current of Ca^{++} through the Ca^{++} channels. These ionic events closely resemble those that occur during the plateau of fast-response action potentials.

■ CONDUCTION IN CARDIAC FIBERS

An action potential traveling down a cardiac muscle fiber is propagated by local circuit currents, similar to the process that occurs in nerve and skeletal muscle fibers. In Figure 2-17, consider that the left half of the cardiac fiber has already been depolarized, whereas the right half is still in the resting state. The fluids normally in contact with the external and internal surfaces of the membrane are essentially solutions of electrolytes and thus are good conductors of electricity. Hence, current (in the abstract sense) will flow from regions of higher to those of lower potential, denoted by the plus and minus signs, respectively. In the external fluid, current will flow from right to left between the active and resting zones, and it will flow in the reverse direction intracellularly. In electrolyte solutions, the true current is carried by a movement of cations in one direction and anions in the opposite direction. At the cell exterior, for example, cations will flow from right to left, and anions from left to right (Figure 2-17). In the cell interior, the opposite migrations will occur. These local currents will tend to depolarize the region of the resting fibers adjacent to the border. Repetition of this process constitutes propagation of the excitation wave along the length of the cardiac fiber.

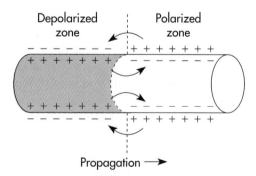

Figure 2-17 ■ The role of local currents in the propagation of a wave of excitation down a cardiac fiber.

Conduction of the Fast Response

In the fast response, the fast Na^+ channels will be activated when the transmembrane potential is suddenly brought from a resting value of about -90 mV to the threshold value of about -70 mV. The inward Na^+ current will then depolarize the cell very rapidly at that site. This portion of the fiber will become part of the depolarized zone, and the border will be displaced accordingly (to the right in Figure 2-17). The same process will then begin at the new border.

At any given point on the fiber, the greater the **amplitude** of the action potential and the greater the **rate of change of potential** (dV_m/dt) during phase 0, the more rapid is the conduction down the fiber. The amplitude of the action potential equals the difference in potential between the fully depolarized and the fully polarized regions of the cell interior (Figure 2-17). The magnitude of the local currents is proportional to this potential difference. Because these local currents shift the potential of the resting zone toward the threshold value, they are the local stimuli that depolarize the adjacent resting portion of the fiber to its threshold potential. *The greater the potential difference between the depolarized and polarized regions* (i.e., the greater the amplitude of the action potential), *the more efficacious are the local stimuli, and the more rapidly the wave of depolarization is propagated down the fiber.*

The rate of change of potential (dV_m/dt) *during phase 0 is also an important determinant of the conduction velocity.* The reason can be appreciated by referring again to Figure 2-17. If the active portion of the fiber depolarized very gradually, the local currents across the border between the depolarized and polarized regions would be very small. Thus, the resting region adjacent to the active zone would be depolarized very slowly, and consequently each new section of the fiber would require more time to reach threshold.

The level of the resting membrane potential is also an important determinant of conduction velocity. This factor operates through its influence on the amplitude and maximal slope of the action potential. The resting potential may vary for several reasons: (1) it can be altered experimentally by varying $[K^+]_o$ (Figure 2-6); (2) in cardiac fibers that are intrinsically automatic, V_m becomes progressively less negative during phase 4 (Figure 2-16, *B*); and (3) during a premature contraction, repolarization may not have been completed when the next excitation arrives (Figure 2-10). In general, the less negative the level of V_m, the less is the velocity of impulse propagation, regardless of the reason for the change in V_m.

The V_m level affects conduction velocity because the inactivation, or h, gates (Figure 2-8) in the fast Na^+ channels are voltage dependent. The less negative the V_m, the greater is the number of h gates that tend to close. During the normal process of excitation, depolarization proceeds so rapidly during phase 0 that the comparatively slow h gates do not close until the end of that phase. If partial depolarization is produced by a more gradual process, however, such as by elevating the level of external K^+, the h gates have ample time to close and thereby inactivate some of the Na^+ channels. When the cell is partially depolarized, many of the Na^+ channels will already be inactivated, and only a fraction of these channels will be available to conduct the inward Na^+ current during phase 0.

The results of an experiment in which the resting V_m of a bundle of Purkinje fibers was varied by altering the value of $[K^+]_o$ are shown in Figure 2-18. When $[K^+]_o$ was 3 mM (panels *A* and *F*), the resting V_m was -82 mV and the slope of phase 0 was steep. At the end of phase 0, the overshoot attained a value of 30 mV. Hence, the amplitude of the action potential was 112 mV. The fiber bundle was stimulated at some distance from the impaled cell, and the stimulus artifact (St) appears as a diphasic deflection just before phase 0. The time from this artifact to the

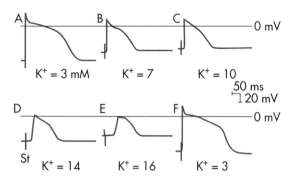

Figure 2-18 ■ **The effect of changes in external potassium concentration on the transmembrane action potentials recorded from a Purkinje fiber. The stimulus artifact (St) appears as a biphasic spike to the left of the upstroke of the action potential. The horizontal lines near the peaks of the action potentials denote 0 mV.** (From Myerburg RJ, Lazzara R. In Fisch E, editor: *Complex electrocardiography,* Philadelphia, 1973, FA Davis.)

Most of the experimentally induced changes in transmembrane potential shown in Figure 2-18 also take place in patients with **coronary artery disease.** When blood flow to a region of the myocardium is diminished, the supply of oxygen and metabolic substrates delivered to the ischemic tissues is insufficient. The Na^+,K^+-ATPase in the membrane of the cardiac myocytes requires considerable metabolic energy to maintain the normal transmembrane exchanges of Na^+ and K^+. When blood flow is inadequate, the activity of the Na^+,K^+-ATPase is impaired, and the ischemic myocytes gain excess Na^+ and lose K^+ to the surrounding interstitial space. Consequently, the K^+ concentration in the extracellular fluid surrounding the ischemic myocytes is elevated, and therefore the myocytes are affected by the elevated K^+ concentration in much the same way as was the myocyte depicted in Figure 2-18. Such changes may lead to serious aberrations of cardiac rhythm and conduction.

beginning of phase 0 is inversely proportional to the conduction velocity.

When $[K^+]_o$ was increased gradually to 16 mM (panels *B* to *E*), the resting V_m became progressively less negative. Concomitantly, the amplitudes and durations of the action potentials and the steepness of the upstrokes all diminished. As a consequence, the conduction velocity diminished progressively, as indicated by the distances from the stimulus artifacts to the upstrokes.

At the $[K^+]_o$ levels of 14 and 16 mM (panels *D* and *E*), the resting V_m had attained levels sufficient to inactivate all the fast Na^+ channels. The action potentials in panels *D* and *E* are characteristic slow responses, presumably mediated by the inward current of Ca^{++}. When the $[K^+]_o$ concentration of 3 mM was reestablished (panel *F*), the action potential was again characteristic of the normal fast response (as in panel *A*).

Conduction of the Slow Response

Local circuits (Figure 2-17) are also responsible for propagation of the slow response. However,

the characteristics of the conduction process differ quantitatively from those of the fast response. The threshold potential is about -40 mV for the slow response, and conduction is much slower than for the fast response. The conduction velocities of the slow responses in the SA and AV nodes are about 0.02 to 0.1 m/s. The fast-response conduction velocities are about 0.3 to 1 m/s for myocardial cells and 1 to 4 m/s for the specialized conducting fibers in the atria and ventricles. Slow responses are more likely to be blocked than are fast responses. Also, the former cannot be conducted at such rapid repetition rates.

■ CARDIAC EXCITABILITY

Currently, detailed knowledge of cardiac excitability is essential because of the rapid development of artificial pacemakers and other electrical devices for correcting serious disturbances of rhythm. The excitability characteristics of cardiac cells differ considerably, depending on whether the action potentials are fast or slow responses.

Fast Response

Once the fast response has been initiated, the depolarized cell will no longer be excitable until about the middle of the period of final repolarization (Figure 2-1, *A*). The interval from the beginning of the action potential until the fiber is able to conduct another action potential is called the **effective refractory period.** In the fast response, this period extends from the beginning of phase 0 to a point in phase 3 where repolarization has reached about -50 mV (time *c* to time *d* in Figure 2-1, *A*). At about this value of V_m the electrochemical gates (m and h) for many of the fast Na$^+$ channels have been reset.

Full excitability is not regained until the cardiac fiber has been fully repolarized (time *e* in Figure 2-1, *A*). During period *d* to *e* in the figure, an action potential may be evoked, but only when the stimulus is stronger than that which could elicit a response during phase 4. Period *d* to *e* is called the **relative refractory period.**

When a fast response is evoked during the relative refractory period of a previous excitation, its characteristics vary with the membrane potential that exists at the time of stimulation. The nature of this voltage dependency is illustrated in Figure 2-10. As the fiber is stimulated later and later in the relative refractory period, the amplitude of the response and the rate of rise of the upstroke increase progressively. Presumably, the number of fast Na$^+$ channels that have recovered from inactivation increases as repolarization proceeds during phase 3. As a consequence of the greater amplitude and upstroke slope of the evoked response, the propagation velocity increases as the cell is stimulated later in the relative refractory period. Once the fiber is fully repolarized, the response is constant no matter

what time in phase 4 the stimulus is applied. By the end of phase 3, the m and h gates of all channels are in their final positions and no further change in excitability occurs.

Slow Response

The relative refractory period during the slow response frequently extends well beyond phase 3 (Figure 2-1, *B*). Even after the cell has completely repolarized, it may be difficult to evoke a propagated response for some time. This characteristic is called **post-repolarization refractoriness.**

Action potentials evoked early in the relative refractory period are small and the upstrokes are not very steep (Figure 2-19). The amplitudes and upstroke slopes gradually improve as action potentials are elicited later and later in the relative refractory period. The recovery of full excitability is much slower than for the fast response. Impulses that arrive early in its relative refractory period are conducted much more slowly than those that arrive late in that period. The lengthy refractory periods also lead to conduction blocks. Even when slow responses recur at a low repetition rate, the fiber may be able to conduct only a fraction of those impulses.

In a patient who has occasional **premature depolarizations** (defined in detail on pp 45 and 46), the timing of these early beats may determine their clinical consequence. If they occur very late in the relative refractory period of the preceding depolarization or after full repolarization, the premature depolarization will probably be inconsequential. However, if they originate early in the relative refractory period, conduction of the premature impulse from the site of origin will be slow, and hence reentry is more likely to occur. If that reentry is very irregular (i.e., if **fibrillation** ensues), the consequence may be very grave, as explained on page 47.

Figure 2-19 ■ The effects of excitation at various times after the initiation of an action potential in a slow-response fiber. In this fiber, excitation very late in phase 3 (or early in phase 4) induces a small, nonpropagated (local) response *(a)*. Later in phase 4, a propagated response *(b)* may be elicited; its amplitude is small and the up-stroke is not very steep. This response, which displays post-repolarization refractoriness, will be conducted very slowly. Still later in phase 4, full excitability will be regained, and the response *(c)* will display its normal characteristics. (Modified from Singer DH et al: *Prog Cardiovasc Dis* 24:97, 1981.)

Figure 2-20 ■ The effect of changes in cycle length *(CL)* on the action potential duration *(APD)* of canine Purkinje fibers. (Modified from Singer D, Ten Eick RE: *Am J Cardiol* 28:381, 1971.)

Effects of Cycle Length

Changes in cycle length alter the action potential duration of cardiac cells and thus change their refractory periods. Consequently, the changes in cycle length are often important factors in the initiation or termination of certain arrhythmias. The changes in action potential durations produced by stepwise reductions in cycle length from 2000 to 200 ms in a Purkinje fiber are shown in Figure 2-20. Note that as the cycle length is diminished, the action potential duration decreases.

This direct correlation between action potential duration and cycle length is ascribable mainly to changes in g_K that involve the delayed rectifier K^+ channels. The i_K current activates slowly, remains activated for hundreds of milliseconds before it is inactivated, and inactivates very slowly. Consequently, as the basic cycle length is diminished, each action potential tends to occur earlier in the inactivation period of the i_K current

initiated by the preceding action potential. Therefore, the shorter the basic cycle length, the greater will be the outward K^+ current during phase 2, and hence the briefer will be the action potential.

■ NATURAL EXCITATION OF THE HEART

The nervous system controls various aspects of cardiac behavior, including the frequency at which the heart beats and the vigor of each contraction. However, cardiac function certainly does not require intact nervous pathways. Indeed, a patient with a completely denervated heart (a cardiac transplant patient) can adapt well to stressful situations.

The properties of **automaticity** (the ability to initiate its own beat) and of **rhythmicity** (the regularity of such pacemaking activity) are intrinsic to cardiac tissue. *The heart will continue to beat even when it is completely removed from the body.* If the coronary vasculature is artificially perfused, rhythmic cardiac contraction will persist for considerable periods. Apparently, at least some cells in the walls of all four cardiac chambers are capable of initiating beats; such cells probably reside in the nodal tissues or specialized conducting fibers of the heart.

The region of the mammalian heart that ordinarily generates impulses at the greatest frequency is the SA node; it is called the **natural pacemaker** of the heart.

Detailed mapping of the electrical potentials on the surface of the right atrium has revealed that two or three sites of automaticity, located 1 or 2 cm from the SA node itself, serve along with the SA node as an **atrial pacemaker complex.** At times, all of these loci initiate impulses simultaneously. At other times, the site of earliest excitation shifts from locus to locus, depending on such conditions as the level of autonomic neural activity.

Ectopic pacemakers may serve as a safety mechanism when the normal pacemaking centers cease functioning. However, if an ectopic center fires while the normal pacemaking center still functions, the ectopic activity may induce either sporadic rhythm disturbances, such as **premature depolarizations,** or continuous rhythm disturbances, such as **paroxysmal tachycardias.** These **arrhythmias** are discussed at the end of this chapter.

When the SA node and the other components of the atrial pacemaker complex are excised or destroyed, pacemaker cells in the AV node are usually the next most rhythmic, and they become the pacemakers for the entire heart. After some time, which may vary from minutes to days, automatic cells in the atria usually become dominant.

Purkinje fibers in the specialized conduction system of the ventricles also possess automaticity. Characteristically, they fire at a very slow rate.

Regions of the heart other than the SA node may initiate beats under special circumstances; such sites are called **ectopic foci,** or **ectopic pacemakers.** Ectopic foci may become pacemakers when (1) their own rhythmicity becomes enhanced, (2) the rhythmicity of the higher-order pacemakers becomes depressed, or (3) all conduction pathways between the ectopic focus and those regions with greater rhythmicity become blocked.

When the AV junction is unable to conduct the cardiac impulse from the atria to the ventricles, such **idioventricular pacemakers** in the Purkinje fiber network initiate the ventricular contractions. Such contractions occur at a frequency of only 30 to 40 beats per minute.

Sinoatrial Node

The SA node is the phylogenetic remnant of the sinus venosus of lower vertebrate hearts. In humans it is about 8 mm long and 2 mm thick. It lies in the groove where the superior vena cava joins the right atrium (Figure 2-21). The sinus node artery runs lengthwise through the center of the node.

The SA node contains two principal types of cells: (1) small, round cells, which have few organelles and myofibrils; and (2) slender, elongated cells, which are intermediate in appearance between the round and the ordinary atrial myocardial cells. The round cells are probably the pacemaker cells, whereas the transitional cells probably conduct the impulses within the node and to the nodal margins.

A typical transmembrane action potential recorded from a cell in the SA node is depicted in Figure 2-16, *B*. Compared with the transmembrane potential recorded from a ventricular myocardial cell (Figure 2-16, *A*), the resting potential of the SA node cell is usually less, the upstroke of the action potential (phase 0) is less steep, a

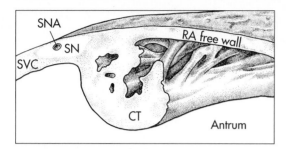

Figure 2-21 ■ **The location of the SA node** *(SN)* **near the junction between the superior vena cava** *(SVC)* **and right atrium** *(RA). SNA,* **Sinoatrial artery;** *CT,* **crista terminalis.** (Redrawn from James TN: *Am J Cardiol* 40:965, 1977.)

These mechanisms of decreasing heart rate operate when vagal activity is predominant. An extreme example is **vasovagal syncope,** which is a brief period of lightheadedness or loss of consciousness caused by an intense burst of vagal activity. This type of syncope is induced reflexly in response to pain or to certain psychological stimuli. With regard to the last of the mechanisms for altering heart rate displayed in Figure 2-22, shifts in the threshold potential of the automatic cells to less negative values are produced by certain antiarrhythmic drugs, such as **quinidine** and **procainamide.**

plateau is not sustained, and repolarization (phase 3) is more gradual. These are all characteristic of the slow response.

The transmembrane potential during phase 4 is much less negative in SA (and AV) nodal automatic cells than in atrial or ventricular myocytes because the i_{K1} type of K$^+$ channel is very sparse in the nodal cells. Therefore, the ratio of g_K/g_{Na} during phase 4 is much less in the nodal cells than in the myocytes. Hence, during phase 4, V_m much more closely approaches the K$^+$ equilibrium potential (E_K) in myocytes than it does in nodal cells.

Under ordinary conditions, tetrodotoxin has no influence on the SA nodal action potential. This indicates that the upstroke of the action potential is not produced by an inward current of Na$^+$ through the fast channels.

However, the principal distinguishing feature of a pacemaker fiber resides in phase 4. In nonautomatic cells the potential remains constant during this phase, whereas in a pacemaker fiber there is a slow depolarization, called the **pacemaker potential,** throughout phase 4. Depolarization proceeds at a steady rate until a threshold is attained, and then an action potential is triggered.

The discharge frequency of pacemaker cells may be varied by a change in (1) the rate of de-

Ordinarily, the frequency of pacemaker firing is controlled by the activity of both divisions of the autonomic nervous system. Increased sympathetic nervous activity, through the release of norepinephrine, raises the heart rate principally by increasing the slope of the pacemaker potential. This mechanism of increasing heart rate operates during physical exertion, anxiety, or certain illnesses, such as **febrile infectious diseases.** Increased vagal activity, through the release of acetylcholine, diminishes the heart rate by hyperpolarizing the pacemaker cell membrane and by reducing the slope of the pacemaker potential (Figure 2-23).

polarization during phase 4, (2) the threshold potential, or (3) the maximal diastolic potential (Figure 2-22). With an increase in the rate of depolarization (*b* to *a* in Figure 2-22, *A*) the threshold potential will be attained earlier, and the heart rate will increase. A rise in the threshold potential (from *TP-1* to *TP-2* in Figure 2-22, *B*) will delay the onset of phase 0 (from time *b* to time *c*), and the heart rate will be reduced accordingly. Similarly, when the diastolic potential at the end

Figure 2-22 ■ **Mechanisms involved in changes of frequency of pacemaker firing. In section A a reduction in the slope of the pacemaker potential from *a* to *b* will diminish the frequency. In section B an increase in the threshold (from *TP-1* to *TP-2*) or an increase in the magnitude of the resting potential (from *a* to *d*) will also diminish the frequency.** (Redrawn from Hoffman BF, Cranefield PF: *Electrophysiology of the heart,* New York, 1960, McGraw-Hill.)

Figure 2-23 ■ **Effect of a brief vagal stimulus (*arrow*) on the transmembrane potential recorded from an SA node pacemaker cell in an isolated cat atrium preparation. The cardiac cycle lengths, in milliseconds are denoted by the numbers at the top of the figure.** (Modified from Jalife J, Moe GK: *Circ Res* 45:595, 1979.)

of phase 3 becomes more negative (from *a* to *d*), more time will be required to reach threshold *TP-2* when the slope of phase 4 remains unchanged, and the heart rate will diminish.

Changes in autonomic neural activity often also induce a **pacemaker shift,** where the site of initiation of the cardiac impulse may shift to a different locus within the SA node or to a different component of the atrial pacemaker complex.

Ionic Basis of Automaticity

Several ionic currents contribute to the slow depolarization that occurs during phase 4 in automatic cells in the heart. In the pacemaker cells of the SA node, the diastolic depolarization is mediated by at least three ionic currents: (1) an inward current, i_f, induced by hyperpolarization;

(2) a calcium current, i_{Ca}; and (3) an outward K^+ current, i_K (Figure 2-24).

The inward **hyperpolarization** current, i_f, is carried mainly by Na^+; the current is conducted through specific channels that differ from the fast Na^+ channels. This current becomes activated during the repolarization phase of the action potential, as the membrane potential becomes more negative than about -50 mV. The more negative the membrane potential becomes at the end of repolarization, the greater will be the activation of the i_f current.

The second current responsible for diastolic depolarization is the calcium current i_{Ca}. This current becomes activated toward the end of phase 4, as the transmembrane potential reaches a value of about -55 mV (Figure 2-24).

Once the Ca^{++} channels become activated, the influx of Ca^{++} into the cell increases. The influx of Ca^{++} accelerates the rate of diastolic depolarization, which then leads to the upstroke of the action potential. A decrease in the external Ca^{++} concentration (Figure 2-25) or the addition of a

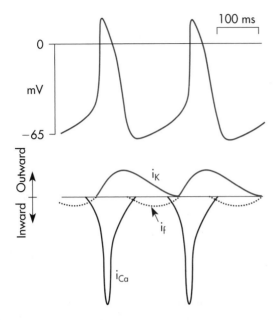

Figure 2-24 ■ The transmembrane potential changes *(top half)* that occur in SA node cells are produced by three principal currents *(bottom half):* (1) the current, i_{Ca}; (2) a hyperpolarization-induced inward current, i_f; and (3) an outward K^+ current, i_K. (Redrawn from Brown HF: *Physiol Rev* 61:644, 1981.)

Figure 2-25 ■ Transmembrane action potentials recorded from an SA node pacemaker cell in an isolated rabbit atrium preparation. The concentration of Ca^{++} in the bath was changed from 2 to **0.2 mM.** (Modified from Kohlhardt M, Figulla HR, Tripathi O: *Basic Res Cardiol* 71:17, 1976.)

calcium channel antagonist (Figure 2-26) diminishes the amplitude of the action potential and the slope of the pacemaker potential in SA node cells.

The progressive diastolic depolarization mediated by the two inward currents, i_f and i_{Ca}, is

opposed by a third current, an outward K^+ current, i_K. This efflux of K^+ tends to repolarize the cell after the upstroke of the action potential. The outward K^+ current continues well beyond the time of maximal repolarization, but it diminishes throughout phase 4 (Figure 2-24). Hence, the opposition of i_K to the depolarizing effects of the two inward currents (i_{Ca} and i_f) gradually decreases.

The ionic basis for automaticity in the AV node pacemaker cells is identical to that in the SA node cells. Similar mechanisms also account for automaticity in Purkinje fibers, except that the calcium current is not involved. Hence, the **slow diastolic depolarization** is mediated principally by the imbalance between the hyperpolarization-induced inward current, i_f and the outward K^+ current, i_K.

The autonomic neurotransmitters affect automaticity by altering the ionic currents across the cell membranes. The adrenergic transmitters increase all three currents involved in SA nodal automaticity. The adrenergically mediated increase in the slope of diastolic depolarization indicates that the augmentations of i_f and i_{Ca} must exceed the enhancement of i_K.

The hyperpolarization (Figure 2-23) induced by the acetylcholine released at the vagus endings in the heart is achieved by an increase in g_K. This change in conductance is mediated through activation of specific K^+ channels that are controlled by the cholinergic receptors. Acetylcholine also depresses the i_f and i_{Ca} currents.

Overdrive Suppression

The automaticity of pacemaker cells becomes depressed after a period of excitation at a high frequency. This phenomenon is known as **overdrive suppression.** Because of the greater intrinsic rhythmicity of the SA node than of the other latent pacemaking sites in the heart, the firing of the SA node tends to suppress the automaticity in the other loci.

Figure 2-26 ■ **The effects of nifedipine (5.6×10^{-7} M), a Ca^{++} channel antagonist, on the transmembrane potentials recorded from a rabbit SA node cell.** (From Ning W, Wit AL: *Am Heart J* 106:345, 1983.)

If an ectopic focus in one of the atria suddenly began to fire at a high rate (e.g., 150 impulses per minute) in an individual with a normal heart rate of 70 beats per minute, the ectopic center would become the pacemaker for the entire heart. When that rapid ectopic focus suddenly stopped firing, the SA node might remain quiescent briefly because of overdrive suppression. The interval from the end of the period of overdrive until the SA node resumes firing is called the **sinus node recovery time.** In patients with the so-called **sick sinus syndrome,** the sinus node recovery time may be markedly prolonged. The resultant period of **asystole** (cardiac standstill) might cause loss of consciousness.

The mechanism responsible for overdrive suppression appears to be based on the activity of the membrane pump (Na^+,K^+-ATPase) that actively extrudes Na^+ from the cell, in partial exchange for K^+. During each depolarization, a certain quantity of Na^+ enters the cell. Therefore, the more frequently it is depolarized, the greater is the amount of Na^+ that enters the cell per minute. At high excitation frequencies the Na^+ pump becomes more active in extruding this larger quantity of Na^+ from the cell interior. The quantity of Na^+ extruded by the pump exceeds the quantity of K^+ that enters the cell; the ratio is 3:2. This enhanced activity of the pump hyperpolarizes the cell, because of the net loss of

cations from the cell interior. Because of the hyperpolarization, the slow diastolic depolarization requires more time to reach the threshold, as shown in Figure 2-22, *B*. Furthermore, when the overdrive suddenly ceases, the Na^+ pump may not decelerate instantaneously but may continue to operate at an accelerated rate for some time. This excessive extrusion of Na^+ opposes the gradual depolarization of the pacemaker cell during phase 4 and thereby suppresses its intrinsic automaticity temporarily.

Atrial Conduction

From the SA node, the cardiac impulse spreads radially throughout the right atrium (Figure 2-27) along ordinary atrial myocardial fibers, at a conduction velocity of approximately 1 m/s. A special pathway, the **anterior interatrial myocardial band** (or **Bachmann's bundle**) conducts the impulse from the SA node directly to the left atrium. Three tracts, the **anterior, middle,** and **posterior internodal pathways,** have been described. These tracts consist of a mixture of ordinary myocardial cells and specialized conducting fibers. Some authorities assert that these pathways constitute the principal routes for conduction of the cardiac impulse from the SA to the AV node.

The configuration of the atrial action potential is depicted in Figure 2-16, *C*. Compared with the potential recorded from a typical ventricular fiber (Figure 2-16, *A*), the plateau (phase 2) is not

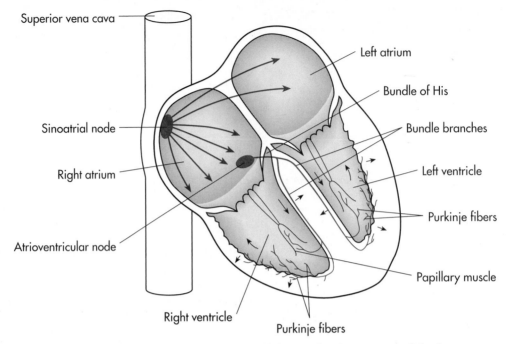

Figure 2-27 ■ Schematic representation of the conduction system of the heart.

as well developed, repolarization (phase 3) occurs as a slower rate, and the duration of the action potential is shorter.

Atrioventricular Conduction

The cardiac action potential proceeds along the internodal pathways in the atrium and ultimately reaches the AV node. This node is approximately 22 mm long, 10 mm wide, and 3 mm thick in adult humans. The node is situated posteriorly on the right side of the interatrial septum near the ostium of the coronary sinus. The AV node contains the same two cell types as the SA node, but the round cells are more sparse and the elongated cells preponderate.

The AV node has been divided into three functional regions: (1) the AN region, the transitional zone between the atrium and the remainder of the node; (2) the N region, the midportion of the AV node; and (3) the NH region, the zone in which nodal fibers gradually merge with the **bundle of His,** which is the upper portion of the specialized conducting system for the ventricles. Normally, the AV node and bundle of His constitute the only pathways for conduction from atria to ventricles.

Several features of AV conduction are of physiologic and clinical significance. The principal delay in the passage of the impulse from the atria to the ventricles occurs in the AN and N regions of the AV node. The conduction velocity is actually less in the N region than in the AN region. However, the path length is substantially greater in the AN than in the N region. The conduction times through the AN and N zones account for the delay between the onsets of the **P wave** (the electrical manifestation of the spread of atrial excitation) and the **QRS complex** (spread of ventricular excitation) in the electrocardiogram (see

Accessory AV pathways are present in some people. Such pathways often serve as a part of a reentry loop (Figure 2-28), which could lead to serious cardiac rhythm disturbances in these patients. The **Wolff-Parkinson-White syndrome,** a congenital disturbance, is the most common clinical disorder in which a bypass tract of myocardial fibers serves as an accessory pathway between atria and ventricles. Ordinarily, the syndrome causes no functional abnormality. It is easily detected in the electrocardiographic reading, because preexcitation of a portion of the ventricular myocardium via the bypass tract just before the normal excitation of the remainder of the ventricular myocardium via the AV node and His-Purkinje system imparts a bizarre configuration to the ventricular (QRS) complex of the **electrocardiogram.** Occasionally, however, a reentry loop develops in which the atrial impulse travels to the ventricle via one of the two AV pathways (AV node or bypass tract), and then back to the atria through the other of the two pathways. Continuous circling around the loop leads to a very rapid rhythm **(supraventricular tachycardia),** which may be incapacitating because the rapid rate may not allow sufficient time for ventricular filling. Transient block of the AV node (by intravenous injection of adenosine or by pressing on the neck over the carotid sinus region to increase activity in the efferent vagus nerve fibers) usually abolishes the tachycardia and restores a normal sinus rhythm.

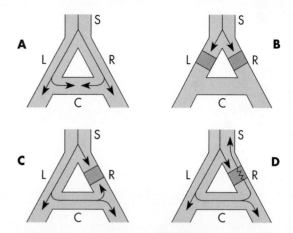

Figure 2-28 ■ **The role of unidirectional block in reentry. In panel A, an excitation wave traveling down a single bundle *(S)* of fibers continues down the left *(L)* and right *(R)* branches. The depolarization wave enters the connecting branch *(C)* from both ends and is extinguished at the zone of collision. In panel B, the wave is blocked in the *L* and *R* branches. In panel C, bidirectional block exists in branch *R.* In panel D, unidirectional block exists in branch *R.* The antegrade impulse is blocked, but the retrograde impulse is conducted through and reenters bundle *S.***

Figure 2-29). *Functionally, this delay between atrial and ventricular excitation permits optimal ventricular filling during atrial contraction.*

In the N region, slow-response action potentials prevail. The resting potential is about −60 mV, the upstroke velocity is very low (about 5 V/s), and the conduction velocity is about 0.05 m/s. Tetrodotoxin, which blocks the fast Na^+ channels, has virtually no effect on the action potentials in this region. Conversely, the Ca^{++} chan-

nel antagonists decrease the amplitude and duration of the action potentials (Figure 2-30) and depress AV conduction. The shapes of the action potentials in the AN region are intermediate between those in the N region and atria. Similarly, the action potentials in the NH region are transitional between those in the N region and bundle of His.

The relative refractory period of the cells in the N region extends well beyond the period of complete repolarization; i.e., these cells display post-repolarization refractoriness (Figure 2-19). *As the repetition rate of atrial depolarizations is increased, conduction through the AV junction slows.* An abnormal prolongation of AV conduction time is called **first-degree AV block** (Figure 2-31, *A*). Most of the prolongation of AV conduction induced by an increase in repetition rate takes place in the N region.

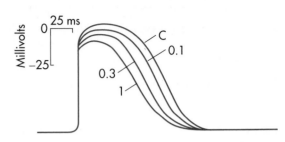

Figure 2-30 ■ Transmembrane potentials recorded from a rabbit AV node cell under control conditions *(C)* and in the presence of the calcium channel blocking drug, diltiazem, in concentrations of 0.1, 0.3, and 1 μmol/L. (Redrawn from Hirth C, Borchard U, Hafner D: *J Mol Cell Cardiol* 15:799, 1983.)

Figure 2-29 ■ Configuration of a typical scalar electrocardiogram, illustrating the important deflections and intervals.

A, First-degree heart block; P-R interval is 0.28 s.

B, Second-degree heart block (2:1).

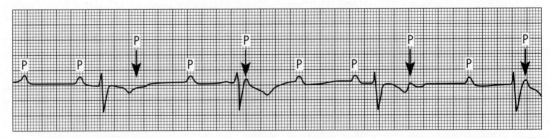

C, Third-degree heart block; note the dissociation between the P waves and the QRS complexes.

Figure 2-31 ■ Atrioventricular (AV) blocks.

Impulses tend to be blocked in the AV node at stimulus repetition rates that are easily conducted in other regions of the heart. If the atria are depolarized at a high frequency, only a fraction (e.g., one half) of the atrial impulses might be conducted through the AV junction to the ventricles. The conduction pattern in which only a fraction of the atrial impulses are conducted to the ventricles is called **second-degree AV block** (Figure 2-31, *B*). This type of block may protect the ventricles from excessive contraction frequencies, wherein the filling time between successive ventricular contractions might be inadequate.

Retrograde conduction can occur through the AV node. However, the propagation time is significantly longer, and the impulse is blocked at lower repetition rates during conduction in the retrograde than in the antegrade direction. Finally, the AV node is a common site for reentry; the underlying mechanisms are explained on pages 38 and 39.

The autonomic nervous system regulates AV conduction. Weak vagal activity may simply prolong the AV conduction time. Stronger vagal activity may cause some or all of the impulses arriving from the atria to be blocked in the node. The conduction pattern in which none of the atrial impulses reach the ventricles for a substantial time is called **third-degree,** or **complete, AV block** (Figure 2-31, *C*). The delayed conduction or block induced by vagal stimulation occurs largely in the N region of the node.

The acetylcholine released by the vagal nerve fibers hyperpolarizes the conducting fibers in the N region (Figure 2-32). The greater the hy-

---

Three degrees of AV block can be distinguished, as shown in Figure 2-31. First-degree AV block is characterized by a prolonged P-R interval. In Figure 2-31, *A,* the P-R interval is 0.28 s; an interval greater than 0.2 s is abnormal. In most cases of first-degree block the A-H interval of the His bundle electrogram is prolonged and the H-V interval is normal. Hence, the delay is located above the bundle of His, that is, in the AV node.

In second-degree AV block, all QRS complexes are preceded by P waves, but not all P waves are followed by QRS complexes. The ratio of P waves to QRS complexes is usually the ratio of two small integers (such as 2:1, 3:1, 3:2). Figure 2-31, *B,* illustrates a typical 2:1 block.

First- and second-degree AV blocks are most frequently caused by inflammatory processes (acute rheumatic fever), drugs (calcium channel antagonists), or rapid atrial rates (supraventricular tachycardias). Third-degree AV block is most often caused by a degenerative process of unknown cause or by severe myocardial ischemia (inadequate coronary blood supply).

His bundle electrograms have demonstrated that the site of block may be above or below the bundle of His. A block below the bundle is more serious than one above the bundle, because it more often evolves into a third-degree block. Hence, an artificial pacemaker is frequently implanted when the block is found to be below the bundle.

Third-degree AV block is often referred to as **complete heart block** because the impulse is unable to traverse the AV conduction pathway from atria to ventricles. His bundle electrograms reveal that the most common sites of complete block are distal to the bundle of His. In complete heart block the atrial and ventricular rhythms are entirely independent. A typical example is displayed in Figure 2-31, *C,* where the QRS complexes bear no fixed relationship to the P waves. Because of the slow ventricular rhythm (32 beats per minute in this example), circulation of blood is often inadequate, especially during muscular activity. Third-degree block is often associated with syncope (so-called **Stokes-Adams** attacks) caused principally by insufficient cerebral blood flow. Third-degree block is one of the most common conditions requiring treatment by artificial pacemakers.

Figure 2-32 ■ **Effects of a brief vagal stimulus** *(St)* **on the transmembrane potential recorded from an AV nodal fiber from a rabbit. Note that shortly after vagal stimulation, the membrane of the fiber was hyperpolarized. The atrial excitation** (A_2) **that arrived at the AV node when the cell was hyperpolarized failed to be conducted, as denoted by the absence of a depolarization in the His electrogram** *(H)*. **The atrial excitations that preceded** (A_1) **and followed** (A_3) **excitation** A_2 **were conducted to the His bundle region.** (Redrawn from Mazgalev T et al: *Am J Physiol* 251:H631, 1986.)

perpolarization at the time of arrival of the atrial impulse, the more impaired the AV conduction will be. In the experiment shown in Figure 2-32, vagus nerve fibers were stimulated intensely (at St) shortly before the second atrial depolarization (A_2). That atrial impulse arrived at the AV node cell when its cell membrane was maximally hyperpolarized. The absence of a corresponding depolarization of the His bundle (H) shows that the second atrial impulse was not conducted through the AV node. Only a small, nonpropagated response to the second atrial impulse is evident in the recording from the conducting fiber.

The cardiac sympathetic nerves, on the other hand, facilitate AV conduction. They decrease AV conduction time and enhance the rhythmicity of the latent pacemakers in the AV junction. The norepinephrine released at the sympathetic nerve terminals increases the amplitude and slope of the upstroke of the AV nodal action potentials, principally in the AN and N regions of the node.

Ventricular Conduction

The bundle of His passes subendocardially down the right side of the interventricular septum for about 1 cm and then divides into the right and left **bundle branches** (Figures 2-27 and 2-33). The right bundle branch is a direct continuation of the bundle of His and proceeds down the right side of the interventricular septum. The left bundle branch, which is considerably thicker than the right, arises almost perpendicularly from the bundle of His and perforates the interventricular septum. On the subendocardial surface of the left side of the interventricular septum, the main left bundle branch splits into a thin **anterior division** and a thick **posterior division.**

The right bundle branch and the two divisions of the left bundle branch ultimately subdivide into a complex network of conducting fibers called Purkinje fibers, which ramify over the subendocardial surfaces of both ventricles. In certain mammalian species, such as cattle, the Purkinje fiber network is arranged in discrete, encapsulated bundles (Figure 2-33).

Purkinje fibers are the broadest cells in the heart, 70 to 80 μm in diameter, compared with 10 to 15 μm for ventricular myocytes. The large diameter accounts in part for the greater conduction velocity in Purkinje than in myocardial fibers. Purkinje cells have abundant, linearly arranged sarcomeres, just as do myocardial cells. However, the T-tubular system is absent in the Purkinje cells of many species, but it is well developed in the myocardial cells.

The conduction of the action potential over the Purkinje fiber system is the fastest of any tissue within the heart; estimates vary from 1 to 4 m/s. This permits a rapid activation of the entire endocardial surface of the ventricles.

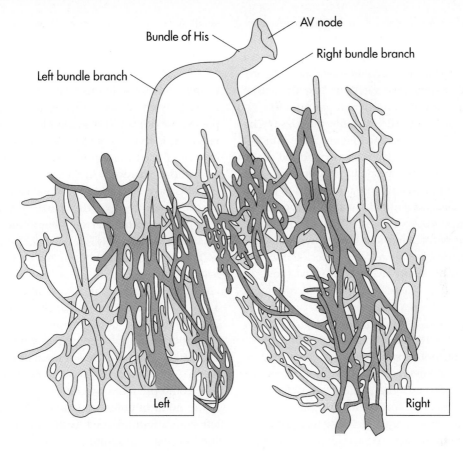

Figure 2-33 ■ **AV and ventricular conduction system of the calf heart.** (Redrawn from DeWitt LM: *Anat Rec* 3:475, 1909.)

Impulse conduction in the right bundle branch, the main left bundle branch, or either division of the left bundle branch may be impaired as a consequence of a degenerative process or of coronary artery disease. Conduction blocks in one or more of these pathways give rise to characteristic electrocardiographic patterns. Block of either of the main bundle branches is known as right or left **bundle branch block.** Block of either division of the left bundle branch is called **left anterior hemiblock** or **left posterior hemiblock.**

The action potentials recorded from Purkinje fibers resemble those of ordinary ventricular myocardial fibers (Figure 2-16, *A*). In general, phase 1 is more prominent in Purkinje fiber action potentials (Figure 2-3) than in those recorded from ventricular fibers (especially endocardial fibers), and the duration of the plateau (phase 2) is longer.

Because of the long refractory period of the Purkinje fibers, many premature activations of the atria are conducted through the AV junction but are blocked by the Purkinje fibers.

Therefore, they fail to evoke a premature contraction of the ventricles. This function of protecting the ventricles against the effects of premature atrial depolarizations is especially pronounced at slow heart rates, because the action potential duration, and hence the effective refractory period of the Purkinje fibers, vary inversely with the heart rate (Figure 2-20). At slow heart rates, the effective refractory period of the Purkinje fibers is especially prolonged; as the heart rate increases, the refractory period diminishes. Similar directional changes in the refractory period occur in most of the other cells in the heart with changes in rate. However, in the AV node, the effective refractory period does not change appreciably over the normal range of heart rates, and it actually increases at very rapid heart rates. Therefore, *at high heart rates, it is the AV node that protects the ventricles when impulses arrive at excessive repetition rates.*

The first portions of the ventricles to be excited are the interventricular septum (except its basal portion) and the papillary muscles. The wave of activation spreads into the substance of the septum from both its left and its right endocardial surfaces. Early contraction of the septum tends to make it more rigid and allows it to serve as an anchor point for the contraction of the remaining ventricular myocardium. Also, early contraction of the papillary muscles prevents eversion of the AV valves during ventricular systole.

The endocardial surfaces of both ventricles are activated rapidly, but the wave of excitation spreads from endocardium to epicardium at a slower velocity (about 0.3 to 0.4 m/s). Because the right ventricular wall is appreciably thinner than the left, the epicardial surface of the right ventricle is activated earlier than that of the left ventricle. Also, apical and central epicardial regions of both ventricles are activated somewhat earlier than are their respective basal regions. The last portions of the ventricles to be excited are the posterior basal epicardial regions and a

small zone in the basal portion of the interventricular septum.

■ REENTRY

Under certain conditions, a cardiac impulse may reexcite some region through which it had passed previously. This phenomenon, known as **reentry,** is responsible for many clinical disturbances of cardiac rhythm. The reentry may be **ordered** or **random.** In the ordered variety, the impulse traverses a fixed anatomic path, whereas in the random type the path continues to change. The principal example of random reentry is **fibrillation** (p 47).

The conditions necessary for reentry are illustrated in Figure 2-28. In each of the four panels, a single bundle *(S)* of cardiac fibers splits into a left *(L)* and a right *(R)* branch. A connecting bundle *(C)* runs between the two branches. Normally, the impulse coming down bundle *S* is conducted along the *L* and *R* branches (panel *A*). As the impulse reaches connecting link *C,* it enters from both sides and becomes extinguished at the point of collision. The impulse from the left side cannot proceed further because the tissue beyond is absolutely refractory, because it had just been depolarized from the other direction. The impulse cannot pass through bundle *C* from the right either, for the same reason.

It is obvious from panel *B* that the impulse cannot make a complete circuit if antegrade block exists in the two branches (*L* and *R*) of the fiber bundle. Furthermore, if bidirectional block exists at any point in the loop (e.g., branch *R* in panel *C*), the impulse will not be able to reenter.

A necessary condition for reentry is that at some point in the loop the impulse is able to pass in one direction but not in the other. This phenomenon is called **unidirectional block.** As shown in panel *D,* the impulse may travel down branch *L* normally and may be blocked in the antegrade direction in branch *R.* The impulse that had been conducted down branch *L* and through the connecting branch *C* may be able to penetrate the depressed region in branch *R* from the retrograde direction, even though the antegrade impulse had been blocked previously at this same site. The antegrade impulse will arrive at the depressed region in branch *R* earlier than the impulse that traverses a longer path and enters branch *R* from the opposite direction. The antegrade impulse may be blocked simply because it arrives at the depressed region during its effective refractory period. If the retrograde impulse is delayed sufficiently, the refractory period may have ended, and the impulse will be conducted back into bundle *S*.

Unidirectional block is a necessary condition for reentry, but not a sufficient one. *The effective refractory period of the reentered region must also be less than the propagation time around the loop.* In panel *D*, if the retrograde impulse is conducted through the depressed zone in branch *R* and if the tissue just beyond is still refractory from the antegrade depolarization, branch *S* will not be reexcited. Therefore, the conditions that promote reentry are those that prolong conduction time or shorten the effective refractory period.

The functional components of reentry loops responsible for specific arrhythmias in intact hearts are diverse. Some loops are very large and involve entire specialized conduction bundles; others are microscopic. The loop may include myocardial fibers, specialized conducting fibers, nodal cells, and junctional tissues, in almost any conceivable arrangement. Also, the cardiac cells in the loop may be normal or deranged.

■ TRIGGERED ACTIVITY

Triggered activity is so named because it is always coupled to a preceding action potential. Consequently, arrhythmias induced by triggered activity are difficult to distinguish from those induced by reentry. Triggered activity is caused by **afterdepolarizations.** Two types of afterdepo-

larizations are recognized: **early afterdepolarizations (EADs)** and **delayed afterdepolarizations (DADs).** EADs occur at the end of the plateau (phase 2) or about midway through repolarization (phase 3), whereas DADs occur near the very end of repolarization or just after full repolarization (phase 4).

Early Afterdepolarizations

EADs are more likely to occur when the prevailing heart rate is slow; rapid pacing suppresses EADs. In the experiment shown in Figure 2-34, EADs were induced by cesium in an isolated Purkinje fiber preparation. No afterdepolarizations were evident when the preparation was driven at a cycle length of 2 s. When the cycle length was increased to 4 s, EADs appeared.

Figure 2-34 ■ Effect of pacing at different cycle lengths *(CL)* on cesium-induced early afterdepolarizations (EADs) in a canine Purkinje fiber. **A,** EADs not evident. **B,** EADs first appear *(arrows).* The third EAD reaches threshold and triggers an action potential *(third arrow).* **C,** EADs that appear after each driven depolarization trigger an action potential. **D,** Triggered action potentials occur in salvos. (Modified with permission from Damiano BP, Rosen M: *Circulation* 69:1013, 1984. By permission of the American Heart Association, Inc.)

Most were subthreshold (first two arrows), but one of the EADs did reach threshold and triggered an action potential. When the cycle length was increased to 6 s, each driven action potential generated an EAD that triggered a second action potential. Furthermore, when the cycle length was increased to 10 s, each driven action potential triggered a salvo of four or five additional action potentials.

EADs may be produced experimentally by interventions that prolong the action potential. Because EADs may be initiated at either of two distinct levels of transmembrane potential, namely, at the end of the plateau and about midway through repolarization, two different mechanisms may be involved in generating them.

Considerable information has been obtained about the mechanism responsible for those EADs that appear at the end of the plateau. The more prolonged the action potential, the more EADs are more likely to occur. For those action potentials that trigger EADs, the plateau appears to be prolonged enough that those Ca^{++} channels that were activated at the beginning of the plateau and then inactivated would have sufficient time to be activated again before the plateau had expired. This secondary activation would trigger an afterdepolarization. Less information is available about the cellular mechanisms responsible for those EADs that appear midway through repolarization.

Delayed Afterdepolarizations

In contrast to EADs, DADs tend to appear when the heart rate is high. The salient characteristics of DADs are shown in Figure 2-35. The transmembrane potentials were recorded from Purkinje fibers that were exposed to a high concentration of **acetylstrophanthidin,** a digitalis-like substance. In the absence of driving stimuli, these fibers were quiescent. In each panel, a sequence of six driven depolarizations was induced at various basic cycle lengths.

Figure 2-35 ▪ Transmembrane action potentials recorded from isolated canine Purkinje fibers. Acetylstrophanthidin was added to the bath, and sequences of six driven beats (denoted by the dots) were produced at basic cycle lengths *(BCL)* of 800, 700, 600, and 500 ms. Note that delayed afterpotentials occurred after the driven beats, and that these afterpotentials reached threshold after the last driven beat in panels B to D, but not in panel A. (From Ferrier GR, Saunders JH, Mendez C: *Circ Res* 32:600, 1973. By permission of the American Heart Association, Inc.)

When the cycle length was 800 ms (panel *A*), the last driven depolarization was followed by a brief DAD that did not reach threshold. Once that afterdepolarization had subsided, the transmembrane potential remained constant until another driving stimulus was given. The upstroke of a DAD can be detected after each of the first five driven depolarizations.

When the basic cycle length was diminished to 700 ms (panel *B*), the DAD that followed the last driven beat did reach threshold, and a nondriven depolarization (or **extrasystole**) ensued. This extrasystole was itself followed by an afterpotential that was subthreshold. Diminution of the basic cycle length to 600 ms (panel C) also evoked an extrasystole after the last driven depolarization. The afterpotential that followed the extrasystole did reach threshold, however, and a second extrasystole occurred. A sequence of three extrasystoles followed the six driven depolarizations that were separated by intervals of 500 ms (panel D). Slightly shorter basic cycle lengths or slightly greater concentrations of acetylstrophanthidin evoked a continuous sequence of nondriven beats, resembling a paroxysmal tachycardia (described on p 47).

DADs are associated with elevated intracellular Ca^{++} concentrations. The amplitudes of the DADs are increased by interventions that raise intracellular Ca^{++} concentrations. Such interventions include elevated extracellular Ca^{++} concentrations and toxic levels of digitalis glycosides. The elevated levels of intracellular Ca^{++} provoke the oscillatory release of Ca^{++} from the sarcoplasmic reticulum. Hence, in myocardial cells, the DADs are accompanied by small changes in developed force. The high intracellular Ca^{++} concentrations also activate certain membrane channels that permit the passage of Na^+ and K^+. The net flux of these cations constitutes a **transient inward current,** i_{ti}, that is at least partly responsible for the afterdepolarization of the cell membrane. The elevated intracellular Ca^{++} may also activate Na^+/Ca^{++} exchange. This electrogenic exchanger brings into the cell three Na^+ for each Ca^{++} it ejects. This process creates a net inward current of cations that would contribute to the DAD.

■ ELECTROCARDIOGRAPHY

The electrocardiograph is a valuable instrument, because it enables the physician to infer the course of the cardiac impulse simply by recording the variations in electrical potential at various loci on the surface of the body. By analyzing the details of these potential fluctuations, the physician gains valuable insight concerning (1) the anatomic orientation of the heart; (2) the relative sizes of its chambers; (3) a variety of disturbances of rhythm and conduction; (4) the extent, location, and progress of ischemic damage to the myocardium; (5) the effects of altered electrolyte concentrations; and (6) the influence of certain drugs (notably digitalis and its derivatives). The science of electrocardiography is extensive and complex, but only the elementary basis of electrocardiography is considered here.

Scalar Electrocardiography

The systems of leads used to record routine electrocardiograms are oriented in certain planes of the body. The diverse electromotive forces that exist in the heart at any moment can be represented by a three-dimensional vector. A system of recording leads oriented in a given plane detects only the projection of the three-dimensional vector on that plane. Furthermore, the potential difference between two recording electrodes represents the projection of the vector on the line between the two leads. Components of vectors projected on such lines are not vectors but **scalar quantities** (having magnitude but not direction). Hence, a recording of the changes with time of the differences of potential between two points on the surface of the skin is called a **scalar electrocardiogram.**

Configuration of the Scalar Electrocardiogram The scalar electrocardiogram detects the changes with time of the electrical potential between some point on the surface of the skin and an indifferent electrode or between pairs of points on the skin surface. The cardiac impulse progresses through the heart in a complex three-dimensional pattern. Hence, the precise configuration of the electrocardiogram varies from individual to individual, and in any given individual the pattern varies with the anatomic location of the leads.

In general, the pattern consists of P, QRS, and

T waves (Figure 2-29). The P-R interval (or more precisely, the P-Q interval) is a measure of the time from the onset of atrial activation to the onset of ventricular activation; it normally ranges from 0.12 to 0.20 s. A considerable fraction of this time involves passage of the impulse through the AV conduction system. Pathologic prolongations of this interval are associated with disturbances of AV conduction produced by inflammatory, circulatory, pharmacologic, or nervous mechanisms.

The configuration and amplitude of the QRS complex vary considerably among individuals. The duration is usually between 0.06 and 0.10 s. Abnormal prolongation may indicate a block in the normal conduction pathways through the ventricles (such as a block of the left or right bundle branch). During the ST interval the entire ventricular myocardium is depolarized. Therefore, the ST segment lies on the **isoelectric line** under normal conditions. Any appreciable deviation from the isoelectric line is noteworthy and may indicate ischemic damage of the myocardium. The Q-T interval is sometimes referred to as the period of "electrical systole" of the ventricles. Its duration is about 0.4 s, but it varies inversely with the heart rate, mainly because the myocardial cell action potential duration varies inversely with the heart rate (Figure 2-20).

In most leads the T wave is deflected in the same direction from the isoelectric line as the major component of the QRS complex, although biphasic or oppositely directed T waves are perfectly normal in certain leads. When the T wave and QRS complex deviate in the same direction from the isoelectric line, it indicates that the repolarization process proceeds in a direction counter to the depolarization process. T waves that are abnormal in either direction or amplitude may indicate myocardial damage, electrolyte disturbances, or cardiac hypertrophy.

Standard Limb Leads The original electrocardiographic lead system was devised by

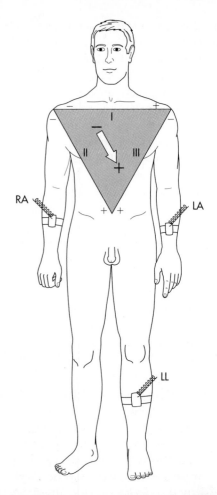

Figure 2-36 ■ Einthoven triangle, illustrating the galvanometer connections for standard limb leads I, II, and III.

Einthoven. In his lead system the **resultant cardiac vector** (the vector sum of all electrical activity occurring in the heart at any given moment) was considered to lie in the center of a triangle (assumed to be equilateral) formed by the left and right shoulders and the pubic region (Figure 2-36). This triangle, called the **Einthoven triangle,** is oriented in the frontal plane of the body. Hence, only the projection of the resultant cardiac vector on the frontal plane is detected by this system of leads. For convenience, the electrodes are connected to the right and left forearms rather than to the corresponding shoulders, because the arms represent simple extensions of the leads from the shoulders. Similarly, the leg is taken as an extension of the lead system from the pubis, and the third electrode is connected to the left leg (by convention).

Certain conventions dictate the manner in which these **standard limb leads** are connected to the galvanometer. Lead I records the potential difference between the left arm (LA) and right arm (RA). The galvanometer connections are such that when the potential at LA (V_{LA}) exceeds the potential at RA (V_{RA}), the galvanometer is deflected upward from the isoelectric line. In Figures 2-36 and 2-37 this arrangement of the galvanometer connections for lead I is designated by a (+) at LA and by a (−) at RA. Lead II records the potential difference between RA and LL (left leg) and yields an upward deflection when V_{LL} exceeds V_{RA}. Finally, lead III registers the potential difference between LA and LL and yields an upward deflection when V_{LL} exceeds V_{LA}. These galvanometer connections were arbitrarily chosen so that the QRS complexes will be upright in all three standard limb leads in most normal individuals.

Let the frontal projection of the resultant cardiac vector at some moment be represented by an arrow (tail negative, head positive), as in Figure 2-36. Then, the potential difference, $V_{LA} - V_{RA}$, recorded in lead I will be represented by the component of the vector projected along the horizontal line between LA and RA, as shown in Figure 2-37. If the cardiac vector makes an angle, θ, of 60 degrees with the horizontal (as in panel A of Figure 2-37), the magnitude of the potential recorded by lead I will equal the vector magnitude times cosine 60 degrees. The deflection recorded in lead I will be upward, because the positive arrowhead lies closer to LA than to RA. The deflection in lead II will also be upright, be-

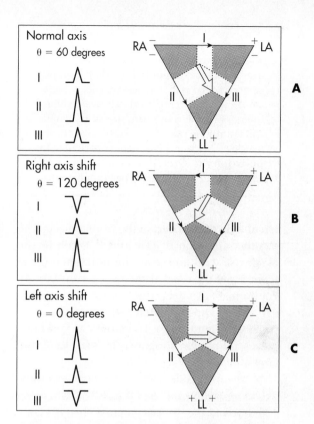

Figure 2-37 ■ **Magnitude and direction of the QRS complexes in limb leads I, II, and III, when the mean electrical axis (θ) is 60 degrees (A), 120 degrees (B), and 0 degrees (C).**

cause the arrowhead lies closer to LL than to RA. The magnitude of the lead II deflection will be greater than that in lead I, because in this example the direction of the vector parallels that of lead II; therefore, the magnitude of the projection on lead II exceeds that on lead I. Similarly, in lead III the deflection will be upright, and in this example, where θ = 60 degrees, its magnitude will equal that in lead I.

If the vector in panel A of Figure 2-37 is the resultant of the electrical events occurring during the peak of the QRS complex, the orientation of this vector is said to represent the **mean elec-**

> Changes in the mean electrical axis may occur with alterations in the anatomic position of the heart or with changes in the relative preponderance of the right and left ventricles. For example, the axis tends to shift toward the left (more horizontal) in short, stocky individuals and toward the right (more vertical) in tall, thin persons. Also, with left or right **ventricular hypertrophy** (increased myocardial mass), the axis will shift toward the hypertrophied side.

trical axis of the heart in the frontal plane. The positive direction of this axis is taken in the clockwise direction from the horizontal plane (contrary to the usual mathematical convention). For normal individuals the average mean electrical axis is approximately +60 degrees (as in panel A of Figure 2-37). Therefore, the QRS complexes are usually upright in all three leads and largest in lead II.

With appreciable shift of the mean electrical axis to the right (panel B of Figure 2-37, where θ = 120 degrees), the displacements of the QRS complexes in the standard leads will change considerably. In this case the largest upright deflection will be in lead III and the deflection in lead I will be inverted, because the arrowhead will be closer to RA than to LA. With left axis shift (panel C of Figure 2-37, where θ = 0 degrees), the largest upright deflection will be in lead I, and the QRS complex in lead III will be inverted.

As is evident from this discussion, the standard limb leads I, II, and III are oriented in the frontal plane at 0, 60, and 120 degrees, respectively, from the horizontal plane. Other limb leads, which are also oriented in the frontal plane, are usually recorded in addition to the standard leads. These "unipolar limb leads" lie along axes at angles of +90, −30, and −150 degrees from the horizontal plane. Such lead systems are described in all textbooks on electrocardiography and are not considered further here.

To obtain information concerning the projections of the cardiac vector on the sagittal and transverse planes of the body in scalar electrocardiography, the **precordial leads** are usually recorded. Most commonly, each of six selected points on the anterior and lateral surfaces of the chest in the vicinity of the heart is connected in turn to the galvanometer. The other galvanometer terminal is usually connected to a **central terminal,** which is composed of a junction of three leads from LA, RA, and LL, each in series with a 5000-ohm resistor. The voltage of this central terminal remains at a theoretical zero potential throughout the cardiac cycle.

■ ARRHYTHMIAS

Cardiac arrhythmias reflect disturbances of either **impulse propagation** or **impulse initiation.** The principal disturbances of impulse propagation are conduction blocks and reentrant rhythms. Disturbances of impulse initiation include those that arise from the SA node and those that originate from various ectopic foci.

Altered Sinoatrial Rhythms

The frequency of pacemaker discharge varies by the mechanisms described earlier in this chapter (Figure 2-22). Changes in SA nodal discharge frequency are usually produced by the cardiac autonomic nerves. Examples of electrocardiograms of sinus tachycardia and sinus bradycardia are shown in Figure 2-38. The P, QRS, and T deflections are all normal, but the duration of the cardiac cycle (the **P-P interval**) is altered. Characteristically, when sinus bradycardia or tachycardia develops, the cardiac frequency changes gradually and requires several beats to attain its new steady-state value. Electrocardiographic evidence of **respiratory cardiac arrhythmia** is common and is manifested as a rhythmic variation in the P-P interval at the respiratory frequency (p 90).

A, Normal sinus rhythm.

B, Sinus tachycardia.

C, Sinus bradycardia.

Figure 2-38 ■ **Sinoatrial rhythms.**

Figure 2-39 ■ **His bundle electrogram (*lower tracing,* retouched) and lead II of the scalar electrocardiogram (*upper tracing*). The deflection, *H,* which represents the impulse conduction over the bundle of His, is clearly visible between the atrial, *A,* and ventricular, *V,* deflections. The conduction time from the atria to the bundle of His is denoted by the A-H interval; that from the bundle of His to the ventricles, by the H-V interval.**

Atrioventricular Transmission Blocks

Various physiologic, pharmacologic, and pathologic processes can impede impulse transmission through the AV conduction tissue. The site of block can be localized more precisely by recording the **His bundle electrogram** (Figure 2-39). To obtain such tracings, an electrode catheter is introduced into a peripheral vein and threaded centrally until the tip containing the electrodes lies in the AV junctional region between the right atrium and ventricle. When the electrodes are properly positioned, a distinct deflection (Figure 2-39, *H*) is registered, which represents the passage of the cardiac impulse down the bundle of His. The time intervals required for propagation from the atrium to the bundle of His **(A-H interval)** and from the bundle of His to the ventricles **(H-V interval)** may be measured accurately. Abnormal prolongation of the former or latter interval indicates block above or below the bundle of His, respectively.

Premature Depolarizations

Premature depolarizations occur at times in most normal individuals but are more common under certain abnormal conditions. They may originate in the atria, AV junction, or ventricles. One type of premature depolarization is coupled to a normally conducted depolarization by a constant **coupling interval.** If the normal depolarization is suppressed temporarily (e.g., by vagal stimulation), the premature depolarization will also be suppressed. Such premature depolarizations are called **coupled extrasystoles,** or simply extrasystoles, and they probably reflect a reentry phenomenon (Figure 2-28). A second type of premature depolarization occurs as the result of enhanced automaticity in some ectopic focus. This ectopic center may fire regularly and be protected from depolarization by the normal cardiac impulse. If this premature depolarization occurs at a regular interval or at a simple multiple of that interval, the disturbance is called **parasystole.**

A **premature atrial depolarization** is shown in the electrocardiogram in Figure 2-40, *A*. The normal interval between beats was 0.89 s (heart rate, 68 beats per minute). The premature atrial depolarization (second P wave in the figure) followed the preceding P wave by only 0.56 s. The configuration of the premature P wave differs from the configuration of the other, normal P waves because the course of atrial excitation, originating at some ectopic focus in the atrium, is different from the normal spread of excitation that originates in the SA node. The QRS complex of the premature depolarization is usually normal in configuration because the spread of ventricular excitation occurs over the usual pathways.

A **premature ventricular depolarization** appears in Figure 2-40, *B*. Because the premature excitation originated at some ectopic focus in the ventricles, the impulse spread was aberrant, and the configurations of the QRS and T waves were entirely different from the normal deflections. The premature QRS complex followed the preceding normal QRS complex by only 0.47 s. The interval after the premature excitation was 1.28 s, considerably longer than the normal interval between beats (0.89 s). The interval (1.75 s) from the QRS complex just before the premature excitation to the QRS complex just after it was virtually equal to the duration of two normal cardiac cycles (1.78 s).

The prolonged interval that usually follows a premature ventricular depolarization is called a **compensatory pause.** The reason for the compensatory pause after a premature ventricular depolarization is that the ectopic ventricular impulse does not disturb the natural rhythm of the SA node. Either the ectopic ventricular impulse is not conducted retrograde through the AV conduction system or, if it is, the time required is such that the SA node has already fired at its natural interval before the ectopic impulse could have reached it. Likewise, the SA nodal impulse usually does not affect the ventricle, because the

Figure 2-40 ■ **A premature atrial depolarization (A) and a premature ventricular depolarization (B). The premature atrial depolarization (second beat in the top tracing) is followed by normal QRS and T waves. The interval following the premature depolarization is not much longer than the usual interval between beats. The brief rectangular deflection just before the last depolarization is a standardization signal. The premature ventricular depolarization (B) is characterized by bizarre QRS and T waves and is followed by a compensatory pause.**

AV junction and perhaps also the ventricles are still refractory from the premature excitation. In Figure 2-40, *B*, the P wave originating in the SA node at the time of the premature depolarization occurred at the same time as the T wave of the premature cycle and therefore cannot easily be identified in the tracing.

Ectopic Tachycardias

When a tachycardia originates from some ectopic site in the heart, the onset and termination are typically abrupt, in contrast to the more gradual changes in heart rate in sinus tachycardia. Be-

Episodes of ectopic tachycardia may persist for only a few beats or for many hours or days, and the episodes often recur. Paroxysmal tachycardias may occur as the result of (1) the rapid firing of an ectopic pacemaker, (2) triggered activity secondary to afterpotentials that reach threshold, or (3) an impulse circling a reentry loop repetitively.

In atrial fibrillation, the AV node is activated at intervals that may vary considerably from cycle to cycle. Hence, there is no constant interval between QRS complexes and therefore between ventricular contractions. Because the strength of ventricular contraction depends on the interval between beats (as explained on p 99), the volume and rhythm of the pulse are very irregular. In many patients the atrial reentry loop and the pattern of AV conduction are more regular. The rhythm is then referred to as **atrial flutter.**

cause of the sudden appearance and abrupt cessation, such ectopic tachycardias are usually called paroxysmal tachycardias.

Such tachycardias may cause lightheadedness or even transient loss of consciousness (syncope), because the very rapid contraction frequency does not permit adequate time for ventricular filling between heartbeats.

Paroxysmal tachycardias originating in the atria or in the AV junctional tissues (Figure 2-41, *A*) are usually indistinguishable, and therefore both are included in the term **paroxysmal supraventricular tachycardia.** The tachycardia often results from an impulse repetitively circling a reentry loop that includes atrial tissue, the AV junction, or both. The QRS complexes are often normal, because ventricular activation proceeds over the normal pathways.

Paroxysmal ventricular tachycardia originates from an ectopic focus in the ventricles. The electrocardiogram is characterized by repeated, bizarre QRS complexes that reflect the aberrant intraventricular impulse conduction (Figure 2-41, *B*). Paroxysmal ventricular tachycardia is much more ominous than supraventricular tachycardia because it is frequently a precursor of ventricular fibrillation, a lethal arrhythmia described in the next section.

Fibrillation

Under certain conditions, cardiac muscle undergoes an irregular type of contraction that is entirely ineffectual in propelling blood. Such an arrhythmia is termed **fibrillation** and may involve either the atria or the ventricles. Fibrillation probably represents a reentry phenomenon in which the reentry loop fragments into multiple, irregular circuits.

The tracing in Figure 2-42, *A,* illustrates the electrocardiographic changes in **atrial fibrillation.** This condition occurs in various types of chronic heart disease. The atria do not contract and relax sequentially during each cardiac cycle and hence do not contribute to ventricular filling. Instead, the atria undergo a continuous, uncoordinated, rippling type of activity. In the electrocardiogram there are no P waves; they are replaced by continuous irregular fluctuations of potential, called **f waves.**

Although atrial fibrillation and flutter are compatible with life and even with full physical activity, the onset of **ventricular fibrillation** leads to loss of consciousness within a few seconds. The irregular, continuous, uncoordinated twitchings of the ventricular muscle fibers pump no blood. In the electrocardiogram (Figure 2-42, *B*), irregular fluctuations of potential are manifest.

Fibrillation is often initiated when a premature impulse arrives during the **vulnerable period.** In the ventricles, this period coincides with the downslope of the T wave. During this period, the excitability of the cardiac cells varies. Some

A, Supraventricular tachycardia.

B, Ventricular tachycardia.

Figure 2-41 ■ **Paroxysmal tachycardias.**

A, Atrial fibrillation.

B, Ventricular fibrillation.

Figure 2-42 ■ **Atrial and ventricular fibrillation.**

Death ensues in ventricular fibrillation unless immediate, effective resuscitation is achieved or unless the rhythm reverts to normal spontaneously, which rarely occurs. Ventricular fibrillation may supervene when the entire ventricle, or some portion of it, is deprived of its normal blood supply. It may also occur as a result of electrocution or in response to certain drugs and anesthetics.

Atrial fibrillation may be reverted to a normal sinus rhythm by drugs that prolong the refractory period. As the cardiac impulses complete the numerous reentry loops, these impulses may then find the myocardial fibers no longer excitable, because of the extended refractory period.

Patients may live many years with atrial fibrillation, and therefore this condition does not usually constitute a medical emergency. However, immediate therapy is required in ventricular fibrillation. Conversion to a normal sinus rhythm is accomplished by means of a strong electrical current that places the entire myocardium briefly in a refractory state. Techniques have been developed to safely transmit the current through the intact chest wall. In successful cases the SA node again takes over as the normal pacemaker for the entire heart.

fibers are still in their effective refractory periods, others have almost fully recovered their excitability, and still others are able to conduct impulses, but only at very slow conduction velocities. As a consequence, the action potentials are propagated over the chambers in multiple wavelets that travel along circuitous paths and at various conduction velocities. As a region of cardiac cells becomes excitable again, it will ultimately be reentered by one of the wave fronts traveling about the chamber. The process is self-sustaining.

Electric shock is sometimes also used to treat atrial fibrillation, especially when the disturbance does not respond optimally to drugs. The timing of the shock is coordinated with the absolute refractory period of the ventricles (i.e., during or shortly after the QRS deflection of the electrocardiogram), so that the shock does not affect ventricular excitation. However, the shock will render all the atrial myocytes temporarily refractory, and thereby interrupt the prevailing reentry circuits.

■ SUMMARY
Transmembrane Action Potentials
The transmembrane action potentials that can be recorded from cardiac myocytes comprise five phases (0 to 4):

1. Phase 0, upstroke. A suprathreshold stimulus rapidly depolarizes the membrane by activating the fast Na^+ channels.
2. Phase I, early partial repolarization. Achieved by the efflux of K^+ through channels that conduct the transient outward current, i_{to}.
3. Phase 2, plateau. Achieved by a balance between the influx of Ca^{++} through Ca^{++} channels and the efflux of K^+ through several types of K^+ channels.
4. Phase 3, final repolarization. Initiated when the efflux of K^+ exceeds the influx of Ca^{++}. The resulting partial repolarization rapidly increases the K^+ conductance and rapidly restores full repolarization.
5. Phase 4, resting potential. The transmembrane potential of the fully repolarized cell is determined mainly by the conductance of the cell membrane to K^+.

Types of Action Potentials
Two principal types of action potentials may be recorded from cardiac cells:

1. Fast-response action potential. Recorded from atrial and ventricular myocardial fibers and from specialized conducting (Purkinje) fibers.

The action potential is characterized by a large-amplitude, steep upstroke, which is produced by the activation of the fast Na^+ channels. The effective refractory period begins at the upstroke of the action potential and persists until about midway through phase 3. The fiber is relatively refractory during the remainder of phase 3, but it regains full excitability as soon as it is fully repolarized (phase 4).

2. Slow-response action potential. Recorded from normal SA and AV nodal cells and from abnormal myocardial cells that have been partially depolarized. The action potential is characterized by a less negative resting potential, a smaller amplitude, and a less steep upstroke than is the fast-response action potential. The upstroke is produced by the activation of Ca^{++} channels. The fiber becomes absolutely refractory at the beginning of the upstroke, but partial excitability may not be regained until very late in phase 3 or after the fiber is fully repolarized. The fiber remains relatively refractory for a significant time after the fiber has fully repolarized.

Automaticity

Automaticity is characteristic of certain cells in the heart, notably those in the SA and AV nodes and in the specialized conducting system. Automaticity is achieved by a slow depolarization of the membrane during phase 4. Ultimately, the transmembrane potential reaches threshold; this leads to the upstroke of the action potential and the firing of the automatic cell.

Cardiac Excitation

1. Normally, the SA node initiates the impulse that induces cardiac contraction. This impulse is propagated from the SA node to the atria, and the wave of excitation ultimately reaches the AV node.

2. Because the cells in the AV node are slow-response fibers, the impulse travels very slowly through the AV node. The consequent delay between atrial and ventricular depolarization provides adequate time for atrial contraction to help fill the ventricles.

Disturbances of Impulse Initiation

Impulses may be initiated abnormally (a) by slow diastolic depolarization of automatic cells in ectopic sites or (b) by afterdepolarizations that reach threshold.

1. Ectopic foci. Automatic cells in the atrium, AV node, or His-Purkinje system may initiate propagated cardiac impulses either because the ordinarily more rhythmic, normal pacemaker cells are suppressed, or because the rhythmicity of the ectopic foci is abnormally enhanced.

2. Afterdepolarizations. Under abnormal conditions, afterdepolarizations may appear early in phase 3 of a normally initiated beat, or they may be delayed until near the end of phase 3 or the beginning of phase 4. Such afterdepolarizations may themselves trigger propagated impulses.

   a. Early afterdepolarization. More likely to occur when the basic cycle length of the initiating beats is very long and when the cardiac action potentials are abnormally prolonged.

   b. Delayed afterdepolarizations. More likely to occur when the basic cycle length of the initiating beats is short and when the cardiac cells are overloaded with Ca^{++}.

Disturbances of Impulse Conduction

Disturbances of impulse conduction consist mainly of simple conduction block and reentry.

1. Simple conduction block. Failure of propagation in a cardiac fiber as the result of a disease process (ischemia, inflammation) or a drug.

2. Reentry. A cardiac impulse may traverse a loop of cardiac fibers and reenter previously

excited tissue when (a) the impulse is conducted slowly around the loop and (b) the impulse is blocked unidirectionally in some section of the loop.

Electrocardiogram

The electrocardiogram is recorded from the surface of the body and traces the conduction of the cardiac impulse through the heart. The component waves of the electrocardiogram are

1. P wave. Spread of excitation over the atria.
2. QRS interval. Spread of excitation over the ventricles.
3. T wave. Spread of repolarization over the ventricles.

The electrocardiogram may be used to detect and analyze certain cardiac arrhythmias, such as altered sinoatrial rhythms, atrioventricular conduction blocks, premature depolarizations, ectopic tachycardias, and atrial and ventricular fibrillation.

■ KEY WORDS AND CONCEPTS

- Transmembrane potentials
- Action potential
- Fast-response action potential
- Slow-response action potential
- Purkinje fibers
- Sinoatrial (SA) node
- Atrioventricular (AV) node
- Ischemia
- Ion channels
- Ion current
- Resting membrane potential
- Action potential upstroke
- Depolarization
- Repolarization
- Nernst equation
- Na^+,K^+-ATPase
- Chord conductance equation
- Electrogenic pump
- Activation gate
- Inactivation gate
- Ionic conductance
- Effective refractory period
- Relative refractory period
- Patch-clamping technique
- Ion channel antagonists
- Adenylyl cyclase
- Cyclic AMP
- Congestive heart failure
- Inward rectification
- Conduction of the cardiac impulse
- Rate dependence of refractoriness
- Post-repolarization refractoriness
- Ectopic pacemakers
- Idioventricular pacemakers
- Pacemaker potential
- Slow diastolic depolarization
- Vasovagal syncope
- Wolff-Parkinson-White syndrome
- Hyperpolarization
- Overdrive suppression
- Asystole
- Atrial internodal pathways
- Bundle of His
- Bundle branches
- Bundle branch block
- Atrioventricular block
- Accessory AV pathways
- Reentry
- Unidirectional block
- Triggered activity
- Early afterdepolarizations (EADs)
- Delayed afterdepolarizations (DADs)
- Electrocardiogram
- Einthoven triangle
- Resultant cardiac vector
- Mean electrical axis
- His bundle electrogram
- Extrasystole
- Bradycardia
- Tachycardia
- Fibrillation

■ SELF-STUDY PROBLEMS

1. What major movements of ions account for each phase of the action potential of a typical fast-response myocardial cell?
2. Why is the cardiac action potential propagated more slowly in an AV node cell than in an atrial or ventricular myocyte?
3. By what pathways does a cardiac impulse that originates in the SA node arrive in the ventricular myocardium?
4. What electrophysiologic conditions might lead to reentry?
5. What electrocardiographic changes would occur in first-, second-, and third-degree AV block?

■ BIBLIOGRAPHY

Journal articles

Antzelevitch C, Sicouri S: Clinical relevance of cardiac arrhythmias generated by afterdepolarization: role of M cells in the generation of U waves, triggered activity and torsade de pointes, *J Am Coll Cardiol* 23:259, 1994.

Antzelevitch C, Sicouri S, Litovsky SH et al: Heterogeneity within the ventricular wall: electrophysiology and pharmacology of epicardial, endocardial and M cells, *Circ Res* 69:1427, 1991.

Balke CW, Rose WC, O'Rourke B et al: Biophysics and physiology of cardiac calcium channels, *Circulation* 87:VII-49, 1993.

Bean BP: Multiple types of calcium channels in heart muscle and neurons, *Ann NY Acad Sci* 560:334, 1989.

Beaumont J, Michaels DC, Delmar M et al: A model study of changes in excitability of ventricular muscle cells: inhibition, facilitation, and hysteresis, *Am J Physiol* 268:H1181, 1995.

Billette J, Nattel S: Dynamic behavior of the atrioventricular node: a functional model of interaction between recovery, facilitation, and fatigue, *J Cardiovasc Electrophysiol* 5:90, 1994.

Bonke FIM, Kirchhof CJHJ, Allessie MA, Wit AL: Impulse propagation from the SA-node to the ventricles, *Experientia* 43:1044, 1987.

Delmar M: Role of potassium currents on cell excitability in cardiac ventricular myocytes, *J Cardiovasc Electrophysiol* 3:474, 1993.

Demir SS, Clark JW, Murphey CR, Giles WR: A mathematical model of a rabbit sinoatrial node cell, *Am J Physiol* 266:C832, 1994.

DiFrancesco D: Pacemaker mechanisms in cardiac tissue, *Annu Rev Physiol* 55:455, 1993.

Grant AO: Evolving concepts of cardiac sodium channel function, *J Cardiovasc Electrophysiol* 1:53, 1990.

Irisawa H, Brown HF, Giles W: Cardiac pacemaking in the sinoatrial node, *Physiol Rev* 73:197, 1993.

January CT, Shorofsky S: Early afterdepolarizations: newer insights into cellular mechanisms, *J Cardiovasc Electrophysiol* 1:161, 1990.

Levy MN: Role of calcium in arrhythmogenesis, *Circulation* 80:IV-23, 1989.

Meijler FL, Janse MJ: Morphology and electrophysiology of the mammalian atrioventricular node, *Physiol Rev* 68:608, 1988.

Nichols CG, Makhina EN, Pearson WL et al: Inward rectification and implications for cardiac excitability, *Circ Res* 78:1, 1996.

Opthof T: Mammalian sinoatrial node, *Cardiovasc Drugs Ther* 1:573, 1988.

Reiter M: Calcium mobilization and cardiac inotropic mechanisms, *Pharmacol Rev* 40:189, 1988.

Rosen MR: Links between basic and clinical cardiac electrophysiology, *Circulation* 77:251, 1988.

Sicouri S, Antzelevitch C: Electrophysiologic characteristics of M cells in the canine left ventricular free wall, *J Cardiovasc Electrophysiol* 6:591, 1995.

Spach MS, Josephson ME: Initiating reentry: the role of nonuniform anisotropy in small circuits, *J Cardiovasc Electrophysiol* 5:182, 1994.

Tseng GN, Boyden PA: Multiple types of Ca^{2+} currents in single canine Purkinje cells, *Circ Res* 65:1735, 1989.

Waldo AL, Wit AL: Mechanisms of cardiac arrhythmias, *Lancet* 341:1189, 1993.

Books and monographs

Armour JA, Ardell JL: *Neurocardiology,* New York, 1994, Oxford University Press.

Cranefield PF, Aronson RS: *Cardiac arrhythmias: the role of triggered activity and other mechanisms,* Mt. Kisco, NY, 1988, Futura.

Dangman KH, Miura DS: *Electrophysiology and pharmacology of the heart: a clinical guide,* New York, 1991, Marcel Dekker.

Levy MN, Schwartz PJ: *Vagal control of the heart: experimental basis and clinical implications,* Armonk, NY, 1994, Futura.

Levy MN, Vassalle M: *Excitation and neural control of the heart,* Bethesda, MD, 1982, American Physiological Society.

Mazgalev T, Dreifus LS, Michelson EL: *Electrophysiology of the sinoatrial and atrioventricular nodes,* New York, 1988, Alan R Liss.

Nathan RD: *Cardiac muscle: regulation of excitation and contraction,* Orlando, 1986, Academic Press.

Noble D, Powell T: *Electrophysiology of single cardiac cells,* Orlando, 1987, Academic Press.

Sakmann B, Neher E: *Single channel recording,* New York, 1983, Plenum Press.

Sperelakis N: *Physiology and pathophysiology of the heart,* ed 3, Boston, 1995, Kluwer Academic.

Spooner PM, Brown AM, Catterall WA, Kaczorowski GJ,

Strauss HC: *Ion channels in the cardiovascular system: function and dysfunction,* Armonk, NY, 1994, Futura.

Wit AL, Janse MJ: *Ventricular arrhythmias of ischemia and infarction: electrophysiological mechanisms,* Armonk, NY, 1993, Futura.

Zipes DP, Jalife J: *Cardiac electrophysiology: from cell to bedside,* ed 2, Philadelphia, 1995, WB Saunders.

The Cardiac Pump

It is nearly impossible to contemplate the pumping action of the heart without being struck by its simplicity of design, its wide range of activity and functional capacity, and the staggering amount of work it performs relentlessly over the lifetime of an individual. To understand how the heart accomplishes its important task, it is first necessary to consider the relationships between the structure and function of its components.

■ STRUCTURE OF THE HEART IN RELATION TO FUNCTION

Myocardial Cell

A number of important morphologic and functional differences exist between myocardial and skeletal muscle cells. However, the contractile elements within the two types of cells are quite similar; each skeletal and cardiac muscle cell is made up of **sarcomeres** (from Z line to Z line) containing thick filaments composed of myosin (in the A band) and thin filaments containing actin. The thin filaments extend from the point where they are anchored to the Z line (through the I band) to interdigitate with the thick filaments. As in the case of skeletal muscle, shortening occurs by the sliding filament mechanism. Actin filaments slide along adjacent myosin filaments by cycling of the intervening crossbridges, thereby bringing the Z lines closer together.

Skeletal and cardiac muscle show similar length-force relationships. The sarcomere length has been determined with electron microscopy in papillary muscles and intact ventricles rapidly fixed during systole or diastole. The developed force is maximal when the muscle begins its contractions at resting sarcomere lengths of 2 to 2.4 μm. At such lengths, there is optimal overlap of thick and thin filaments, and a maximal number of crossbridge attachments. Stretch of the myocardium and increases in load enhance the affinity of troponin C for Ca^{++}. Just how an increase in sarcomere length increases the sensitivity of the myofilaments to calcium remains to be determined. One concept is that the thick and thin filaments are brought closer to each other as the diameter of the muscle fiber narrows during stretch. Developed force of cardiac muscle is less than the maximal value when the sarcomeres are stretched beyond the optimal length, because of less overlap of the filaments, and hence less cycling of the crossbridges. At resting sarcomere lengths shorter than optimal value, the thin filaments overlap each other, which diminishes contractile force.

In general, the fiber length-force relationship for the papillary muscle also holds true for fibers in the intact heart. This relationship may be expressed graphically, as in Figure 3-1, by substituting ventricular systolic pressure for force and end-diastolic ventricular volume for myocardial resting fiber (and hence sarcomere) length. The lower curve in Figure 3-1 represents the increment in pressure produced by each increment in volume when the heart is in diastole. The upper curve represents the peak pressure developed by the ventricle during systole at each degree of filling, and illustrates the **Frank-Starling relationship** of initial myocardial fiber length (or initial volume) to force (or pressure) development by the ventricle.

Note that the pressure-volume curve in diastole is initially quite flat, indicating that large increases in volume can be accommodated with only small increases in pressure, yet systolic pressure development is considerable at the lower filling pressures. However, the ventricle becomes much less distensible with greater filling, as evidenced by the sharp rise of the diastolic curve at large intraventricular volumes. In the normal intact heart, peak force may be attained at a filling pressure of 12 mm Hg. At this intraventricular diastolic pressure, which is about the upper limit observed in the normal heart, the sarcomere length is 2.2 μm. However, developed force peaks at filling pressures as high as 30 mm Hg in the isolated heart; even at higher diastolic pressures (>50 mm Hg), the sarcomere length is not greater than 2.6 μm. This resistance to stretch of the myocardium at high filling pressures probably resides in the noncontractile constituents of the tissue (connective tissue) and may serve as a safety factor against overloading of the heart in diastole. Usually, ventricular diastolic pressure is about 0 to 7 mm Hg, and the average diastolic sarcomere length is about 2.2 μm. Thus, *the normal heart operates on the ascending portion of the Frank-Starling curve* depicted in Figure 3-1.

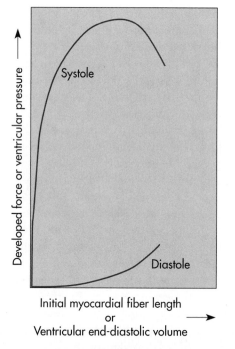

Figure 3-1 ■ Relationship of myocardial resting fiber length (sarcomere length) or end-diastolic volume to developed force or peak systolic ventricular pressure during ventricular contraction in the intact dog heart. (Redrawn from Patterson SW, Piper H, Starling EH: *J Physiol* 48:465, 1914.)

If the heart becomes greatly distended with blood during diastole, as may occur in cardiac failure, it is less efficient; more energy is required (greater wall tension) for the distended heart to eject the same volume of blood per beat than for the normal undilated heart. This is an example of Laplace's law (p 155), which states that the tension in the wall of a vessel (in this case the ventricles) equals the transmural pressure (pressure across the wall, or distending pressure) times the radius of the vessel or chamber. The Laplace relationship applies to infinitely thin-walled vessels but can be applied to the heart if correction is made for wall thickness. The equation is $\tau = Pr/w$ where τ = wall stress, P = transmural pressure, r = radius, and w = wall thickness.

A striking difference in the appearance of cardiac and skeletal muscle is the semblance of a syncytium in cardiac muscle with branching interconnecting fibers (Figures 3-2 and 3-3). However, the myocardium is not a true anatomic syncytium, because laterally the myocardial fibers are separated from adjacent fibers by their respective sarcolemmas, and the end of each fiber is separated from its neighbor by dense structures, **intercalated disks,** that are continuous with the sarcolemma (Figures 3-2 to 3-4). Nevertheless, *cardiac muscle functions as a syncytium,* because a wave of depolarization followed by contraction of the entire myocardium (an *all-or-none*

response) occurs when a suprathreshold stimulus is applied to any one focus.

As the wave of excitation approaches the end of a cardiac cell, the spread of excitation to the next cell depends on the electrical conductance of the boundary between the two cells. **Gap junctions (nexi)** with high conductances are present in the intercalated disks between adjacent cells (Figures 3-2 to 3-4). These gap junctions, which facilitate the conduction of the cardiac impulse from one cell to the next, are made up of **connexons,** hexagonal structures that connect the cytosol of adjacent cells. Each connexon consists of six polypeptides surrounding a

A band

I band

Invagination of sarcolemma by transverse tubule

Transverse tubule

Mitochondria

M line in H zone

Z line

Sarcomere

Red cell in capillary

Capillary endothelium

Connective tissue

Intercalated disk

Gap junction

Sarcolemma

Sarcoplasmic reticulum

Figure 3-2 ■ Diagram of an electron micrograph of cardiac muscle showing large numbers of mitochondria and the intercalated disks with nexi (gap junctions), transverse tubules, and longitudinal tubules.

Figure 3-3 ■ For legend see opposite page.

core channel approximately 1.6 to 2.0 nm wide, which serves as a low-resistance pathway for cell-to-cell conductance.

Impulse conduction in cardiac tissues progresses more rapidly in a direction parallel to the long axes of the constituent fibers than in a direction perpendicular to the long axes of those fibers. Gap junctions exist in the borders between myocardial fibers that are in contact with each other longitudinally; they are very sparse or absent in the borders between myocardial fibers that lie side by side.

Another difference between cardiac and fast skeletal muscle fibers is in the number of mitochondria (**sarcosomes**) in the two tissues. Fast skeletal muscle, which is called on for relatively short periods of repetitive or sustained contraction and which can metabolize anaerobically and build up a substantial oxygen debt, has relatively few mitochondria in the muscle fibers. In contrast, cardiac muscle, which contracts repetitively for a lifetime and requires a continuous supply of oxygen, is very rich in mitochondria (Figures 3-2 to 3-4). Rapid oxidation of substrates with the synthesis of adenosine triphosphate (ATP) can keep pace with the myocardial energy require-

ments because of the large numbers of mitochondria containing the respiratory enzymes necessary for oxidative phosphorylation.

To provide adequate oxygen and substrate for its metabolic machinery, the myocardium is also endowed with a rich capillary supply, about one capillary per fiber. Thus, diffusion distances are short, and oxygen, carbon dioxide, substrates, and waste material can move rapidly between myocardial cell and capillary. With respect to exchange of substances between the capillary blood and the myocardial cells, electron micrographs of myocardium show deep invaginations of the sarcolemma into the fiber at the Z lines (Figures 3-2 to 3-4). These sarcolemmal invaginations constitute the **transverse-tubular,** or **T-tubular, system.** The lumina of these T tubules are continuous with the bulk interstitial fluid, and they play a key role in excitation-contraction coupling.

In mammalian ventricular cells, adjacent T tubules are interconnected by longitudinally running or axial tubules, thus forming an extensively interconnected lattice of "intracellular" tubules (Figure 3-4). This T-tubule system is open to the interstitial fluid, is lined with a basement mem-

---

Figure 3-3 ■ A, Low-magnification electron micrograph of a monkey heart (ventricle). Typical features of myocardial cells include the elongated nucleus *(Nu),* striated myofibrils *(MF)* with columns of mitochondria *(Mit)* between the myofibrils, and intercellular junctions (intercalated disks, *ID).* A blood vessel *(BV)* is located between two myocardial cells. B, Medium-magnification electron micrograph of monkey ventricular cells showing details of ultrastructure. The sarcolemma *(SL)* is the boundary of the muscle cells and is thrown into multiple folds where the cells meet at the intercalated disk region *(ID).* The prominent myofibrils *(MF)* show distinct banding patterns, including the A band *(A),* dark Z lines *(Z),* I band regions *(I),* and M lines *(M)* at the center of each sarcomere unit. Mitochondria *(Mit)* occur either in rows between myofibrils or in masses just underneath the sarcolemma. Regularly spaced transverse tubules *(TT)* appear at the Z line levels of the myofibrils. C, High-magnification electron micrograph of a specialized intercellular junction between two myocardial cells of the mouse. Called a gap junction *(GJ)* or nexus, this attachment consists of very close apposition of the sarcolemmal membranes of the two cells and appears in thin section to consist of seven layers. D, Freeze-fracture replica of mouse myocardial gap junction, showing distinct arrays of characteristic intramembranous particles. Large particles *(P)* belong to the inner half of the sarcolemma of one myocardial cell, whereas the "pitted" membrane face *(E)* is formed by the outer half of the sarcolemma of the cell above.

Figure 3-4 ■ For legend see opposite page.

brane continuous with that of the surface sarcolemma, and contains micropinocytotic vesicles. Thus, in ventricular cells the myofibrils and mitochondria have ready access to a space that is continuous with the interstitial fluid. The T-tubular system is absent or poorly developed in atrial cells of many mammalian hearts.

A network of **sarcoplasmic reticulum** (Figure 3-4) consisting of small-diameter sarcotubules is also present surrounding the myofibrils; these sarcotubules are believed to be "closed," because colloidal tracer particles (2 to 10 nm in diameter) do not enter them. They do not contain basement membrane. Flattened elements of the sarcoplasmic reticulum are often found in close proximity to the T-tubular system, as well as to the surface sarcolemma, forming "diads."

Excitation-Contraction Coupling

The earliest studies on isolated hearts perfused with isotonic saline solutions indicated the need for optimal concentrations of Na^+, K^+, and Ca^{++}. In the absence of Na^+ the heart is not excitable and will not beat, because the action potential depends on extracellular Na ions. In contrast, the resting membrane potential is independent of the Na ion gradient across the membrane (see Figure 2-8). Under normal conditions the extracellular K^+ concentration is about 4 mM. A reduction in extracellular K^+ has little effect on myocardial excitation and contraction. However, increases in extracellular K^+, if great enough, produce depolarization, loss of excitability of the myocardial cells, and cardiac arrest in diastole. *Ca^{++} is also essential for cardiac contraction;* removal of Ca^{++} from the extracellular fluid results in decreased contractile force and eventual arrest in diastole. Conversely, an increase in extracellular Ca^{++} enhances contractile force, and very high Ca^{++} concentrations induce cardiac arrest in systole (rigor). *The free intracellular Ca^{++} is the agent responsible for the contractile state of the myocardium.*

Initially a wave of excitation spreads rapidly along the myocardial sarcolemma from cell to cell via gap junctions. Excitation also spreads into the interior of the cells via the T tubules (Figures 3-2 to 3-4), which invaginate the cardiac fibers at the Z lines. Electrical stimulation at the Z line or the application of ionized Ca to the Z lines in the skinned (sarcolemma removed) cardiac fiber elicits a localized contraction of adjacent myofibrils. During the plateau (phase 2) of the action potential, Ca^{++} permeability of the sarcolemma increases. Ca^{++} flows down its electrochemical gradient and is largely responsible for the slow inward current (p 17). Ca^{++} enters the cell through Ca^{++} channels in the sarcolemma and in the invaginations of the sarcolemma, the T tubules. Opening of the Ca^{++} channels is be-

Figure 3-4 ■ A, Low-magnification electron micrograph of the right ventricular wall of a mouse heart. Tissue was fixed in a phosphate-buffered glutaraldehyde solution and postfixed in ferrocyanide-reduced osmium tetroxide. This procedure has resulted in the deposition of electron-opaque precipitate in the extracellular space, thus outlining the sarcolemmal borders *(SL)* of the muscle cells and delineating the intercalated disks *(ID)* and transverse tubules *(TT)*. *Nu,* Nucleus of the myocardial cell. **B,** Mouse cardiac muscle in longitudinal section, treated as in panel A. The path of the extracellular space is traced through the intercalated disk region *(ID),* and sarcolemmal invaginations that are oriented transverse to the cell axis (transverse tubules, *TT*) or parallel to it (axial tubules, *AT*) are clearly identified. Gap junctions *(GJ)* are associated with the intercalated disk. Mitochondria are large and elongated and lie between the myofibrils. **C,** Mouse cardiac muscle. Tissue treated with ferrocyanide-reduced osmium tetroxide to identify the internal membrane system (sarcoplasmic reticulum, *SR*). Specific staining of the SR reveals its architecture as a complex network of small-diameter tubules that are closely associated with the myofibrils and mitochondria.

lieved to be caused by phosphorylation of the channel proteins by a cyclic AMP (cAMP)–dependent protein kinase. The primary source of extracellular Ca^{++} is the interstitial fluid (10^{-3}M Ca^{++}). Some Ca^{++} also may be bound to the sarcolemma and to the **glycocalyx,** a mucopolysaccharide that covers the sarcolemma. The amount of calcium entering the cell interior from the extracellular space is not sufficient to induce contraction of the myofibrils, but it serves as a trigger **(trigger Ca^{++})** to release Ca^{++} from the intracel-

lular Ca^{++} stores, the sarcoplasmic reticulum (Figure 3-5). The cytosolic free Ca^{++} increases from a resting level of about 10^{-7}M to levels of 10^{-6} to 10^{-5}M during excitation, and the Ca^{++} binds to the protein troponin C. The Ca^{++}-troponin complex interacts with tropomyosin to unblock active sites between the actin and myosin filaments, which allows crossbridge cycling and hence contraction of the myofibrils (systole).

Mechanisms that raise cystolic Ca^{++} increase the developed force, and those that lower Ca^{++}

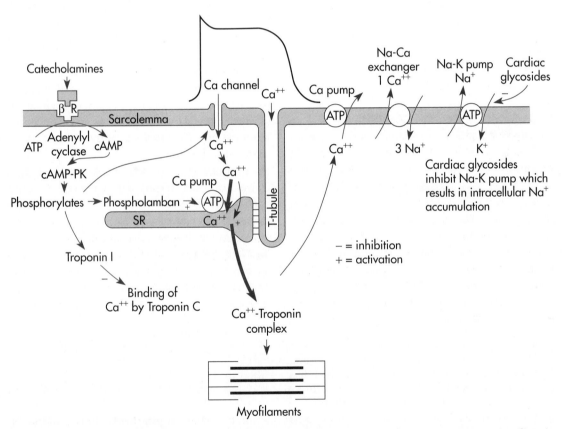

Figure 3-5 ■ Schematic diagram of the movements of calcium in excitation-contraction coupling in cardiac muscle. The influx of Ca^{++} from the interstitial fluid during excitation triggers the release of Ca^{++} from the sarcoplasmic reticulum (*SR*). The free cytosolic Ca^{++} activates contraction of the myofilaments (systole). Relaxation (diastole) occurs as a result of uptake of Ca^{++} by the sarcoplasmic reticulum, by extrusion of intracellular Ca^{++} by $Na^+–Ca^{++}$ exchange, and to a limited degree by the Ca pump. βR, beta-adrenergic receptor; *cAMP*, cyclic adenosine monophosphate; *cAMP-PK,* cyclic AMP–dependent protein kinase.

decrease the developed force. For example, catecholamines increase the movement of Ca^{++} into the cell by phosphorylation of the Ca^{++} channels via a cAMP-dependent protein kinase. In addition, catecholamines, like other agonists, enhance myocardial contractile force by increasing the sensitivity of the contractile machinery to Ca^{++}. An increase in cystolic Ca^{++} is also achieved by increasing extracellular Ca^{++} or decreasing the Na^+ gradient across the sarcolemma.

The sodium gradient can be reduced by increasing intracellular Na^+ or decreasing extracellular Na^+. Cardiac glycosides increase intracellular Na^+ by poisoning the Na-K pump, which results in an accumulation of Na^+ in the cells. The elevated cytosolic Na^+ reverses the Na-Ca exchanger so that less Ca^{++} is removed from the cell. A lowered extracellular Na^+ results in a reduction in Na^+ entry into the cell and hence less exchange of Na^+ for Ca^{++} (Figure 3-5).

Developed tension is diminished by a reduction in extracellular Ca^{++}, by an increase in the Na^+ gradient across the sarcolemma, or by administration of Ca^{++} blockers that prevent Ca^{++} from entering the myocardial cell (see Figure 2-15).

At the end of systole the Ca^{++} influx ceases and the sarcoplasmic reticulum is no longer stimulated to release Ca^{++}. In fact, the sarcoplasmic reticulum avidly takes up Ca^{++} by means of an ATP-energized calcium pump that is stimulated by **phospholamban** after the phospholamban

---

A patient in heart failure with a dilated heart, low cardiac output, fluid retention, high venous pressure, an enlarged liver, and peripheral edema is often treated with digitalis and a diuretic. The digitalis increases cardiomyocyte intracellular calcium, thereby enhancing contractile force, and the diuretic reduces extracellular fluid volume, thereby lessening the volume load (preload) on the heart and reducing venous pressure, liver congestion, and edema.

---

is phosphorylated by cAMP-dependent protein kinase. Phosphorylation of troponin I inhibits the Ca^{++} binding of troponin C, which permits tropomyosin to again block the sites for interaction between the actin and myosin filaments, and relaxation (diastole) occurs. Cardiac contraction and relaxation are both accelerated by catecholamines and adenylyl cyclase activation. The resulting increase in cAMP activates the cAMP-dependent protein kinase, which phosphorylates the Ca channel in the sarcolemma. This allows a greater influx of Ca^{++} into the cell and thereby accelerates contraction. However, it also accelerates relaxation by phosphorylating phospholamban, which enhances Ca^{++} uptake by the sarcoplasmic reticulum, and by phosphorylating troponin I, which inhibits the Ca^{++} binding of troponin C. Thus, the phosphorylations by cAMP-dependent protein kinase serve to increase both the speed of contraction *and* the speed of relaxation.

Mitochondria also take up and release Ca^{++}, but the process is too slow to be involved in excitation-contraction coupling. Only at very high intracellular Ca^{++} levels (pathologic states) do the mitochondria take up a significant amount of Ca^{++}.

The Ca^{++} that enters the cell to initiate contraction must be removed during diastole. The removal is primarily accomplished by the exchange of 3 Na^+ for 1 Ca^{++} (Figure 3-5). Ca^{++} is also removed from the cell by an electrogenic pump that utilizes ATP to transport Ca^{++} across the sarcolemma (Figure 3-5).

Myocardial Contractile Machinery and Contractility

Velocity and force (afterload) of contraction are functions of the intracellular concentration of free Ca ions. *Afterload and velocity are inversely related, so that with no load, velocity is maximal. In an isometric contraction, where no external shortening occurs, total load is maximal and velocity is zero* (Figure 3-6).

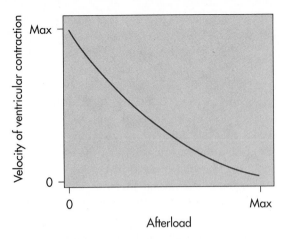

Figure 3-6 ■ Effect of increasing afterload on the velocity of contraction at constant preload.

The sequence of events in a **preloaded** and **afterloaded** isotonic contraction of a papillary muscle is illustrated in Figure 3-7. Point *A* represents the resting state in which the preload is responsible for the existing initial stretch. With stimulation the **contractile element** begins to shorten, and at point *B* the **elastic element** has been stretched, but the load has not yet been lifted because the overall length of the muscle has not changed; the muscle fibers have shortened at the expense of the elastic element.

This stretch of the elastic element (an expression of the muscle extensibility) consumes a certain amount of energy. To this energy is added the energy of shortening to obtain the total energy expenditure of a single contraction. Stretch of the elastic element is represented in the diagram (Figure 3-7) as a progressive rise in force with no external shortening. At point *B* the force developed by the contractile element has equaled the load

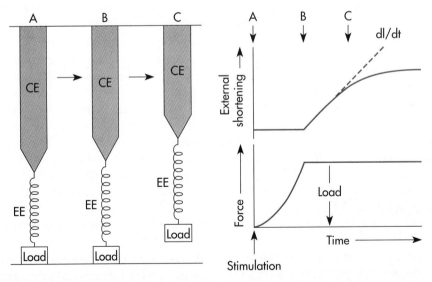

Figure 3-7 ■ Model for a preloaded (isometric) and afterloaded (isotonic) contraction of papillary muscle. A, Muscle at rest. Preload is represented by partial stretch of the elastic element *(EE)*. B, Partial contraction of the contractile element *(CE)* with stretch of the elastic element and no external shortening (the isometric phase of the contraction). C, Further contraction of the contractile element with external shortening and lifting of the afterload. The tangent *(dl/dt)* to the initial slope of the shortening curve on the right is the velocity of initial shortening. (Redrawn from Sonnenblick EH: *The myocardial cell,* Philadelphia, 1966, University of Pennsylvania Press.)

(the afterload), and the load begins to rise without further stretch of the elastic element. This is represented in the diagram (Figure 3-7) as external shortening of the muscle without a further increase in force (points *B* to *C*).

When these observations on papillary muscle are applied to the whole heart, the preload refers to the stretch of the left ventricle just before the onset of contraction (the so-called **end-diastolic volume**), and the afterload refers to the aortic pressure during the period when the aortic valve is open.

The preload can be increased by greater filling of the left ventricle during diastole (Figure 3-1). At lower end-diastolic volumes, increments in filling pressure during diastole elicit a greater systolic pressure during the subsequent contraction until a maximal systolic pressure is reached at the optimal preload (Figure 3-1). Further diastolic filling beyond this point results in no further increase in developed pressure; at very high filling pressures, peak pressure development in systole is reduced. At a constant preload, a higher systolic pressure can be reached during ventricular contractions by raising the afterload (e.g., increasing aortic pressure by restricting the runoff of blood to the periphery during diastole). Increments in afterload produce progressively higher peak systolic pressures until the afterload is so great that the ventricle can no longer generate enough force to open the aortic valve (Figure 3-8). At this point, ventricular systole is totally isometric; there is no ejection of blood, and hence no change in volume of the ventricle during systole. The maximal pressure developed by the left ventricle under these conditions is the maximal isometric force of which the ventricle is capable at a given preload. At preloads below the optimal filling volume, an increase in preload can yield a greater maximal isometric force (Figure 3-1).

The preloads and afterloads depend on the characteristics of the vascular system and the behavior of the heart. With respect to the vascula-

Figure 3-8 ■ Effect of increasing afterload on developed pressure at constant preload. At the arrow, maximal developed pressure is reached. Further increments in afterload prevent opening of the aortic valve.

In contrast to the normal heart, strips of papillary muscle from the terminally failing human heart show no increase in developed force with increases in preload.

ture, the degree of venomotor tone and peripheral resistance influence preload and afterload. With respect to the heart, a change in rate or stroke volume can also alter preload and afterload. Hence, the cardiac and vascular factors are interactive in their effect on preload and afterload (see Chapter 9 for a full explanation).

If the phospholamban gene is ablated in mice, myocardial contractility is enhanced, as evidenced by increased work at a given preload, afterload, and heart rate, and by a greater dP/dt (see p 66).

Contractility represents the performance of the heart at a given preload and afterload. *It is the change in peak isometric force (isovolumic pressure) at a given initial fiber length (end-diastolic volume).* Augmentation of contractil-

In rare instances, patients have accidentally received excessive doses of epinephrine subcutaneously for severe asthmatic attacks. They develop marked tachycardia and increases in myocardial contractility, cardiac output, and total peripheral resistance. The result is dangerously high blood pressure. Treatment consists of a tourniquet on the injected limb, with intermittent brief releases of the tourniquet, and the use of adrenergic blocking drugs.

ity is observed with certain drugs, such as norepinephrine or digitalis, and with an increase in contraction frequency **(tachycardia).** The increase in contractility **(positive inotropic effect)** produced by any of these interventions is reflected by increments in developed force and velocity of contraction.

Indices of Contractility

A reasonable index of myocardial contractility can be obtained from the contour of ventricular pressure curves (Figure 3-9). A hypodynamic heart is characterized by elevated end-diastolic pressure, slowly rising ventricular pressure, and a somewhat reduced ejection phase (curve C, Figure 3-9). A normal ventricle under adrenergic stimulation shows reduced end-diastolic pressure, fast-rising ventricular pressure, and a brief ejection phase (curve B, Figure 3-9). The slope of the ascending limb of the ventricular pressure curve indicates the maximal rate of force development by the ventricle (maximal rate of change in pressure with time; maximal dP/dt, as illustrated by the tangents to the steepest portion of the ascending limbs of the ventricular pressure curves in Figure 3-9). The slope is maximal during the isovolumic phase of systole (Figure 3-10) and, at any given degree of ventricular filling, provides an index of the initial contraction velocity and hence of contractility.

Similarly, one can obtain an indication of the contractile state of the myocardium from the ini-

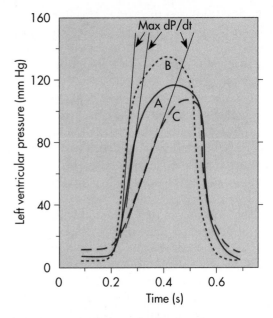

Figure 3-9 ■ **Left ventricular pressure curves with tangents drawn to the steepest portions of the ascending limbs to indicate maximal dP/dt values.** *A,* **Control;** *B,* **hyperdynamic heart, as with norepinephrine administration;** *C,* **hypodynamic heart, as in cardiac failure.**

tial velocity of blood flow in the ascending aorta (the initial slope of the aortic flow curve) (Figure 3-10). Also, the **ejection fraction,** which is the ratio of the volume of blood ejected from the left ventricle per beat **(stroke volume)** to the volume of blood in the left ventricle at the end of diastole, is widely used clinically as an index of contractility. Other measurements or combinations of measurements that in general are concerned with the magnitude or velocity of the ventricular contraction have been used to assess the contractile state of the cardiac muscle. There is no index that is entirely satisfactory at present, and this undoubtedly accounts for the several indices currently in use.

Cardiac Chambers

The atria are thin-walled, low-pressure chambers that function more as large reservoir conduits of

Figure 3-10 ■ Left atrial, aortic, and left ventricular pressure pulses correlated in time with aortic flow, ventricular volume, heart sounds, venous pulse, and the electrocardiogram for a complete cardiac cycle in the dog.

blood for their respective ventricles than as important pumps for the forward propulsion of blood. The ventricles were once thought to be made up of bands of muscle. However, it now appears that they are formed by a continuum of muscle fibers that take origin from the fibrous skeleton at the base of the heart (chiefly around the aortic orifice). These fibers sweep toward the apex at the epicardial surface, and also pass toward the endocardium as they gradually undergo a 180-degree change in direction to lie parallel to the epicardial fibers and form the endocardium and papillary muscles (Figure 3-11). At the apex of the heart the fibers twist and turn inward to form papillary muscles, whereas at the base and around the valve orifices they form a thick powerful muscle that not only decreases ventricular circumference for ejection of blood but also narrows the atrioventricular valve orifices as an aid to valve closure. In addition to a reduction in circumference, ventricular ejection is accomplished by a decrease in the longitudinal axis with descent of the base of the heart. The earlier contraction of the apical part of the ventricles, coupled with approximation of the ventricular walls, propels the blood toward the outflow tracts. The right ventricle, which develops a mean pressure about one seventh that developed by the left ventricle, is considerably thinner than the left.

Cardiac Valves

The cardiac valves consist of thin flaps of flexible, tough, endothelium-covered fibrous tissue firmly attached at the base to the fibrous valve rings. Movements of the valve leaflets are essentially passive, and the orientation of the cardiac valves is responsible for unidirectional flow of blood through the heart. There are two types of valves in the heart: the **atrioventricular (AV) valves** and the **semilunar valves** (Figures 3-12 and 3-13).

Atrioventricular Valves The valve between the right atrium and right ventricle is made up of three cusps **(tricuspid valve)**, whereas that

Endocardium

Midwall

100 μm

Epicardium

Figure 3-11 ■ Sequence of photomicrographs showing fiber angles in successive sections taken from the middle of the free wall of the left ventricle from a heart in systole. The sections are parallel to the epicardial plane. The fiber angle is 90 degrees at the endocardium, running through 0 degrees at the midwall to −90 degrees at the epicardium. (From Streeter DD Jr, Spotnitz HM, Patel DP, Ross J Jr, Sonnenblick EH: *Circ Res* 24:339, 1969. By permission of the American Heart Association, Inc.)

between the left atrium and left ventricle has two cusps **(mitral valve).** The total area of the cusps of each AV valve is approximately twice that of the respective AV orifice so that there is considerable overlap of the leaflets in the closed position (Figures 3-12 and 3-13). Attached to the

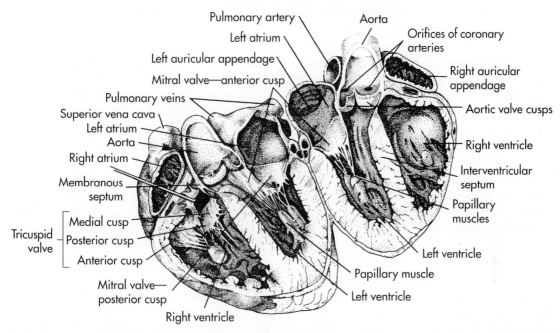

Figure 3-12 ■ Drawing of a heart split perpendicular to the interventricular septum to illustrate the anatomic relationships of the leaflets of the atrioventricular and aortic valves.

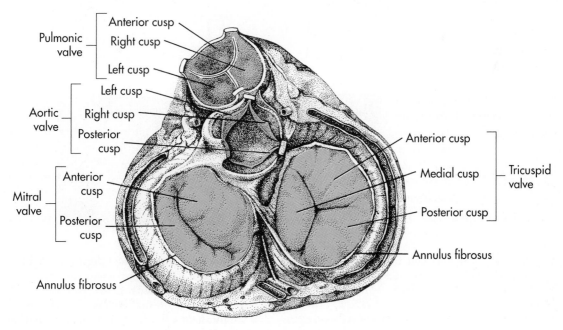

Figure 3-13 ■ Four cardiac valves as viewed from the base of the heart. Note how the leaflets overlap in the closed valves.

free edges of these valves are fine, strong ligaments **(chordae tendineae),** which arise from the powerful papillary muscles of the respective ventricles and prevent eversion of the valves during ventricular systole.

In the normal heart the valve leaflets are relatively close during ventricular filling and provide a funnel for the transfer of blood from atrium to ventricle. This partial approximation of the valve surfaces during diastole is caused by eddy currents behind the leaflets and also by some tension on the free edges of the valves, exerted by the chordae tendineae and papillary muscles that are stretched by the filling ventricle. Movements of the mitral valve leaflets throughout the cardiac cycle are shown in an **echocardiogram** (Figure 3-14). Echocardiography consists of sending short pulses of high-frequency sound waves (ultrasound) through the chest tissues and the heart and recording the echoes reflected from the various structures. The timing and pat-

tern of the reflected waves provide such information as the diameter of the heart, the ventricular wall thickness, and the magnitude and direction of the movements of various components of the heart.

In Figure 3-14 the echocardiograph is positioned to depict movement of the anterior leaflet of the mitral valve. The posterior leaflet moves in a pattern that is a mirror image of the anterior leaflet, but in the projection shown in Figure 3-14 the excursions appear much smaller. At point *D* the mitral valve opens, and during rapid filling (*D* to *E*) the anterior leaflet moves toward the ventricular septum. During the reduced filling phase (*E* to *F*) the valve leaflets float toward each other, but the valve does not close. The ventricular filling contributed by atrial contraction (*F* to *A*) forces the leaflets apart, and a second approximation of the leaflets follows (*A* to *C*). At point *C* the valve is closed by ventricular contraction. The valve leaflets, which bulge toward

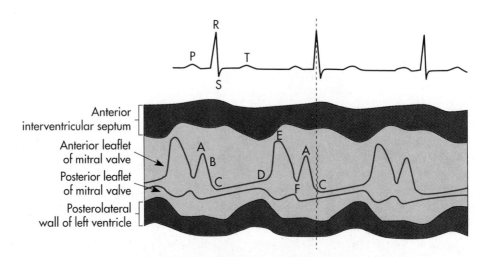

Figure 3-14 ■ **Drawing made from an echocardiogram showing movements of the mitral valve leaflets (particularly the anterior leaflet) and the changes in the diameter of the left ventricular cavity and the thickness of the left ventricular walls during cardiac cycles in a normal person.** *D* **to** *C,* **Ventricular diastole;** *C* **to** *D,* **ventricular systole;** *D* **to** *E,* **rapid filling;** *E* **to** *F,* **reduced filling (diastasis);** *F* **to** *A,* **atrial contraction. The mitral valve closes at** *C* **and opens at** *D.* **Simultaneously recorded electrocardiogram at top.**

the atrium, stay pressed together during ventricular systole (*C* to *D*).

Semilunar Valves The valves between the right ventricle and the pulmonary artery and between the left ventricle and the aorta consist of three cuplike cusps attached to the valve rings (Figures 3-12 and 3-13). At the end of the reduced ejection phase of ventricular systole, there is a brief reversal of blood flow toward the ventricles (shown as a negative flow in the phasic aortic flow curve in Figure 3-10) that snaps the cusps together and prevents regurgitation of blood into the ventricles. During ventricular systole the cusps do not lie back against the walls of the pulmonary artery and aorta but float in the bloodstream approximately midway between the vessel walls and their closed position. Behind the semilunar valves are small outpocketings of the pulmonary artery and aorta **(sinuses of Valsalva),** where eddy currents develop that tend to keep the valve cusps away from the vessel walls. The orifices of the right and left coronary arteries are behind the right and the left cusps, respectively, of the aortic valve. Were it not for the presence of the sinuses of Valsalva and the eddy currents developed therein, the coronary ostia could be blocked by the valve cusps.

The Pericardium

The pericardium is an epithelized fibrous sac. It closely invests the entire heart and the cardiac portion of the great vessels and is reflected onto the cardiac surface as the epicardium. The sac normally contains a small amount of fluid, which provides lubrication for the continuous movement of the enclosed heart. The distensibility of the pericardium is small, so that it strongly resists a large, rapid increase in cardiac size. Because of this characteristic, the pericardium plays a role in preventing sudden overdistension of the chambers of the heart. However, in congenital absence of the pericardium or after its surgical removal, cardiac function is within physiologic lim-

> With slow, progressive, and sustained enlargement of the heart, as occurs in cardiac hypertrophy, or with a slow progressive increase in pericardial fluid, as occurs in pericarditis with pericardial effusion, the intact pericardium is gradually stretched.

its. Nevertheless, with the pericardium intact, an increase in diastolic pressure in one ventricle increases the pressure and decreases the compliance of the other ventricle.

Heart Sounds

There are usually four sounds produced by the heart, but only two are ordinarily audible through a stethoscope. With electronic amplification the less intense sounds can be detected and recorded graphically as a **phonocardiogram.** This means of registering heart sounds that may be inaudible to the human ear helps to delineate the precise timing of the heart sounds relative to other events in the cardiac cycle.

The first heart sound is initiated at the onset of ventricular systole (Figure 3-10) and consists of a series of vibrations of mixed, unrelated, low frequencies (a noise). It is the loudest and longest of the heart sounds, has a crescendo-decrescendo quality, and is heard best over the apical region of the heart. The tricuspid valve sounds are heard best in the fifth intercostal space just to the left of the sternum; the mitral sounds are heard best in the fifth intercostal space at the cardiac apex.

The first heart sound is chiefly caused by oscillation of blood in the ventricular chambers and vibration of the chamber walls. The vibrations are engendered in part by the abrupt rise of ventricular pressure with acceleration of blood back toward the atria, but primarily by sudden tension and recoil of the AV valves and adjacent structures with deceleration of the blood resulting from closure of the AV valves. The vibrations of the ventricles and the contained blood are transmitted through surrounding tissues and reach the chest wall, where they may be heard or recorded. The intensity of the first sound is a function of the force of ventricular contraction and of the distance between the valve leaflets. The first sound is loudest when the leaflets are farthest apart, as occurs when the interval between atrial and ventricular systoles is prolonged (AV valve leaflets float apart) or when ventricular systole immediately follows atrial systole.

The second heart sound, which occurs with closure of the semilunar valves (Figure 3-10), is composed of higher-frequency vibrations (higher pitch), is of shorter duration and lower intensity, and has a more snapping quality than the first heart sound. The second sound is caused by abrupt closure of the semilunar valves, which initiates oscillations of the columns of blood and the tensed vessel walls by the stretch and recoil of the closed valve. The second sound caused by closure of the pulmonic valve is heard best in the second thoracic interspace just to the left of the sternum, whereas that caused by closure of the aortic valve is heard best in the same intercostal space but to the right of the sternum. Conditions that bring about a more rapid closure of the semilunar valves, such as increases in pulmonary artery or aortic pressure (e.g., pulmonary or systemic hypertension), increase the intensity of the second heart sound. In adults the aortic valve sound is usually louder than the pulmonic, but in cases of pulmonary hypertension the reverse is often true.

A normal phonocardiogram taken simultaneously with an electrocardiogram is illustrated in Figure 3-15. Note that the first sound, which starts just beyond the peak of the R wave, is composed of irregular waves and is of greater intensity and duration than the second sound, which appears at the end of the T wave. A third and fourth heart sound do not appear on this record.

The third heart sound, which is sometimes

Figure 3-15 ■ Phonocardiogram illustrating the first and second heart sounds and their relationship to the P, R, and T waves of the electrocardiogram. (Time lines = 0.04 s.)

In overloaded hearts, as in congestive heart failure, when the ventricular volume is very large and the ventricular walls are stretched to the point where distensibility abruptly decreases, a third heart sound may be heard. A third heart sound in patients with heart disease is usually a grave sign.

heard in children with thin chest walls or in patients with left ventricular failure, consists of a few low-intensity, low-frequency vibrations heard best in the region of the apex. It occurs in early diastole and is believed to be the result of vibrations of the ventricular walls caused by abrupt cessation of ventricular distension and deceleration of blood entering the ventricles.

A fourth, or atrial, sound, consisting of a few low-frequency oscillations, is occasionally heard in normal individuals. It is caused by oscillation of blood and cardiac chambers created by atrial contraction (Figure 3-10).

Because the onset and termination of right

Mitral insufficiency and mitral stenosis produce, respectively, systolic and diastolic murmurs heard best at the cardiac apex, whereas aortic insufficiency and aortic stenosis produce, respectively, diastolic and systolic murmurs heard best in the second intercostal space just to the right of the sternum. The heart sounds may also be altered by deformities of the valves; **murmurs** may be produced, and the character of the murmur serves as an important guide in the diagnosis of valvular disease.

When the third and fourth (atrial) sounds are accentuated, as occurs in certain abnormal conditions, triplets of sounds may occur, resembling the sound of a galloping horse. These **gallop rhythms** are essentially of two types: **presystolic gallop** caused by accentuation of the atrial sound, and **protodiastolic gallop** caused by accentuation of the third heart sound.

and left ventricular systoles are not precisely synchronous, differences in the time of vibration of the two AV valves or two semilunar valves can sometimes be detected with the stethoscope. Such asynchrony of valve vibrations, which may sometimes indicate abnormal cardiac function, is manifested as a **split sound** over the apex of the heart for the AV valves and over the base for the semilunar valves.

■ CARDIAC CYCLE
Ventricular Systole

Isovolumic Contraction The onset of ventricular contraction coincides with the peak of the R wave of the electrocardiogram and the initial vibration of the first heart sound. It is indicated on the ventricular pressure curve as the earliest rise in ventricular pressure after atrial contraction. The interval of time between the start of ventricular systole and the opening of the semilunar valves (when ventricular pressure rises abruptly) is termed **isovolumic contraction,**

because ventricular volume is constant during this brief period (Figure 3-10).

The increment in ventricular pressure during isovolumic contraction is transmitted across the closed valves. Isovolumic contraction has also been referred to as isometric contraction. However, some fibers shorten and others lengthen, as evidenced by changes in ventricular shape; it is therefore not a true isometric contraction.

Ejection Opening of the semilunar valves marks the onset of the ejection phase, which may be subdivided into an earlier, shorter phase **(rapid ejection)** and a later, longer phase **(reduced ejection).** The rapid ejection phase is distinguished from the reduced ejection phase by (1) the sharp rise in ventricular and aortic pressures that terminates at the peak ventricular and aortic pressures, (2) a more abrupt decrease in ventricular volume, and (3) a greater aortic blood flow (Figure 3-10). The sharp decrease in the left atrial pressure curve at the onset of ejection results from the descent of the base of the heart and stretch of the atria. During the reduced ejection period, runoff of blood from the aorta to the periphery exceeds ventricular output, and therefore aortic pressure declines. Throughout ventricular systole the blood returning to the atria produces a progressive increase in atrial pressure. Note that during approximately the first third of the ejection period left ventricular pressure slightly exceeds aortic pressure and flow accelerates (continues to increase), whereas during the last two thirds of ventricular ejection the reverse holds true. This reversal of the ventricular-aortic pressure gradient in the presence of continued flow of blood from the left ventricle to the aorta (caused by the momentum of the forward blood flow) is the result of the storage of potential energy in the stretched arterial walls, which produces a deceleration of blood flow into the aorta. The peak of the flow curve coincides in time with the point at which the left ventricular pressure curve intersects the aortic pressure curve during ejection. Thereafter, flow decelerates (continues to decrease) because the pressure gradient has been reversed.

With right ventricular ejection, there is shortening of the free wall of the right ventricle (descent of the tricuspid valve ring) in addition to lateral compression of the chamber. However, with left ventricular ejection, there is very little shortening of the base-to-apex axis, and ejection is accomplished chiefly by compression of the left ventricular chamber.

The effect of ventricular systole on left ventricular diameter is shown in an echocardiogram (Figure 3-14). During ventricular systole (Figure 3-14, C to D) the septum and the free wall of the left ventricle become thicker and move closer to each other.

The venous pulse curve shown in Figure 3-10 has been taken from a jugular vein, and the c wave is caused by the impact of the adjacent common carotid artery and to some extent by transmission of a pressure wave produced by the abrupt closure of the tricuspid valve in early ventricular systole. Note that except for the c wave, the venous pulse closely follows the atrial pressure curve.

At the end of ejection, a volume of blood approximately equal to that ejected during systole remains in the ventricular cavities. This **residual volume** is fairly constant in normal hearts but is smaller with increased heart rate or reduced outflow resistance and larger when the opposite conditions prevail.

An increase in myocardial contractility, as produced by catecholamines or by digitalis in a patient with a depressed heart, may decrease residual volume and increase stroke volume and ejection fraction. With severely hypodynamic and dilated hearts, as in **heart failure,** the residual volume can become many times greater than the stroke volume.

In addition to serving as a small adjustable blood reservoir, the residual volume to a limited degree can permit transient disparities between the outputs of the two ventricles.

Ventricular Diastole

Isovolumic Relaxation Closure of the aortic valve produces the **incisura** on the descending limb of the aortic pressure curve and the second heart sound (with some vibrations evident on the atrial pressure curve), and marks the end of ventricular systole. The period between closure of the semilunar valves and opening of the AV valves is termed **isovolumic** relaxation and is characterized by a precipitous fall in ventricular pressure without a change in ventricular volume.

Rapid Filling Phase The major part of the ventricular filling occurs immediately on opening of the AV valves when the blood that had returned to the atria during the previous ventricular systole is abruptly released into the relaxing ventricles. This period of ventricular filling is called the **rapid filling phase.** In Figure 3-10 the onset of the rapid filling phase is indicated by the decrease in left ventricular pressure below left atrial pressure, resulting in the opening of the mitral valve. The rapid flow of blood from atria to relaxing ventricles produces a decrease in atrial and ventricular pressures and a sharp increase in ventricular volume.

The decrease in pressure from the peak of the v wave of the venous pulse in Figure 3-10 is caused by transmission of the pressure decrease incident to the abrupt transfer of blood from the right atrium to the right ventricle with opening of the tricuspid valve. Elastic recoil of the previous ventricular contraction may aid in drawing blood into the relaxing ventricle when residual volume is small, especially when ventricular contractility is enhanced, as produced by catecholamines. However, this mechanism probably does not play a significant role in ventricular filling under most normal conditions.

Diastasis   The rapid filling phase is followed by a phase of slow filling, called **diastasis.** During diastasis, blood returning from the periphery flows into the right ventricle and blood from the lungs into the left ventricle. This small, slow addition to ventricular filling is indicated by a gradual rise in atrial, ventricular, and venous pressures and in ventricular volume (Figure 3-10).

Atrial Systole   The onset of atrial systole occurs soon after the beginning of the P wave of the electrocardiogram (curve of atrial depolarization) and the transfer of blood from atrium to ventricle made by the peristalsis-like wave of atrial contraction completes the period of ventricular filling. Atrial systole is responsible for the small increases in atrial, ventricular, and venous (*a* wave) pressures, as well as in ventricular volume shown in Figure 3-10. Throughout ventricular diastole, atrial pressure barely exceeds ventricular pressure, indicating a low-resistance pathway across the open AV valves during ventricular filling.

Because there are no valves at the junctions of the venae cavae and right atrium or of the pulmonary veins and left atrium, atrial contraction can force blood in both directions. Actually, little blood is pumped back into the venous tributaries during the brief atrial contraction, mainly because of the inertia of the inflowing blood.

Atrial contraction is not essential for ventricular filling, as can be observed in atrial fibrillation or complete heart block. However, its contribution is governed to a great extent by the heart rate and the structure of the AV valves. At slow heart rates, filling practically ceases toward the end of diastasis, and atrial contraction contributes little additional filling. During tachycardia, diastasis is abbreviated and the atrial contribution can become substantial, especially if it occurs immediately after the rapid filling phase when the AV pressure gradient is maximal. Should tachycardia become so great that the rapid filling phase is encroached on, atrial contraction assumes great importance in rapidly propelling blood into the ventricle during this brief period of the cardiac cycle. Of course, if the period of ventricular relaxation is so brief that filling is seriously impaired, even atrial contraction cannot prevent inadequate ventricular filling. The consequent reduction in cardiac output may result in syncope. Obviously, if atrial contraction occurs simultaneously with ventricular contraction, no atrial contribution to ventricular filling can occur.

Pressure-Volume Relationship   The changes in left ventricular pressure and volume throughout the cardiac cycle are summarized in Figure 3-16. The element of time is not considered in this **pressure-volume loop.** Diastolic filling starts at *A* and terminates at *C,* when the mitral valve closes. The initial decrease in left ventricular pressure (*A* to *B*), despite the rapid inflow of blood from the atrium, is attributed to progressive ventricular relaxation and distensibility. During the remainder of diastole (*B* to *C*) the increase in ventricular pressure reflects ventricular filling and the passive elastic characteristics of the ventricle. Note that only a small increase in pressure occurs with the increase in ventricular volume during diastole (*B* to *C*). The small increase in pressure just to the left of *C* is caused by the contribution of atrial contraction to ventricular filling. With isovolumic contraction (*C* to *D*), there is a steep rise in pressure and no change in ventricular volume. At *D* the aortic valve opens, and during the first phase of ejection (rapid ejection, *D* to *E*), the large reduction in volume is associated with a continued but less

> In certain disease states, the AV valves may be markedly narrowed (**stenotic**). Under such conditions, atrial contraction plays a much more important role in ventricular filling than it does in the normal heart.

Figure 3-16 ■ Pressure-volume loop of the left ventricle for a single cardiac cycle *(ABCDEF).*

steep increase in ventricular pressure than that which occurred during isovolumic contraction. This volume reduction is followed by reduced ejection (*E* to *F*) and a small decrease in ventricular pressure. The aortic valve closes at *F,* and this event is followed by isovolumic relaxation (*F* to *A*), characterized by a sharp drop in pressure and no change in volume. The mitral valve opens at *A* to complete one cardiac cycle.

■ MEASUREMENT OF CARDIAC OUTPUT
Fick Principle

In 1870 the German physiologist Adoph Fick contrived the first method for measuring cardiac output in intact animals and people. The basis for this method, called the **Fick principle,** is simply an application of the law of conservation of mass. It is derived from the fact that the quantity of oxygen (O_2) delivered to the pulmonary capillaries via the pulmonary artery, plus the quantity of O_2 that enters the pulmonary capillaries from the alveoli, must equal the quantity of O_2 that is carried away by the pulmonary veins.

This is depicted schematically in Figure 3-17. The rate, q_1, of O_2 delivery to the lungs equals the O_2 concentration in the pulmonary arterial blood, $[O_2]_{pa}$, times the pulmonary arterial blood flow, Q, which equals the cardiac output; that is,

$$\dot{q}_1 = Q[O_2]_{pa} \qquad (1)$$

Let q_2 be the net rate of O_2 uptake by the pulmonary capillaries from the alveoli. At equilibrium, q_2 equals the **O_2 consumption** of the body. The rate, q_3, at which O_2 is carried away by the pulmonary veins equals the O_2 concentration in the pulmonary venous blood, $[O_2]_{pv}$, times the total pulmonary venous flow, which is virtually equal to the pulmonary arterial blood flow, Q; that is,

$$\dot{q}_3 = Q[O_2]_{pv} \qquad (2)$$

From conservation of mass,

$$\dot{q}_1 + \dot{q}_2 = \dot{q}_3 \qquad (3)$$

Therefore,

$$Q[O_2]_{pa} + \dot{q}_2 = Q[O_2]_{pv} \qquad (4)$$

Solving for cardiac output,

$$Q = \dot{q}_2/([O_2]_{pv} - [O_2]_{pa}) \qquad (5)$$

Equation 5 is the statement of the Fick principle.

In the clinical determination of cardiac output, O_2 consumption is computed from measurements of the volume and O_2 content of expired air over a given interval of time. Because the O_2 concentration of peripheral arterial blood is essentially identical to that in the pulmonary veins, $[O_2]_{pv}$ is determined on a sample of peripheral arterial blood withdrawn by needle puncture. Pulmonary arterial blood actually represents mixed systemic venous blood. Samples for O_2 analysis are obtained from the pulmonary artery or right ventricle through a catheter. In the past a relatively stiff catheter was

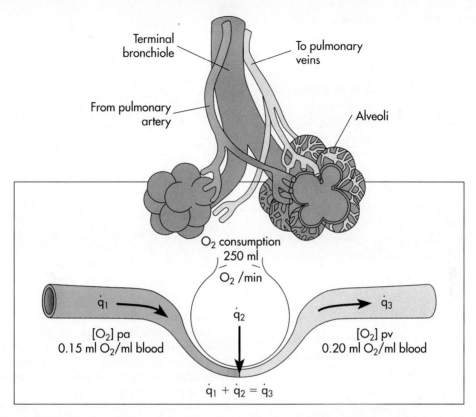

Terminal bronchiole

To pulmonary veins

From pulmonary artery

Alveoli

O_2 consumption 250 ml

O_2 /min

$\dot{q}_1$

$\dot{q}_2$

$\dot{q}_3$

$[O_2]$ pa
0.15 ml O_2/ml blood

$[O_2]$ pv
0.20 ml O_2/ml blood

$\dot{q}_1 + \dot{q}_2 = \dot{q}_3$

Figure 3-17 ■ Schema illustrating the Fick principle for measuring cardiac output. The change in color from pulmonary artery to pulmonary vein represents the change in color of the blood as venous blood becomes fully oxygenated.

used and had to be introduced into the pulmonary artery under fluoroscopic guidance. Today, a very flexible catheter with a small balloon near the tip can be inserted into a peripheral vein. As the tube is advanced, it is carried by the flowing blood toward the heart. By following the pressure changes, the physician is able to advance the catheter tip into the pulmonary artery without the aid of fluoroscopy.

An example of calculation of cardiac output in a normal, resting adult is illustrated in Figure 3-17. With an O_2 consumption of 250 ml/min, an arterial (pulmonary venous) O_2 content of 0.20 ml O_2/ml blood, and a mixed venous (pulmonary arterial) O_2 content of 0.15 ml O_2/ml blood, the

cardiac output would equal 250 ÷ (0.20 − 0.15) = 5000 ml/min.

The Fick principle is also used for estimating the O_2 consumption of organs in situ, when blood flow and the O_2 contents of the arterial and venous blood can be determined. Algebraic rearrangement reveals that O_2 consumption equals the blood flow times the arteriovenous O_2 concentration difference. For example, if the blood flow through one kidney is 700 ml/min, arterial O_2 content is 0.20 ml O_2/ml blood, and renal venous O_2 content is 0.18 ml O_2/ml blood, the rate of O_2 consumption by that kidney must be 700 (0.20 − 0.18) = 14 ml O_2/min.

Indicator Dilution Techniques

The indicator dilution technique for measuring cardiac output is also based on the law of conservation of mass and is illustrated by the model in Figure 3-18. Let a liquid flow through a tube at a rate of Q ml/s, and let q mg of dye be injected as a slug into the stream at point *A*. Let mixing occur at some point downstream. If a small sample of liquid is continually withdrawn from point *B* farther downstream and passed through a densitometer, a curve of the dye concentration, *c*, may be recorded as a function of time, *t*, as shown in the lower half of Figure 3-18.

If no dye is lost between points *A* and *B*, the amount of dye, *q*, passing point *B* between times t_1 and t_2 will be

$$q = \bar{c} Q (t_2 - t_1) \qquad (6)$$

where $\bar{c}$ is the mean concentration of dye. The value of $\bar{c}$ may be computed by dividing the area of the dye concentration by the duration ($t_2 - t_1$) of that curve; that is

$$\bar{c} = \int_{t1}^{t2} c\,dt / (t_2 - t_1) \qquad (7)$$

Substituting this value of $\bar{c}$ into equation 6 and solving for Q yields

$$Q = \frac{q}{\int_{t1}^{t2} c\,dt} \qquad (8)$$

Thus, flow may be measured by dividing the amount of indicator injected upstream by the area under the downstream concentration curve.

This technique has been widely used to estimate cardiac output in humans. A measured quantity of some indicator (a dye or isotope that remains within the circulation) is injected rapidly into a large central vein or into the right side of the heart through a catheter. Arterial blood is continuously drawn through a detector (densitometer or isotope rate counter), and a curve of indicator concentration is recorded as a function of time.

Figure 3-18 ■ **Indicator dilution technique for measuring cardiac output. In this model, in which there is no recirculation, q mg of dye are injected instantaneously at point *A* into a stream flowing at Q ml/min. A mixed sample of the fluid flowing past point *B* is withdrawn at a constant rate through a densitometer. The resulting dye concentration curve at point *B* has the configuration shown in the lower section of the figure.**

Presently the most popular indicator dilution technique is **thermodilution.** The indicator is cold saline. The temperature and volume of the saline are measured accurately before injection. A flexible catheter is introduced into a peripheral vein and advanced so that the tip lies in the pulmonary artery. A small thermistor at the catheter tip records the changes in temperature. The opening in the catheter lies a few inches proximal to the tip. When the tip is in the pulmonary artery, the opening lies in or near the right atrium. The cold saline is injected rapidly into the right atrium through the catheter. The resultant change in temperature downstream is recorded by the thermistor in the pulmonary artery.

The thermodilution technique has the following advantages: (1) an arterial puncture is not necessary; (2) the small volumes of saline used in each determination are innocuous, allowing repeated determinations to be made; and (3) recirculation is negligible. Temperature equilibration takes place as the cooled blood flows through the pulmonary and systemic capillary beds, before it flows by the thermistor in the pulmonary artery the second time.

■ SUMMARY

1. An increase in myocardial fiber length, as occurs with an augmented ventricular filling during diastole (preload), produces a more forceful ventricular contraction. This relation between fiber length and strength of contraction is known as Starling's law of the heart.

2. Although the myocardium is made up of individual cells with discrete membrane boundaries, the cardiac myocytes that comprise the ventricles contract almost in unison, as do those of the atria. The myocardium functions as a syncytium with an all-or-none response to excitation. Cell-to-cell conduction occurs through gap junctions that connect the cytosol of adjacent cells.

3. On excitation, voltage-gated calcium channels open to admit extracellular Ca^{++} into the cell. The influx of Ca^{++} triggers the release of Ca^{++} from the sarcoplasmic reticulum. The elevated intracellular Ca^{++} produces contraction of the myofilaments. Relaxation is accomplished via restoration of the resting cytosolic Ca^{++} level by pumping it back into the sarcoplasmic reticulum and exchanging it for extracellular Na^+ across the sarcolemma.

4. Velocity and force (afterload) of contraction are functions of the intracellular concentration of free Ca ions. Afterload and velocity are inversely related, so that with no load, velocity is maximal. In an isometric contraction, where no external shortening occurs, total load is maximal and velocity is zero.

5. In ventricular contraction the preload is the stretch of the fibers by the blood during ventricular filling and the afterload is the aortic pressure against which the left ventricle ejects the blood.

6. Contractility is an expression of cardiac performance at a given preload and afterload.

7. Simultaneous recording of left atrial, left ventricular, and aortic pressures; ventricular volume; heart sounds; and electrocardiogram graphically portray the sequential and related electrical and cardiodynamic events throughout a cardiac cycle. The first heart sound is caused mainly by abrupt closure of the AV valves; the second heart sound is caused by abrupt closure of the semilunar valves.

8. Cardiac output can be determined, according to the Fick principle, by measuring the oxygen consumption of the body (MVO_2) and the oxygen content of arterial $[O_2]_a$ and mixed venous $[O_2]_v$ blood. Cardiac output = $MVO_2/([O_2]_a - [O_2]_v)$. It can also be measured by dye dilution or thermodilution techniques. The greater the cardiac output, the greater is the dilution of the injected dye or cold saline by the arterial blood.

■ KEY WORDS AND CONCEPTS

- Sarcomeres
- Sarcomere length
- Troponin
- Thick and thin filaments
- Crossbridges
- Calcium sensitivity
- Frank-Starling relationship
- Developed force
- Law of Laplace
- Syncytium
- Intercalated disks
- Gap junctions (nexi)
- Mitochondria

- Connexons
- Transverse tubules
- Sarcoplasmic reticulum
- Excitation-contraction coupling
- Trigger calcium
- Phospholamban
- Preload
- Afterload
- Contractility
- Contractile element
- Elastic element
- dP/dt
- Ejection fraction
- Stroke volume
- Atrioventricular valves
- Semilunar valves
- Echocardiogram
- Pericardium
- Pressure pulses
- Heart sounds
- Phonocardiogram
- Murmurs
- Isovolumic contraction
- Rapid ejection
- Reduced ejection
- Isovolumic relaxation
- Residual volume
- Rapid filling phase
- Diastasis
- Atrial systole
- Pressure-volume relationship
- Cardiac output measurement
- Fick principle
- Indicator dilution techniques

■ SELF-STUDY PROBLEMS

1. Increase of force in skeletal muscle is accomplished by recruitment of muscle fibers via motor nerve activity. How does the heart increase its contractile force?
2. What are cardiac preload and afterload, and how do they affect developed pressure and velocity of contraction?
3. How is myocardial contractility evaluated?
4. What is the function of the pericardium and how can it affect cardiac filling and performance?
5. In a patient with severe mitral stenosis, where precisely in the cardiac cycle does the murmur occur?
6. If the arterial blood oxygen content is 19 ml/dl, the mixed venous oxygen content 12 ml/dl, and the oxygen consumption 280 ml/min, what is the cardiac output? In the same person, if the coronary sinus blood oxygen content is 5 ml/dl and the coronary sinus blood flow 250 ml/min, what is the oxygen consumption of the myocardium drained via the coronary sinus?

■ BIBLIOGRAPHY

Journal articles

Bers DM, Lederer WJ, Berlin JR: Intracellular Ca transients in rat cardiac myocytes: role of Na-Ca exchange in excitation-contraction coupling, *Am J Physiol* 258:C944, 1990.

Brutsaert DL, Sys SU: Relaxation and diastole of the heart, *Physiol Rev* 69:1228, 1989.

Cannell MB, Cheng H, Lederer WJ: The control of calcium release in heart muscle, *Science* 268:1045, 1995.

Carafoli E: Calcium pump of the plasma membrane, *Physiol Rev* 71:129, 1991.

Chapman RA: Control of cardiac contractility at the cellular level, *Am J Physiol* 245:H535, 1983.

Elzinga G, Westerhof N: Matching between ventricle and arterial load, *Circ Res* 68:1495, 1991.

Fabiato A, Fabiato F: Calcium and cardiac excitation-contraction coupling, *Annu Rev Physiol* 41:473, 1979.

Fleischer S, Inui M: Biochemistry and biophysics of excitation-contraction coupling, *Annu Rev Biophys Biophys Chem* 18:333, 1989.

Ford LE: Mechanical manifestations of activation in cardiac muscle, *Circ Res* 68:621, 1991.

Gilbert JC, Glantz SA: Determinants of left ventricular filling and of the diastolic pressure-volume relation, *Circ Res* 64:827, 1989.

Katz AM: Cyclic adenosine monophosphate effects on the myocardium: a man who blows hot and cold with one breath, *J Am Coll Cardiol* 2:143, 1983.

Katz AM: Interplay between inotropic and lusitropic effects of cyclic adenosine monophosphate on the myocardial cell, *Circulation* 82:I-7, 1990.

Landesberg A, Sideman S: Mechanical regulation of cardiac muscle by coupling calcium kinetics with crossbridge cycling: a dynamic model, *Am J Physiol* 267:H779, 1994.

Luo W, Grupp IL, Harrer J, Ponniah S, Grupp G, Duffy JJ, Doetschman T, Kranias EG: Targeted ablation of the phospholamban gene is associated with markedly enhanced myocardial contractility and loss of β-agonist stimulation, *Circ Res* 75:401, 1994.

Sagawa K: The ventricular pressure-volume diagram revisited, *Circ Res* 43:677, 1978.

Schwinger RHG, Bohm M, Koch A, Schmidt U, Morano I, Eissner H-J, Uberfuhr P, Reichart B, Erdmann E: The failing human heart is unable to use the Frank-Starling mechanism, *Circ Res* 74:959, 1994.

Smith JS, Rousseau E, Meissner G: Single sarcoplasmic reticulum Ca^{2+}-release channels from calmodulin modulation of cardiac and skeletal muscle, *Circ Res* 64:352, 1989.

Stern MD, Lakatta EG: Excitation-contraction coupling in the heart: the state of the question, *FASEB J* 6:3092, 1992.

Streeter DD Jr, Spotnitz HM, Patel DP et al: Fiber orientation in the canine left ventricle during diastole and systole, *Circ Res* 24:339, 1969.

Zhang R, Zhao J, Mandveno A, Potter JD: Cardiac troponin I phosphorylation increases the rate of cardiac muscle relaxation, *Circ Res* 76:1028, 1995.

Books and monographs

Brady AJ: *Mechanical properties of cardiac fibers.* In *Handbook of physiology,* section 2: *The cardiovascular system—the heart,* vol I, Bethesda, Md., 1979, American Physiological Society.

Frank GB, Bianchi CP, ten Keurs HEDJ, editors: *Excitation-contraction coupling in skeletal cardiac and smooth muscle,* New York, 1992, Plenum Press.

Gibbons WR, Zygmunt AC: *Excitation-contraction coupling in the heart.* In Fozzard HA et al, editors: *The heart and cardiovascular system,* ed 2, New York, 1991, Raven Press.

Lakatta EG: *Length modulation of muscle performance: Frank-Starling law of the heart.* In Fozzard HA et al, editors: *The heart and cardiovascular system,* ed 2, New York, 1991, Raven Press.

Lytton J, MacLennan DH: *Sarcoplasmic reticulum.* In Fozzard HA et al, editors: *The heart and cardiovascular system,* ed 2, New York, 1991, Raven Press.

Parmley WW, Talbot L: *Heart as a pump.* In *Handbook of physiology,* section 2: *The cardiovascular system—the heart,* vol I, Bethesda, Md., 1979, American Physiological Society.

Ruegg JC: *Calcium in muscle activation,* Heidelberg, 1988, Springer-Verlag.

Sheu SS, Blaustein MP: *Sodium/calcium exchange and control of cell calcium and contractility in cardiac muscle and vascular smooth muscle.* In Fozzard HA et al, editors: *The heart and cardiovascular system,* ed 2, New York, 1991, Raven Press.

Sommer JR, Johnson EA: *Ultrastructure of cardiac muscle.* In *Handbook of physiology,* section 2: *The cardiovascular system—the heart,* vol I, Bethesda, Md., 1979, American Physiological Society.

Regulation of the Heartbeat

The quantity of blood pumped by the heart each minute (i.e., the **cardiac output, CO**) may be varied by changing the frequency of its beats (i.e., **heart rate, HR**) or the volume ejected per stroke (i.e., **stroke volume, SV**). Cardiac output is the product of heart rate and stroke volume; that is,

$$CO = HR \times SV$$

A discussion of the control of cardiac activity may therefore be subdivided into a consideration of the regulation of pacemaker activity and the regulation of myocardial performance. However, in the intact organism, a change in the behavior of one of these features of cardiac activity almost invariably alters the other.

Certain local factors, such as temperature changes and tissue stretch, can affect the discharge frequency of the sinoatrial (SA) node. However, the principal control of heart rate is relegated to the autonomic nervous system, and the discussion is restricted to this aspect of heart rate control. Relative to myocardial performance, intrinsic and extrinsic factors are considered.

■ NERVOUS CONTROL OF HEART RATE

In normal adults the average heart rate at rest is approximately 70 beats per minute, but it is significantly greater in children. During sleep the heart rate diminishes by 10 to 20 beats per minute, but during emotional excitement or muscular activity it may accelerate to rates considerably above 100. In well-trained athletes at rest the rate is usually only about 50 beats per minute.

The SA node is usually under the tonic influence of both divisions of the autonomic nervous system. The sympathetic system enhances automaticity, whereas the parasympathetic system inhibits it. Changes in heart rate usually involve a reciprocal action of the two divisions of the autonomic nervous system. Thus, an increased heart rate is produced by a diminution of parasympathetic activity and concomitant increase in sympathetic activity; deceleration is usually achieved by the opposite mechanisms. Under certain conditions the heart rate may change by selective action of just one division of the autonomic nervous system, rather than by reciprocal changes in both divisions.

Ordinarily, in healthy, resting individuals, parasympathetic tone predominates. Abolition of parasympathetic influences by administration of **atropine** usually increases heart rate substantially, whereas abrogation of sympathetic effects by administration of **propranolol** usually decreases heart rate only slightly (Figure 4-1). When both divisions of the autonomic nervous system are blocked, the heart rate of young adults averages about 100 beats per minute. The rate that prevails after complete autonomic blockade is called the **intrinsic heart rate.**

Parasympathetic Pathways

The cardiac parasympathetic fibers originate in the medulla oblongata, in cells that lie in the **dorsal motor nucleus of the vagus** or in the **nucleus ambiguus.** The precise location varies from species to species. Efferent vagal fibers pass inferiorly through the neck as the cervical vagus nerves (Figure 4-2), which lie close to the common carotid arteries. They then pass through the mediastinum to synapse with postganglionic cells on the epicardial surface or within the walls of the heart itself. Most of the cardiac ganglion cells are located near the SA node and atrioventricular (AV) conduction tissue.

The right and left vagi are distributed differentially to the various cardiac structures. The right vagus nerve affects the SA node predominantly. Stimulation slows SA nodal firing or may even stop it for several seconds. The left vagus nerve mainly inhibits AV conduction tissue, to produce various degrees of AV block. However, the distributions of the efferent vagal fibers overlap, such that left vagal stimulation also depresses the SA node and right vagal stimulation impedes AV conduction.

The SA and AV nodes are rich in **cholinesterase.** Hence, the effects of any given vagal impulse are ephemeral because the acetylcholine released at the nerve terminals is rapidly

Figure 4-1 ■ **Effects of four equal doses of atropine (0.04 mg/kg total) and of propranolol (0.2 mg/kg total) on the heart rate of 10 healthy young men (mean age, 21.9 years). In half of the trials, atropine was given first *(top curve);* in the other half, propranolol was given first *(bottom curve).*** (Redrawn from Katona PG, McLean M, Dighton DH, Guz A: *J Appl Physiol* 52:1652, 1982.)

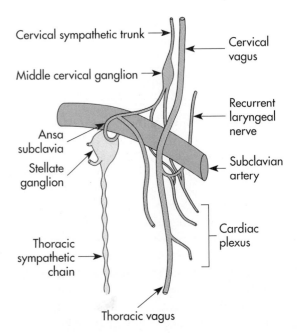

Figure 4-2 ■ **The cardiac autonomic nerves on the right side of the human body.**

hydrolyzed. Furthermore, the effects of vagal activity on SA and AV nodal function have a very short latency (about 50 to 100 ms), because the released acetylcholine activates special K^+ channels in the cardiac cells. Opening of these channels is so prompt because it does not require the operation of a second messenger system, such as the adenylyl cyclase system.

When the vagus nerves are stimulated at a constant frequency for several seconds, the heart rate decreases abruptly and attains a steady-state value within one or two cardiac cycles (Figure 4-3, *A*). Also, when stimulation is discontinued, the heart rate returns very quickly to its basal level. The combination of the brief latency and rapid decay of the response (because of the abundance of cholinesterase) provides the potential for the vagus nerves to exert a beat by beat control of SA and AV nodal function.

Parasympathetic influences preponderate over sympathetic effects at the SA node, as shown in Figure 4-4. As the frequency of sympathetic stimulation in an anesthetized dog was increased from 0 to 4 Hz, the heart rate increased by about 80 beats per minute in the absence of vagal stimulation (Vag = 0 Hz). However, when the vagi were stimulated at 8 Hz, increasing the sympathetic stimulation frequency from 0 to 4 Hz had a negligible influence on heart rate. This vagal preponderance in the regulation of heart rate is mediated mainly by an effective throttling of the release of norepinephrine from the sympathetic nerve endings by the acetylcholine released from neighboring vagus nerve endings. This type of interaction between the two divisions of the autonomic nervous system is discussed more fully below, in association with Figure 4-5.

Figure 4-3 ■ **Changes in heart rate evoked by stimulation *(horizontal bars)* of the vagus (A) and sympathetic (B) nerves in an anesthetized dog.** (Modified from Warner HR, Cox AJ: *J Appl Physiol* 17:349, 1962.)

Figure 4-4 ■ **Changes in heart rate in an anesthetized dog when the vagus and cardiac sympathetic nerves were stimulated simultaneously. The sympathetic nerves were stimulated at 0, 2, and 4 Hz; the vagus nerves at 0, 4, and 8 Hz. The symbols represent the observed changes in heart rate; the curves were derived from a computed regression equation.** (Modified from Levy MN, Zieske H: *J Appl Physiol* 27:465, 1969.)

Cardiac cell

Figure 4-5 ■ Interneuronal and intracellular mechanisms responsible for the interactions between the sympathetic and parasympathetic systems in the neural control of cardiac function. (From Levy MN: In Kulbertus HE, Franck G, editors: *Neurocardiology*, Mt Kisco, NY, 1988, Futura.)

Sympathetic Pathways

The cardiac sympathetic fibers originate in the intermediolateral columns of the upper five or six thoracic and lower one or two cervical segments of the spinal cord. They emerge from the spinal column through the white communicating branches and enter the paravertebral chains of ganglia. The preganglionic and postganglionic neurons synapse mainly in the stellate or middle cervical ganglia (Figure 4-2), depending on the species. The middle cervical ganglia lie close to the vagus nerves in the superior portion of the mediastinum. Sympathetic and parasympathetic fibers then join to form a complex plexus of mixed efferent nerves to the heart (Figure 4-2).

The postganglionic cardiac sympathetic fibers approach the base of the heart along the adventitial surface of the great vessels. On reaching the base of the heart, these fibers are distributed to the various chambers as an extensive epicardial plexus. They then penetrate the myocardium, usually along the coronary vessels. *The adrenergic receptors in the nodal regions and in the myocardium are predominantly of the beta type;* that is, they are responsive to beta-adrenergic agonists, such as **isoproterenol,** and are inhibited by beta-adrenergic blocking agents, such as **propranolol.**

As with the vagus nerves, the left and right sympathetic fibers are distributed differentially. In the dog, for example, the fibers on the left side have more pronounced effects on myocardial contractility than do fibers on the right side, whereas the fibers on the left side have much less effect on heart rate than do the fibers on the right side (Figure 4-6). In some dogs, left cardiac sympathetic nerve stimulation may not affect heart rate at all. This bilateral asymmetry probably also exists in humans. In a group of patients, right stellate ganglion blockade caused a mean reduction in heart rate of 14 beats per minute, whereas left-sided blockade decreased heart rate by only 2 beats per minute.

It is evident from Figures 4-3, *B* and 4-6 that the effects of sympathetic stimulation decay very gradually after the cessation of stimulation, in contrast to the abrupt termination of the response after vagal activity (Figure 4-3, *A*). Most of the norepinephrine released during sympathetic stimulation is taken up again by the nerve terminals, and much of the remainder is carried away by the bloodstream. These processes are relatively slow. Furthermore, at the beginning of sympathetic stimulation, the facilitatory effects on the heart attain steady-state values much more slowly than do the inhibitory effects of vagal stimulation (Figure 4-3).

Figure 4-6 ■ In the dog, stimulation of the left stellate ganglion has a greater effect on ventricular contractility than does right-sided stimulation, but it has a lesser effect on heart rate. In this example, traced from an original record, left stellate ganglion stimulation had no detectable effect at all on heart rate but had a considerable effect on ventricular performance in an isovolumic left ventricle preparation. (From Levy MN: Unpublished tracing.)

At least two factors are responsible for the more gradual onset of the heart rate response to sympathetic activity than to vagal activity. First, the response to sympathetic activity depends mainly on the intracellular buildup of second messengers, mainly **cyclic AMP (cAMP),** in the automatic cells in the SA node. This is a slower process than that which transduces the response to vagal activity. The **muscarinic receptors** that respond to the acetylcholine released from the vagal terminals are coupled directly to the acetylcholine-regulated K^+ channels by a G protein; this direct coupling allows a prompt response. Second, the neurotransmitters are released at different rates from the postganglionic nerve endings of each of the two autonomic divisions. Enough acetylcholine can be released during a

brief period (e.g., 1 second) of intense vagal activity to stop the heartbeat entirely. Conversely, even during intense sympathetic activity, enough **norepinephrine** is released during each cardiac cycle to change cardiac behavior by only a small increment. Thus, the vagus nerves are able to exert beat-by-beat control of heart rate, whereas the sympathetic nerves are not able to alter cardiac behavior very much within one cardiac cycle.

Control by Higher Centers

Dramatic alterations in cardiac rate, rhythm, and contractility have been induced experimentally by stimulation of various regions of the brain. In the cerebral cortex the centers regulating cardiac function are mostly in the anterior half of the brain, principally in the frontal lobe, the orbital cortex, the motor and premotor cortex, the anterior part of the temporal lobe, the insula, and the cingulate gyrus. In the thalamus, tachycardia may be induced by stimulation of the midline, ventral, and medial groups of nuclei. Variations in heart rate also may be evoked by stimulating the posterior and posterolateral regions of the hypothalamus. Stimuli applied to the H_2 fields of Forel in the diencephalon elicit a variety of cardiovascular responses, including tachycardia; such changes simulate closely those observed during muscular exercise. Undoubtedly the cortical and diencephalic centers are responsible for initiating the cardiac reactions that occur during excitement, anxiety, and other emotional states. The hypothalamic centers are also involved in the cardiac response to alterations in environmental temperature. Localized temperature changes in the preoptic anterior hypothalamus alter heart rate and peripheral resistance.

Stimulation of the parahypoglossal area of the medulla activates the cardiac sympathetic and inhibits the cardiac parasympathetic pathways. In certain dorsal regions of the medulla, distinct cardiac accelerator and augmentor sites have been detected in animals with transected vagi. Stimulation of accelerator sites increases heart rate, whereas stimulation of augmentor sites increases cardiac contractility. The accelerator regions were found to be more abundant on the right and the augmentor sites more prevalent on the left. A similar distribution also exists in the hypothalamus. It appears, therefore, that for the most part the sympathetic fibers descend the brainstem ipsilaterally.

Baroreceptor Reflex

Acute changes in arterial blood pressure reflexly elicit inverse changes in heart rate (Figure 4-7) via the baroreceptors located in the aortic arch and carotid sinuses (p 183). The inverse relation between heart rate and arterial blood pressure is usually most pronounced over an intermediate range of arterial blood pressures. In an experiment conducted on conscious, chronically instrumented monkeys (Figure 4-7), this range varied between about 70 and 160 mm Hg. Below the intermediate range of pressures, the heart rate maintains a constant, high value, whereas above this pressure range, it maintains a constant, low value.

The effects of changes in carotid sinus pressure on the activity in the cardiac autonomic nerves of an anesthetized dog are shown in Figure 4-8. Over an intermediate range of arterial pressures (from about 100 to 200 mm Hg), the alterations in heart rate are achieved by reciprocal changes in vagal and sympathetic neural activity. Below this range of arterial blood pressures, the high heart rate is achieved by intense sympathetic activity and the virtual absence of

Figure 4-7 ■ Heart rate as a function of mean arterial pressure in a group of five conscious, chronically instrumented monkeys. The mean control arterial pressure was 114 mm Hg. Pressure was increased above the control value by infusing phenylephrine, and was decreased below the control value by infusing nitroprusside. (Adapted from Cornish KG, Barazanji MW, Yong T et al: *Am J Physiol* 257:R595, 1989.)

Figure 4-8 ■ Changes in neural activity in cardiac vagal and sympathetic nerve fibers induced by changes in pressure in the isolated carotid sinuses in an anesthetized dog. (Adapted from Kollai M, Koizumi K: *Pflugers Arch Ges Physiol* 413:365, 1989.)

vagal activity. Conversely, above the intermediate range of arterial blood pressures, the low heart rate is achieved by intense vagal activity and a constant low level of sympathetic activity.

Bainbridge Reflex and Atrial Receptors

In 1915 Bainbridge reported that infusions of blood or saline accelerated the heart rate in dogs. This increase in heart rate occurred whether arterial blood pressure did or did not rise. Acceleration was observed whenever central venous pressure rose sufficiently to distend the right side of the heart, and the effect was abolished by bilateral transection of the vagi.

Numerous investigators have confirmed Bainbridge's observations. However, the magnitude and direction of the response depend on the prevailing heart rate. When the heart rate is slow, intravenous infusions usually accelerate the heart. At more rapid heart rates, however, infusions ordinarily slow the heart. Increases in blood volume not only evoke the Bainbridge reflex, but they also activate other reflexes (notably the baroreceptor reflex) that tend to change the heart rate in the opposite direction. The actual change in heart rate evoked by an alteration of blood volume is therefore the result of these antagonistic reflex effects (Figure 4-9).

In unanesthetized dogs, volume loading with blood increased heart rate and cardiac output proportionately (Figure 4-10). Consequently, stroke volume remained virtually constant. Conversely, reductions in blood volume diminished the cardiac output but increased heart rate. Undoubtedly, the Bainbridge reflex was prepotent over the baroreceptor reflex when the blood volume was raised, but the baroreceptor reflex prevailed over the Bainbridge reflex when the blood volume was diminished.

Receptors that influence heart rate exist in both atria. They are located principally in the venoatrial junctions—in the right atrium at its junctions with the venae cavae and in the left atrium at its junctions with the pulmonary veins. Distension of these atrial receptors sends impulses centripetally in the vagi. The efferent impulses are carried by fibers from both autonomic divisions to the SA node. The cardiac response is highly selective. Even when the reflex increase in heart rate is large, changes in ventricular contractility have been negligible. Furthermore, the increase in heart rate is unattended by an increase of sympathetic activity to the peripheral arterioles.

Stimulation of the atrial receptors also causes an increase in urine volume. Reduced activity in the renal sympathetic nerve fibers

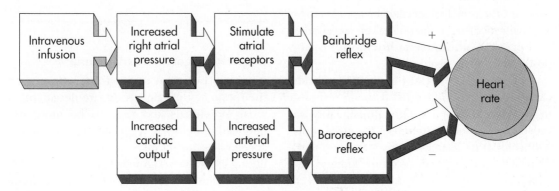

Figure 4-9 ■ **Intravenous infusions of blood or electrolyte solutions tend to increase heart rate via the Bainbridge reflex and to decrease heart rate via the baroreceptor reflex. The actual change in heart rate induced by such infusions is the result of these two opposing effects.**

Figure 4-11 ■ Respiratory sinus arrhythmia in a resting, unanesthetized dog. Note that the cardiac cycle length increases during expiration and decreases during inspiration. (Modified from Warner MR, de Tarnowsky JM, Whitson CC, Loeb JM: *Am J Physiol* 251:H1134, 1986.)

Figure 4-10 ■ Effects of blood transfusion and of bleeding on cardiac output, heart rate, and stroke volume in unanesthetized dogs. (From Vatner SF, Boettcher DH: *Circ Res* 42:557, 1978. By permission of the American Heart Association, Inc.)

In **congestive heart failure,** sodium chloride (NaCl) and water are retained, mainly because of the increased release of aldosterone from the adrenal cortex, consequent to stimulation by the renin-angiotensin system. The plasma level of ANP is also increased in congestive heart failure. This peptide acts to enhance the renal excretion of NaCl and water, and thereby attenuates the fluid retention and consequent elevations of central venous pressure and cardiac preload.

might be partially responsible for this diuresis. However, the principal mechanism appears to be a neurally mediated reduction in the secretion of **vasopressin (antidiuretic hormone)** by the posterior pituitary gland.

A peptide, called **atrial natriuretic peptide (ANP),** is released from atrial tissue in response to increases in blood volume, presumably because of the resultant stretch of the atrial walls. ANP consists of 28 amino acids. It has potent diuretic and natriuretic effects on the kidneys, and it has vasodilator effects on the resistance and capacitance blood vessels. Thus, ANP is an important regulator of blood volume and blood pressure.

Respiratory Cardiac Arrhythmia

Rhythmic variations in heart rate, occurring at the frequency of respiration, are detectable in most individuals and tend to be more pronounced in children. Typically, the cardiac rate accelerates during inspiration and decelerates during expiration (Figure 4-11).

Recordings from the autonomic nerves to the heart reveal that the neural activity increases in the sympathetic fibers during inspiration, whereas the neural activity in the vagal fibers in-

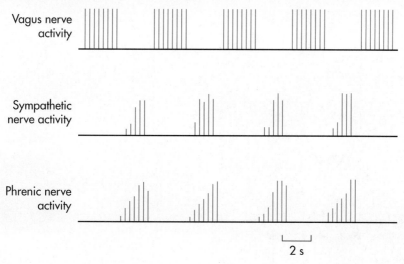

Vagus nerve
activity

Sympathetic
nerve activity

Phrenic nerve
activity

2 s

Figure 4-12 ■ Respiratory fluctuations in efferent neural activity in the cardiac nerves of an anesthetized dog. Note that the sympathetic nerve activity occurs synchronously with the phrenic nerve discharges (which initiate diaphragmatic contraction), whereas the vagus nerve activity occurs between the phrenic nerve discharges. (From Kollai M, Koizumi K: *J Auton Nerv Syst* 1:33, 1979.)

creases during expiration (Figure 4-12). The acetylcholine released at the vagal endings is removed so rapidly that the rhythmic changes in activity are able to elicit rhythmic variations in heart rate. Conversely, the norepinephrine released at the sympathetic endings is removed more slowly, thus damping out the effects of rhythmic variations in norepinephrine release on heart rate. Hence, rhythmic changes in heart rate are ascribable almost entirely to the oscillations in vagal activity. Respiratory sinus arrhythmia is exaggerated when vagal tone is enhanced.

Both reflex and central factors contribute to the genesis of the respiratory cardiac arrhythmia (Figure 4-13). During inspiration, intrathoracic pressure decreases, and therefore venous return to the right side of the heart is accelerated (see p 217), which elicits the Bainbridge reflex (Figure 4-13). After the time delay required for the increased venous return to reach the left side of the heart, left ventricular output increases and raises arterial blood pressure. This in turn re-

duces heart rate reflexly through baroreceptor stimulation (Figure 4-13).

Fluctuations in sympathetic activity to the arterioles cause peripheral resistance to vary at the respiratory frequency. Consequently, arterial blood pressure fluctuates rhythmically, which affects heart rate via the baroreceptor reflex. Stretch receptors in the lungs may also affect heart rate (Figure 4-13). Moderate pulmonary inflation may increase heart rate reflexly. The afferent and efferent limbs of this reflex are located in the vagus nerves.

Central factors are also responsible for respiratory cardiac arrhythmia (Figure 4-13). The respiratory center in the medulla influences the cardiac autonomic centers. In heart-lung bypass experiments conducted on animals, the chest is open, the lungs are collapsed, venous return is diverted to a pump-oxygenator, and arterial blood pressure is maintained at a constant level. In such experiments, rhythmic movements of the rib cage attest to the activity of the medullary respi-

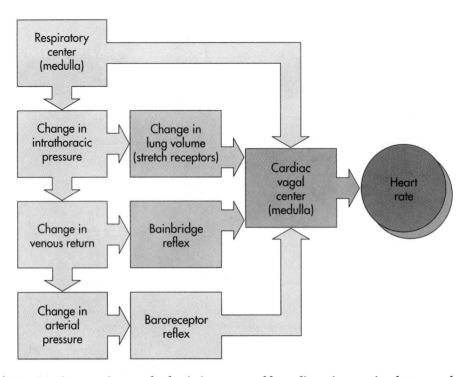

Figure 4-13 ■ **Respiratory sinus arrhythmia is generated by a direct interaction between the respiratory and cardiac centers in the medulla, as well as by reflexes originating from stretch receptors in the lungs, stretch receptors in the right atrium (Bainbridge reflex), and baroreceptors in the carotid sinuses and aortic arch.**

ratory centers, and the movements of the rib cage are often accompanied by rhythmic changes in heart rate at the respiratory frequency. *This respiratory cardiac arrhythmia is almost certainly induced by an interaction between the respiratory and cardiac centers in the medulla* (Figure 4-13).

Chemoreceptor Reflex

The cardiac response to peripheral chemoreceptor stimulation merits special consideration because it illustrates the complexity that may be introduced when one stimulus excites two organ systems simultaneously. In intact animals, stimulation of the carotid chemoreceptors consistently increases ventilatory rate and depth, but heart rate usually changes only slightly.

The directional change in heart rate is related to the enhancement of pulmonary ventilation, as shown in Figure 4-14. When respiratory stimulation is mild, heart rate usually diminishes; when the increase in pulmonary ventilation is more pronounced, heart rate usually accelerates.

The cardiac response to peripheral chemoreceptor stimulation is the result of primary and secondary reflex mechanisms (Figure 4-15). The *primary reflex effect* of carotid chemoreceptor excitation is mainly to facilitate the medullary vagal center and thereby to decrease heart rate. *Secondary effects* are mediated by the respiratory system. Respiratory stimulation by the arterial chemoreceptors tends to inhibit the medullary vagal center. This inhibitory effect varies with concomitant stimulation of respiration.

Figure 4-14 ■ Relationship between the change in heart rate and the change in respiratory minute volume during carotid chemoreceptor stimulation in spontaneously breathing cats and dogs. When respiratory stimulation was relatively slight, heart rate usually diminished; when respiratory stimulation was more pronounced, heart rate usually increased. (Modified from Daly MdeB, Scott MJ: *J Physiol* 144:148, 1958.)

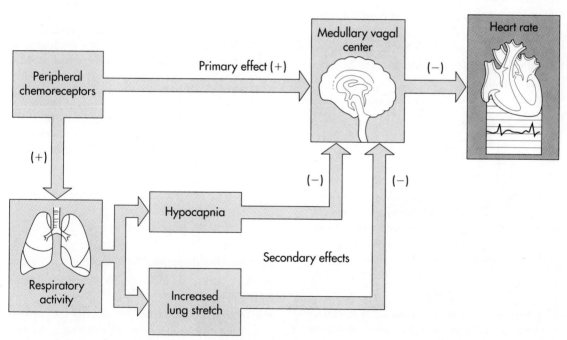

Figure 4-15 ■ The primary effect of stimulation of the peripheral chemoreceptors on heart rate is to excite the cardiac vagal center in the medulla and thus to decrease heart rate. Peripheral chemoreceptor stimulation also excites the respiratory center in the medulla. This effect produces hypocapnia and increases lung inflation, both of which secondarily inhibit the medullary vagal center. Thus, these secondary influences attenuate the primary reflex effect of peripheral chemoreceptor stimulation of heart rate.

An example of the primary inhibitory influence is displayed in Figure 4-16. In this experiment on an anesthetized dog, the lungs were completely collapsed and blood oxygenation was accomplished by an artificial oxygenator. When the carotid chemoreceptors were stimulated, an intense bradycardia and some degree of AV block ensued. Such effects are mediated primarily by efferent vagal fibers.

The pulmonary hyperventilation that is ordinarily evoked by carotid chemoreceptor stimulation influences heart rate secondarily, both by initiating more pronounced pulmonary inflation reflexes and by producing hypocapnia (Figure 4-15). Each of these influences tends to depress the primary cardiac response to chemoreceptor stimulation and thereby to accelerate the heart. Hence, when pulmonary hyperventilation is not prevented, the primary and secondary effects tend to neutralize each other, and carotid chemoreceptor stimulation affects heart rate only minimally.

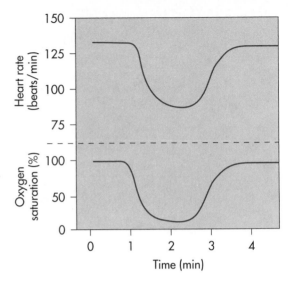

Figure 4-16 ■ Changes in heart rate during carotid chemoreceptor stimulation in an anesthetized dog on total heart bypass. The lungs remain deflated and respiratory gas exchange is accomplished by an artificial oxygenator. The lower tracing represents the oxygen saturation of the blood perfusing the carotid chemoreceptors. The blood perfusing the remainder of the animal, including the myocardium, was fully saturated with oxygen throughout the experiment. (Modified from Levy MN, DeGeest H, Zieske H: *Circ Res* 18:67, 1966.)

The identical primary inhibitory effect also operates in humans. The electrocardiogram shown in Figure 4-17 was recorded from a quadriplegic patient who could not breathe spontaneously but required tracheal intubation and artificial respiration. When the tracheal catheter was briefly disconnected to permit nursing care, the patient quickly developed a profound bradycardia. His heart rate was 65 beats per minute just before the tracheal catheter was disconnected. In less than 10 s after cessation of artificial respiration, his heart rate dropped to about 20 beats per minute. This bradycardia could be prevented by blocking the effects of efferent vagal activity with atropine, and its onset could be delayed considerably by hyperventilating the patient before disconnecting the tracheal catheter.

Ventricular Receptor Reflexes

Sensory receptors near the endocardial surfaces of the ventricular walls initiate reflex effects similar to those elicited by the arterial baroreceptors. Excitation of these endocardial receptors diminishes heart rate and peripheral resistance. Other sensory receptors have been identified in the epicardial regions of the ventricles. Ventricular receptors are excited by a variety of mechanical and chemical stimuli, but their physiologic functions are not clear.

Figure 4-17 ■ **Electrocardiogram of a 30-year-old quadriplegic man who could not breathe spontaneously and required tracheal intubation and artificial respiration. The two strips are continuous. The tracheal catheter was temporarily disconnected from the respirator at the beginning of the top strip.** (Modified from Berk JL, Levy MN: *Eur Surg Res* 9:75, 1977.)

Ventricular receptors are suspected of being involved in the initiation of **vasovagal syncope,** which is lightheadedness or brief loss of consciousness that may be triggered by psychological or orthostatic stress. The ventricular receptors are believed to be stimulated by a reduced ventricular filling volume combined with a vigorous ventricular contraction. In a person standing quietly, ventricular filling is diminished because blood tends to pool in the veins in the abdomen and legs, as explained in Chapter 9. Consequently, the reduction in cardiac output and arterial blood pressure leads to a generalized increase in sympathetic neural activity via the baroreceptor reflex (Figure 4-8). The enhanced sympathetic activity to the heart evokes a vigorous ventricular contraction, which thereby stimulates the ventricular receptors. Excitation of the ventricular receptors is widely believed to initiate the autonomic neural changes that evoke vasovagal syncope, namely, a combination of a profound, vagally mediated bradycardia and a generalized arteriolar vasodilation mediated by a diminution in sympathetic neural activity.

■ INTRINSIC REGULATION OF MYOCARDIAL PERFORMANCE

Just as the heart can initiate its own beat in the absence of any nervous or hormonal control, so also can the myocardium adapt to changing hemodynamic conditions by mechanisms that are intrinsic to cardiac muscle itself. Experiments on denervated hearts reveal that this organ adjusts remarkably well to stress. For example, racing greyhounds with denervated hearts perform almost as well as those with intact innervation. Their maximal running speed was found to be only 5% less after complete cardiac denervation. In these dogs, the three- to fourfold increase in cardiac output during exertion was achieved principally by an increase in stroke volume. In normal dogs the increase of cardiac output with exercise is accompanied by a proportionate increase of heart rate; stroke volume does not change much (see Chapter 12). It is unlikely that the cardiac adaptation in the denervated animals is achieved entirely by intrinsic mechanisms; circulating catecholamines undoubtedly contribute. If the beta-adrenergic receptors are blocked in greyhounds with denervated hearts, their racing performance is severely impaired.

The intrinsic cardiac adaptation that has received the greatest attention involves changes in the resting length of the myocardial fibers. This adaptation is designated **Starling's law of the heart** or the **Frank-Starling mechanism.** The mechanical, ultrastructural, and physiologic bases for this mechanism have been explained in Chapter 3.

Frank-Starling Mechanism

Isolated Hearts In 1895 the German physiologist Otto Frank described the response of the isolated heart of the frog to alterations in the load on the myocardial fibers just before ventricular contraction. He observed that as the load was increased, the heart responded with a more forceful contraction.

In 1914 the English physiologist Ernest Starling described the intrinsic response of the heart to changes in right atrial and aortic pressure in the canine isolated heart-lung preparation. In this preparation the right ventricular filling pressure is varied by altering the height of a reservoir connected to the right atrium. The ventricular filling pressure just before ventricular contraction constitutes the **preload** for the myocardial fibers in the ventricular wall. The right ventricle then pumps this blood through the pulmonary vessels to the left atrium. The lungs are artificially ventilated. Blood is pumped by the left ventricle into the aortic arch and then through some external tubing back to the right atrial reservoir. A resistance device in the external tubing allows the investigator to control the aortic pressure; this pressure constitutes the **afterload** for left ventricular ejection.

When the blood reservoir is abruptly raised to increase the preload, the stroke volume and the end-diastolic ventricular volume increase progressively over the next several beats; heart rate and afterload remain constant. In the brief period during which the stroke volume and ventricular volume gradually increase, a disparity must exist between ventricular inflow during diastole and ventricular output during systole. Thus, during this transient period before equilibrium is attained, the stroke volume must be less than the filling volume. The consequent accumulation of blood dilates the ventricles and lengthens the individual myocardial fibers that make up the walls of the ventricles.

The increased diastolic fiber length somehow facilitates ventricular contraction and enables the ventricles to pump a greater stroke volume, so that at equilibrium cardiac output exactly matches the augmented venous return. Increased fiber length alters cardiac performance in part by changing the number of myofilament cross-bridges that can interact, but mainly by changing the calcium sensitivity of the myofilaments (see Chapter 3). An optimal fiber length apparently exists beyond which contraction is actually impaired. Therefore, excessively high filling pressures may depress rather than enhance the pumping capacity of the ventricles by overstretching the myocardial fibers. Such excessive degrees of stretch are rarely encountered under normal conditions.

The heart is partially or completely denervated in a variety of clinical situations: (1) the surgically transplanted heart is totally decentralized, although the intrinsic, postganglionic parasympathetic fibers persist; (2) atropine blocks vagal effects on the heart, and propranolol blocks sympathetic beta-adrenergic influences; (3) certain drugs, such as reserpine, deplete cardiac norepinephrine stores and thereby restrict or abolish sympathetic control; and (4) in chronic congestive heart failure, cardiac norepinephrine stores are often severely diminished, thereby attenuating any sympathetic influences.

Changes in diastolic fiber length also permit the isolated heart to compensate for an increase in peripheral resistance. In a Starling preparation, when the arterial resistance is abruptly increased but ventricular filling rate is held constant, stroke volume diminishes and arterial pressure and ventricular volume increase for several heartbeats. However, after a brief period the stroke volume increases to equal the constant ventricular filling volume, and the arterial pressure and end-diastolic ventricular volume are greater than the respective values that prevailed before the experimentally induced increase in afterload. Thus, when the afterload is first increased, the stroke volume ejected by the ventricles during systole is less than the filling volume that enters the ventricles during diastole. The consequent excess of volume in the ventricles stretches the myocardial fibers in the ventricular walls, and this increase in myocardial fiber length enables the ventricles to eject a given volume against an increased afterload.

Changes in ventricular volume are also involved in the cardiac adaptation to alterations in heart rate. During bradycardia, for example, the increased duration of diastole permits greater ventricular filling. The consequent augmentation of myocardial fiber length increases stroke volume. Therefore, the reduction in heart rate may be fully compensated by the increase in stroke volume, such that cardiac output may remain constant (see Figure 9-16).

When cardiac compensation involves ventricular dilation, the force required by each myocardial fiber to generate a given intraventricular systolic pressure must be appreciably greater than that developed by the fibers in a ventricle of normal size. The relationship between wall tension and cavity pressure resembles that for cylindric tubes (p 155) in that for a constant internal pressure, wall tension varies directly with the radius. As a consequence, the dilated heart requires considerably more oxygen to perform a given

---

In the cardiac dilation and hypertrophy that accompanies **chronic heart failure,** the pericardium is stretched considerably (Figure 4-18). The pericardial limitation of cardiac filling is exerted at pressures and volumes entirely different from those in normal individuals.

---

amount of external work than does the normal heart.

The relatively rigid pericardium that encloses the heart determines the pressure-volume relationship at high levels of pressure and volume. The pericardium exerts this limitation of volume even under normal conditions, when an individual is at rest and the heart rate is slow.

Intact Preparations The major problem of assessing the role of the Frank-Starling mechanism in intact animals and humans is the difficulty of measuring end-diastolic myocardial fiber length. The Frank-Starling mechanism has been represented graphically by plotting some index of ventricular performance along the ordinate and some index of fiber length along the abscissa. The most commonly used indexes of ventricular performance are cardiac output, stroke volume, and stroke work. The indexes of fiber length include ventricular end-diastolic volume, ventricular end-diastolic pressure, ventricular circumference, and mean atrial pressure.

The Frank-Starling mechanism is better represented by a family of so-called ventricular function curves than by a single curve. To construct a given ventricular function curve, the blood volume of an experimental animal is altered over a range of values, and stroke work and end-diastolic pressure are measured at each step. Similar observations are then made during the desired experimental intervention. For example, the ventricular function curve obtained during a norepinephrine infusion lies above and to the left of a control ventricular function curve (Fig-

Figure 4-18 ■ Pericardial pressure-volume relations in a normal dog and in a dog with experimentally induced chronic cardiac hypertrophy. (Modified from Freeman GL, Le Winter MM: *Circ Res* 54:294, 1984. By permission of the American Heart Association, Inc.)

ure 4-19). It is evident that, for a given level of left ventricular end-diastolic pressure, the left ventricle performs more work during a norepinephrine infusion than during control conditions. Hence a shift of the ventricular function curve to the left usually signifies an improvement of ventricular **contractility** (p 65); a shift to the right usually indicates an impairment of contractility and a consequent tendency toward **cardiac failure.** Contractility is a measure of cardiac performance at a given level of preload and afterload. The end-diastolic pressure is ordinarily a good index of preload, whereas the aortic systolic pressure is a good index of afterload.

The Frank-Starling mechanism is ideally suited for matching cardiac output to venous return. Any sudden, excessive output by one ventricle soon increases the venous return to the other ventricle. The consequent increase in diastolic fiber length augments the output of the second ventricle to correspond with that of its mate. Therefore, *it is the Frank-Starling mechanism that maintains a precise balance between the*

outputs of the right and left ventricles. Because the two ventricles are arranged in series in a closed circuit, even a small, but maintained, imbalance in the outputs of the two ventricles would otherwise be catastrophic.

The curves that relate cardiac output to mean atrial pressure for the two ventricles are not coincident; the curve for the left ventricle usually lies below that for the right, as shown in Figure 4-20. At equal right and left atrial pressures (points *A* and *B*), right ventricular output would exceed left ventricular output. Hence, venous return to the left ventricle (a function of right ventricular output) would exceed left ventricular output, and left ventricular diastolic volume and pressure would rise. By the Frank-Starling mechanism, left ventricular output would therefore increase (from *B* toward *C*). Only when the outputs of both ventricles are identical (points *A* and *C*) would the equilibrium be stable. Under such conditions, however, left atrial pressure *(C)* would exceed right atrial pressure *(A),* and this is precisely the relationship that ordinarily prevails.

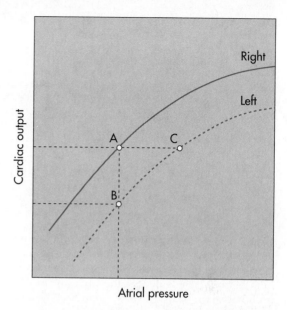

Figure 4-20 ■ Outputs of the right and left ventricles as functions of the mean right and left atrial pressure, respectively. At a given level of cardiac output, mean left atrial pressure (e.g., point *C*) exceeds mean right atrial pressure (point *A*).

Figure 4-19 ■ A constant infusion of norepinephrine in a dog shifts the ventricular function curve to the left. This shift signifies an enhancement of ventricular contractility. (Redrawn from Sarnoff SJ, Brockman SK, Gilmore JP, Linden RJ, Mitchell JH: *Circ Res* 8:1108, 1960.)

This difference in atrial pressures accounts for the observation that in **congenital atrial septal defects,** where the two atria communicate, the direction of the shunt flow is usually from left to right.

Rate-Induced Regulation

The effects of the frequency of contraction on the force developed in an isometrically contracting cat papillary muscle are shown in Figure 4-21. Initially, the strip of cardiac muscle was stimulated to contract only once every 20 s (Figure 4-21, *A*). When the muscle was suddenly made to contract once every 0.63 s, the developed force increased progressively over the next several beats. This progressive increase in developed force induced by a change in contraction frequency is known as the **staircase, or treppe, phenomenon.**

At the new steady state, the developed force was more than five times as great as it was at the larger contraction interval. A return to the larger interval (20 s) had the opposite influence on developed force.

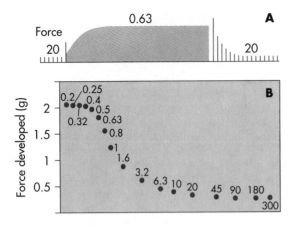

Figure 4-21 ■ Changes in force development in an isolated papillary muscle from a cat as the interval between contractions is varied. The numbers in both panels denote the interval (in seconds) between beats. (Redrawn from Koch-Weser J, Blinks JR: *Pharmacol Rev* 15:601, 1963.)

Figure 4-22 ■ Calcium currents induced in a guinea pig myocyte during the first and seventh depolarizations in a sequence of depolarizations. Arrows indicate the half-times of inactivation. Note that during the seventh depolarization, the maximal inward Ca++ current and the half-time of inactivation were greater than the respective values for the first depolarization. (Modified from Lee KS: *Proc Natl Acad Sci USA* 84:3941, 1987.)

The effect of the interval between contractions on the steady-state level of developed force is shown in Figure 4-21, *B* for a wide range of intervals. As the interval is diminished from 300 s down to about 20 s, developed force changes slightly. As the interval is reduced further, to a value of about 0.5 s, force increases sharply. Further reduction of the interval to 0.2 s has little additional effect on developed force.

The initial progressive rise in developed force when the interval between beats is suddenly decreased (e.g., from 20 to 0.63 s in Figure 4-21, *B*) is achieved by a gradual increase in intracellular Ca++ content. Two mechanisms contribute to the rise in Ca++ content: (1) an increase in the number of depolarizations per minute and (2) an increase in the inward Ca++ current per depolarization.

With respect to the first mechanism, Ca++ enters the myocardial cell during each action potential plateau (see Figure 2-20). As the interval between beats is diminished, the number of plateaus per minute increases. Even though the duration of each action potential (and of each plateau) decreases as the interval between beats is reduced (see Figure 2-20), the overriding effect of the increased number of plateaus per minute on the influx of Ca++ would increase the intracellular content of Ca++.

With respect to the second mechanism, as the interval between beats is suddenly diminished, the inward Ca++ current (i_{Ca}) progressively increases with each successive beat until a new steady state is attained at the new basic cycle length. Figure 4-22 shows that in an isolated ventricular myocyte that was subjected to repetitive depolarizations, the Ca++ current into the myocyte increased on successive beats. For example, the maximal i_{Ca} was considerably greater during the seventh depolarization than it was during the first depolarization. Furthermore, the decay of that current (i.e., its inactivation) was substantially slower during the seventh depolarization than during the first depolarization. Both of these characteristics of the i_{Ca} would result in a greater influx of Ca++ into the myocyte during the sev-

Figure 4-23 ◼ In an isovolumic canine left ventricle preparation a premature ventricular systole (beat *A*) is typically feeble, whereas the postextrasystolic contraction (beat *B*) is characteristically strong, and the enhanced contractility may persist to a diminishing degree over a few beats (e.g., contraction *C*). In this preparation the animal is placed on total heart-lung bypass, and a balloon filled with saline is positioned in the left ventricle. (From Levy MN: Unpublished tracing.)

enth depolarization than during the first depolarization. The greater influx of Ca^{++} would, of course, strengthen the contraction.

Transient changes in the intervals between beats also affect the strength of contraction. When a premature ventricular systole (Figure 4-23, beat *A*) occurs, the premature contraction (extrasystole) itself is feeble, whereas the beat *(B)* after the subsequent pause is very strong. This response depends partly on the Frank-Starling mechanism. Inadequate ventricular filling just before the premature beat accounts partly for the weak premature contraction. The exaggerated degree of filling associated with the subsequent pause explains in part the vigorous postextrasystolic contraction.

Although the Frank-Starling mechanism is certainly involved in the usual ventricular adaptation to a premature beat, it is not the exclusive mechanism. For example, in the ventricular pressure curves recorded from an isovolumic left ventricle preparation (Figure 4-23), in which neither filling nor ejection takes place during the cardiac cycle, the premature beat *(A)* is feeble and the succeeding contraction *(B)* is supernormal. Such enhanced contractility in contraction

B is an example of **postextrasystolic potentiation**, and it may persist for one or more additional beats (e.g., contraction *C*).

The weakness of the premature beat is directly related to the degree of prematurity. Conversely, as the time **(coupling interval)** between the premature beat and the preceding beat is increased, the more nearly normal will be the strength of the premature beat. The curve that relates the strength of contraction of a premature beat to the coupling interval is called a **mechanical restitution curve.** Figure 4-24 shows the restitution curve obtained by varying the coupling intervals of test beats in an isolated ventricular muscle preparation from a guinea pig.

The restitution of contractile strength probably depends on the time course of the intracellular circulation of Ca^{++} during the contraction and relaxation process (see Figure 3-5). During relaxation, the Ca^{++} that dissociates from the contractile proteins is taken up by the sarcoplasmic reticulum for subsequent release. However, about 500 to 800 ms are required before the Ca^{++} that had been taken up becomes available for release in response to the next depolarization.

The premature beat itself (Figure 4-23, beat *A*)

Figure 4-24 ■ Force generated during premature contractions in a guinea pig isolated ventricular muscle preparation. The muscle was driven to contract once per second. Periodically, the muscle was stimulated to contract prematurely. The scale along the abscissa denotes the time between the driven and premature beat. The ordinate denotes the ratio of the contractile force of the premature beat to that of the driven beat. (Modified from Seed WA, Walker JM: *Cardiovasc Res* 22:303, 1988.)

is feeble probably because not enough time has elapsed to allow much of the Ca^{++} taken up by the sarcoplasmic reticulum during the preceding relaxation to become available for release in response to the premature depolarization. The postextrasystolic beat (Figure 4-23, beat *B*), conversely, is considerably stronger than normal. The reason is that after the pause between beats *A* and *B*, the sarcoplasmic reticulum had available for release the Ca^{++} that had been taken up during two heartbeats: the extrasystole (beat *A*) and the preceding normal beat.

■ EXTRINSIC REGULATION OF MYOCARDIAL PERFORMANCE

Although the completely isolated heart can adapt well to changes in preload and afterload, various extrinsic factors also influence the heart in the intact animal. Under many normal conditions these extrinsic regulatory mechanisms may overwhelm the intrinsic mechanisms. These extrinsic regulatory factors may be subdivided into nervous and chemical components.

Nervous Control

Sympathetic Influences Sympathetic nervous activity enhances atrial and ventricular contractility. The effects of increased cardiac sympathetic activity on the ventricular myocardium are asymmetric. The cardiac sympathetic nerves on the left side of the body usually have a much greater effect on left ventricular contraction than do those on the right side (Figure 4-6).

The alterations in left ventricular contraction evoked by electrical stimulation of the left stellate ganglion in a canine isovolumic left ventricle preparation are shown in Figure 4-25. The peak pressure and the maximal rate of pressure rise (dP/dt) during systole are markedly increased. Also, the duration of systole is reduced and the rate of ventricular relaxation is increased during the early phases of diastole. The shortening of systole and more rapid ventricular relaxation would enhance ventricular filling in the intact circulatory system. For a given cardiac cycle length, the abbreviation of systole allows more time for diastole and hence for ventricular filling. In the experiment shown in Figure 4-26, for example, the animal's heart was paced at a constant rapid rate. Sympathetic stimulation (right panel) shortened systole, which allowed substantially more time for ventricular filling.

Sympathetic nervous activity enhances myocardial performance. Neurally released norepinephrine or circulating catecholamines interact with beta-adrenergic receptors on the cardiac cell membranes (Figure 4-5). This reaction activates adenylyl cyclase, which raises the intra-

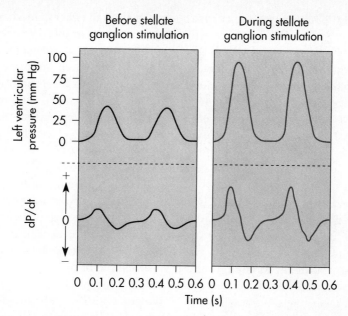

Figure 4-25 ■ In an isovolumic left ventricle preparation, stimulation of cardiac sympathetic nerves evokes a substantial rise in peak left ventricular pressure and in the maximal rates of intraventricular pressure rise and fall *(dP/dt)*. (From Levy MN: Unpublished tracing.)

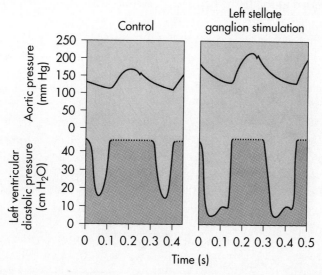

Figure 4-26 ■ Stimulation of the left stellate ganglion of a dog increases arterial pressure, stroke volume, and stroke work despite a concomitant reduction in ventricular end-diastolic pressure. Note also the abridgment of systole, thereby allowing more time for ventricular filling; the heart was paced at a constant rate. In the ventricular pressure tracings the pen excursion is limited at 45 mm Hg; actual ventricular pressures during systole can be estimated from the aortic pressure tracings. (Redrawn from Mitchell JH, Linden RJ, Sarnoff SJ: *Circ Res* 8:1100, 1960.)

cellular levels of cAMP. As a consequence, protein kinases are activated that promote the phosphorylation of various proteins within the myocardial cells. Phosphorylation of specific sarcolemmal proteins activates the calcium channels in the myocardial cell membranes. Phosphorylation of another specific protein, **phospholamban,** facilitates the reuptake of cystolic Ca^{++} by the sarcoplasmic reticulum, and thus it accelerates the relaxation of myocardial cells (see Chapter 3).

Activation of the calcium channels increases the influx of Ca^{++} during the action potential plateau, and more Ca^{++} is released from the sarcoplasmic reticulum in response to each cardiac excitation. The contractile strength of the heart is thereby increased. Figure 4-27 shows the correlation between the contractile force developed by a thin strip of ventricular muscle and the Ca^{++} concentration (as reflected by the aequorin light signal) in the myocytes as the concentration of isoproterenol (a beta-adrenergic agonist) was increased in the tissue bath.

The overall effect of increased cardiac sympathetic activity in intact animals can best be appreciated in terms of families of ventricular function curves. When stepwise increases in the frequency of electrical stimulation are applied to the left stellate ganglion, the ventricular function curves shift progressively to the left. The changes parallel those produced by catecholamine infusions (Figure 4-19). Hence, for any given left ventricular end-diastolic pressure, the ventricle is capable of performing more work as the level of sympathetic nervous activity is raised.

During cardiac sympathetic stimulation the increase in work is usually accompanied by a reduction in left ventricular end-diastolic pressure. An example of the response to stellate ganglion stimulation in a heart paced at a constant frequency is shown in Figure 4-26. In this experiment, stroke work was found to increase by about 50%, despite a reduction in left ventricular end-diastolic pressure (i.e., the preload). Note also the pronounced shortening of ventricular systole, with the consequent lengthening of the

Figure 4-27 ■ **Effects of various concentrations of isoproterenol *(Iso)* on the aequorin light signal (in nA) and contractile force (in mN/mm²) in a rat ventricular muscle injected with aequorin. The aequorin light signal reflects the instantaneous changes in intracellular Ca^{++} concentration.** (Modified from Kurihara S, Konishi M: *Pflugers Arch* 409:427, 1987.)

filling period. The reason for the reduction in ventricular preload is explained on page 196.

Parasympathetic Influences The vagus nerves inhibit the cardiac pacemaker, atrial myocardium, and AV conduction tissue. The vagus nerves also depress the ventricular myocardium, but the effects are less pronounced. In the isovolumic left ventricle preparation, vagal stimulation decreases the peak left ventricular pressure, maximal rate of pressure development (dP/dt), and maximal rate of pressure decline during diastole (Figure 4-28). In pumping heart preparations, vagal stimulation affects the relation between ventricular performance and preload such that the ventricular function curve shifts to the right.

The vagal effects on the ventricular myocardium are achieved by at least two mechanisms, as shown in Figure 4-5. The acetylcholine (ACh) released from the vagal endings can inter-

act with muscarinic (M) receptors in the cardiac cell membrane. This interaction inhibits adenylyl cyclase. The consequent diminution in the intracellular concentration of cAMP diminishes the Ca^{++} conductance of the cell membrane, and hence decreases myocardial contractility.

The ACh released from the vagal endings can also inhibit the release of norepinephrine from neighboring sympathetic nerve endings (Figure 4-5). The experiment illustrated in Figure 4-29 demonstrates that stimulation of the cardiac sympathetic nerves *(S)* results in the overflow of substantial amounts of norepinephrine into the coronary sinus blood. Concomitant vagal stimulation *(S + V)* reduces the overflow of norepinephrine by about 30%. The amount of norepinephrine overflowing into the coronary sinus

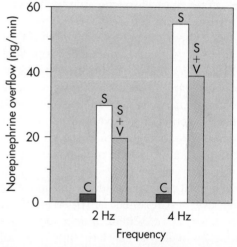

Figure 4-29 ■ Mean rates of overflow of norepinephrine into the coronary sinus blood in a group of seven dogs under control conditions *(C)*, during cardiac sympathetic stimulation *(S)* at 2 or 4 Hz and during combined sympathetic and vagal stimulation *(S + V)*. The combined stimulus consisted of sympathetic stimulation at 2 or 4 Hz, and vagal stimulation at 15 Hz. (Redrawn from Levy MN, Blattberg B: *Circ Res* 38:81, 1976. By permission of the American Heart Association, Inc.)

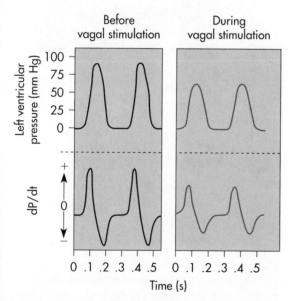

Figure 4-28 ■ In an isovolumic left ventricle preparation, when the ventricle is paced at a constant frequency, vagal stimulation decreases the peak left ventricular pressure and diminishes the maximal rates of pressure rise and fall *(dP/dt)*. (From Levy MN: Unpublished tracing.)

blood probably parallels the amount released at the sympathetic terminals. Thus, vagal activity can decrease ventricular contractility partly by antagonizing the facilitatory effects of any concomitant sympathetic activity to enhance ventricular contractility. The tendency for vagal activity to diminish the release of norepinephrine from neighboring sympathetic nerve endings also accounts for the preponderance of vagal influence over the sympathetic influence on heart rate, as reflected by the experimental results shown in Figure 4-4. Similarly, sympathetic nerves release norepinephrine and certain neuropeptides, including **neuropeptide Y (NPY)**; norepinephrine and NPY both inhibit the release of acetylcholine from neighboring vagal fibers (Figure 4-5).

Baroreceptor Reflex Just as stimulation of the carotid sinus and aortic arch baroreceptors may change heart rate (p 88), so also may it alter myocardial performance. Evidence of reflex alterations of ventricular contractility is presented in Figure 4-30. Ventricular function curves were obtained at four levels of carotid sinus pressure. With each successive rise in pressure, the ventricular function curves were displaced farther and farther to the right, denoting a progressively greater reflex depression of ventricular performance.

In normal, resting individuals and animals, the tonic level of sympathetic activity is usually very low. Under such conditions, moderate changes in baroreceptor activity may have little reflex influence on myocardial contractility. In states of augmented sympathetic neural activity, however, the effects of the baroreceptor reflex on contractility may be substantial.

Chemical Control

Hormones

Adrenomedullary Hormones The adrenal medulla is essentially a component of the autonomic nervous system. The principal hormone

secreted by the adrenal medulla is epinephrine, although some norepinephrine is also released. The rate of secretion of catecholamines by the adrenal medulla is largely regulated by the same mechanisms that control sympathetic nervous activity. The concentrations of catecholamines in the blood rise under the same conditions that activate the sympathoadrenal system. However, the cardiovascular effects of circulating catecholamines are probably minimal under normal conditions.

The changes in myocardial contractility induced by norepinephrine infusions have been tested in resting, unanesthetized dogs. The maximal rate of rise of left ventricular pressure (dP/dt), an index of myocardial contractility, was

Figure 4-30 ■ **As the pressure in the isolated carotid sinus is progressively raised, the ventricular function curves shift to the right. The numbers at the tops of each curve represent the systolic/diastolic perfusion pressures (in millimeters of mercury) in the carotid sinus regions of the dog.** (Redrawn from Sarnoff SJ, Gilmore JP, Brockman SK, Mitchell JH, Linden RJ: *Circ Res* 8:1123, 1960.)

found to be proportional to the norepinephrine concentration in the blood (Figure 4-31). In these same animals, moderate exercise increased the maximal dP/dt by almost 100%, but it raised the circulating catecholamines by only 500 pg/ml. Such a rise in blood norepinephrine concentration, by itself, would have had only a negligible effect on left ventricular dP/dt (Figure 4-31). Hence, the pronounced change in dP/dt observed during exercise must have been achieved mainly by the norepinephrine released from the cardiac sympathetic nerve fibers rather than by the catecholamines released from the adrenal medulla.

Adrenocortical Hormones The influence of adrenocortical steroids on the myocardium is controversial. Cardiac muscle removed from adrenalectomized animals and placed in a tissue bath is more likely to fatigue than that obtained from normal animals. In some species the adrenocortical hormones enhance contractility. Futhermore, hydrocortisone potentiates the car-

diotonic effects of the catecholamines. This potentiation may be mediated in part by an inhibition of the uptake mechanisms for the catecholamines by the adrenocortical steroids.

Thyroid Hormones Numerous studies on intact animals and humans have demonstrated that thyroid hormones enhance myocardial contractility. The rates of Ca^{++} uptake and of ATP hydrolysis by the sarcoplasmic reticulum are increased in response to excess thyroid hormones, and the opposite effects occur when thyroid hormones are inadequate. Thyroid hormones increase protein synthesis in the heart, which leads to cardiac hypertrophy. These hormones also affect the

> Cardiovascular problems are common in adrenocortical insufficiency (**Addison's disease**). The blood volume tends to fall, which may lead to severe hypotension and cardiovascular collapse, the so-called **addisonian crisis**.

Figure 4-31 ■ **Effect of norepinephrine infusions on ventricular contractility in a group of resting, unanesthetized dogs. The plasma concentrations of norepinephrine** *(pg/ml)* **plotted along the abscissa are the increments above the control values. The maximal rate of rise of left ventricular pressure** *(LV dP/dt)* **is plotted along the ordinate as percentage change from the control value; it is an index of contractility.** (Redrawn from Young MA, Hintze TH, Vatner SF: *Am J Physiol* 248:H82, 1985.)

composition of myosin isoenzymes in cardiac muscle. They increase principally those isoenzymes with the greatest ATPase activity, which thereby enhances myocardial contractility.

Insulin Insulin has a prominent, direct, positive inotropic effect on the heart. The effect of insulin is evident even when hypoglycemia is prevented by glucose infusions and when the beta-adrenergic receptors are blocked. In fact, the positive inotropic effect of insulin is potentiated by beta-adrenergic receptor blockade. The enhancement of contractility cannot be explained satisfactorily by concomitant augmentation of glucose transport into the myocardial cells.

Glucagon Glucagon has potent positive inotropic and chronotropic effects on the heart. The endogenous hormone probably plays no significant role in the normal regulation of the cardiovascular system, but it has been used to treat various cardiac conditions. The effects of glucagon on the heart closely resemble those of the catecholamines, and certain metabolic effects are similar. Both glucagon and catecholamines acti-

---

The cardiovascular changes in thyroid dysfunction also depend on indirect mechanisms. Thyroid hyperactivity increases the body's metabolic rate, and this in turn results in arteriolar vasodilation. The consequent reduction in total peripheral resistance increases cardiac output, as explained on page 208. Substantial evidence indicates that hyperthyroidism increases the density of beta-adrenergic receptors in cardiac tissue and it increases the responsiveness of the heart to sympathetic neural activity. Cardiac activity is sluggish in patients with inadequate thyroid function (**hypothyroidism**); that is, the heart rate is slow and cardiac output is diminished. The converse is true in patients with overactive thyroid glands (**hyperthyroidism**). Characteristically, hyperthyroid patients exhibit tachycardia, high cardiac output, palpitations, and arrhythmias (such as atrial fibrillation).

---

vate adenylyl cyclase to increase the myocardial tissue levels of cAMP. The catecholamines activate adenylyl cyclase by interacting with beta-adrenergic receptors, but glucagon activates this enzyme through a different mechanism.

Blood Gases

Oxygen Changes in oxygen tension (Pao_2) of the blood perfusing the brain and the peripheral chemoreceptors affect the heart through nervous mechanisms, as described earlier in this chapter. These indirect cardiac effects of hypoxia are usually prepotent. Moderate degrees of systemic hypoxia characteristically increase heart rate, cardiac output, and myocardial contractility. These changes are largely mediated by the sympathetic nervous system, and they are effectively abolished by beta-adrenergic receptor blockade.

The Pao_2 of the blood perfusing the myocardium also influences myocardial performance directly. Moderate to severe degrees of hypoxia depress myocardial contractility. The principal mechanism for the diminished contractility has not been established. Certain studies indicate that the sensitivity of the contractile proteins to Ca^{++} is reduced; other studies show that the impaired contractility is produced by increased intracellular concentrations of inorganic phosphate and of hydrogen ions.

Carbon Dioxide and Acidosis Changes in $Paco_2$ may also affect the myocardium directly and indirectly. The indirect, neurally mediated effects produced by increased $Paco_2$ are similar to those evoked by a decrease in Pao_2.

With respect to the direct effects on the heart, alterations in myocardial performance elicited by changes of $Paco_2$ in the coronary arterial blood are illustrated in Figure 4-32. In this experiment on an isolated left ventricle preparation, the control $Paco_2$ was 45 mm Hg (arrow *A*). Decreasing the $Paco_2$ to 34 mm Hg (arrow *B*) was stimulatory, whereas increasing $Paco_2$ to 86 mm Hg (arrow *C*) was depressant. In intact animals, systemic hypercapnia activates the sympatho-

Figure 4-32 ■ **Decrease in** Pa_{CO_2} **increases left ventricular systolic pressure (arrow** *B***) in an isovolumic left ventricle preparation; a rise in** Pa_{CO_2} **(arrow** *C***) has the reverse effect. When** Pa_{CO_2} **is returned to the control level (arrow** *D***), left ventricular systolic pressure returns to its original value (arrow** *A***).** (Levy MN: Unpublished tracing.)

Figure 4-33 ■ **Effect of pH on the relationship between relative force and pCa in a "skinned" ventricular fiber from a rat. Relative force is the force developed by the preparation under the various experimental conditions, expressed as a percentage of the maximal force developed by the preparation when intracellular pH was normal (i.e., 7.1) and pCa was less than 4.6. The "skinned" fiber was prepared by treating the preparation with a detergent to solubilize the cell membranes, thus exposing the contractile proteins in the fiber to the concentrations of** H^+ **and of** Ca^{++} **that prevailed in the bathing solution.** (Modified from Mayoux E, Coutry N, Lechêne P et al: *Am J Physiol* 266:H2051, 1994.)

adrenal system, which tends to compensate for the direct depressant effect of the increased Pa_{CO_2} on the heart.

Neither the Pa_{CO_2} nor the blood pH are primary determinants of myocardial behavior. The associated change in intracellular pH is the critical factor. The reduced intracellular pH diminishes the amount of Ca^{++} released from the sarcoplasmic reticulum in response to excitation. The diminished pH also decreases the sensitivity of the myofilaments to Ca^{++}. This effect of acidosis on sensitivity to Ca^{++} is reflected by a shift in the relationship between developed force and pCa (the negative logarithm of the intracellular Ca^{++} concentration). Figure 4-33 illustrates such a shift in an experiment on isolated ventricular fibers immersed in a tissue bath. When the pH of the bath was changed from 7.1 to 6.8, the curve of contractile force as a function of pCa was shifted substantially to the right (normal intra-

cellular pH is about 7.1). Furthermore, in this same preparation, at high intracellular Ca^{++} concentrations (i.e., at values of pCa below about 4.6), a reduction in pH diminishes the maximal developed force. This reduction in maximal force suggests that the low pH depresses the actomyosin interactions.

■ SUMMARY

1. Cardiac function is regulated by various intrinsic and extrinsic mechanisms.

2. Heart rate is regulated mainly by the autonomic nervous system. Sympathetic nervous activity increases heart rate, whereas parasympathetic (vagal) activity decreases heart rate. When both systems are active, the vagal effects usually dominate.

3. The following reflexes regulate heart rate: baroreceptor, chemoreceptor, pulmonary inflation, atrial receptor (Bainbridge), and ventricular receptor reflexes.

4. The principal intrinsic mechanisms that regulate myocardial contraction are the Frank-Starling mechanism and rate-induced regulation.

    a. Frank-Starling mechanism: a change in the resting length of the muscle influences the subsequent contraction in part by altering the affinity of the myofilaments for calcium.

    b. Rate-induced regulation: a sustained change in contraction frequency affects the strength of contraction by altering the influx of Ca^{++} into the cell per minute, whereas a transient change in contraction frequency alters contractile strength because an appreciable delay exists between the time that Ca^{++} is taken up by the sarcoplasmic reticulum and the time that it becomes available again for release.

5. The autonomic nervous system regulates myocardial performance mainly by varying the Ca^{++} conductance of the cell membrane via the adenylyl cyclase system.

6. Various hormones, including epinephrine, adrenocortical steroids, thyroid hormones, insulin, glucagon, and anterior pituitary hormones, regulate myocardial performance.

7. Changes in the blood concentrations of O_2, CO_2, and H^+ alter cardiac function directly and, via the central and peripheral chemoreceptors, reflexly.

■ KEY WORDS AND CONCEPTS

- Cardiac output
- Heart rate
- Stroke volume
- Autonomic nervous system
- Sympathetic nerves
- Parasympathetic nerves
- Vagus nerves
- Norepinephrine
- Isoproterenol
- Acetylcholine
- Adrenergic receptors
- Muscarinic receptors
- Receptor antagonists
- Acetylcholinesterase
- Cyclic AMP
- Baroreceptor reflex
- Carotid sinus baroreceptors
- Aortic arch baroreceptors
- Bainbridge reflex
- Atrial sensory receptors
- Vasopressin
- Atrial natriuretic peptide
- Renin-angiotensin system
- Respiratory cardiac arrhythmia
- Chemoreceptor reflex
- Vasovagal syncope
- Ventricular preload
- Ventricular afterload
- Starling's law of the heart
- Frank-Starling mechanism
- Pericardium
- Cardiac hypertrophy
- Congestive heart failure
- Myocardial contractility
- Atrial septal defect
- Staircase phenomenon (Treppe)
- Postextrasystolic potentiation
- Restitution curve
- Neuropeptide Y
- Epinephrine
- Addison's disease
- Hypothyroidism

- Hyperthyroidism
- Insulin
- Glucagon
- Blood gases
- Acidosis
- Alkalosis

■ SELF-STUDY PROBLEMS

1. What are the temporal characterisics of the changes in heart rate induced by (a) a 1-minute period of vagus nerve stimulation and (b) a 1-minute period of cardiac sympathetic nerve stimulation, and what are the main factors responsible for those characteristics?

2. What changes in heart rate occur when the cardiac sympathetic and vagus nerves are both stimulated strongly and simultaneously, and what factors operate to induce the changes evoked by simultaneous stimulation?

3. What changes in heart rate would occur if a vasoconstrictor drug were given to raise a subject's arterial blood pressure by about 25 mm Hg? What changes in efferent vagal and sympathetic neural activity would be elicited?

4. If 200 ml of blood were rapidly infused intravenously, what would be the temporal sequence of the changes in stroke volume of the right and left ventricles?

5. What changes would take place in the stroke volumes of the right and left ventricles if a substantial opening was made in the interatrial septum in the course of a cardiac catheterization?

6. During a cardiac catheterization, manipulation of the catheter in the right ventricle induced a premature ventricular beat, which was followed by a relatively long pause terminated by a postextrasystolic ventricular beat. Compare the magnitudes of the stroke volumes ejected during a normal beat, during the premature beat, and during the postextrasystolic beat.

■ BIBLIOGRAPHY

Journal articles

Bouchard RA, Bose D: Analysis of the interval-force relationship in rat and canine ventricular myocardium, *Am J Physiol* 257:H2036, 1989.

Cantin M, Genest J: The heart as an endocrine gland, *Hypertension* 10(suppl I):I-118, 1987.

Dampney RAL: Functional organization of central pathways regulating the cardiovascular system, *Physiol Rev* 74:323, 1994.

Endoh M, Blinks JR: Actions of sympathomimetic amines on the Ca^{2+} transients and contractions of rabbit myocardium: reciprocal changes in myofibrillar responsiveness to Ca^{2+} mediated through α- and β-adrenoceptors, *Circ Res* 62:247, 1988.

Farah AE: Glucagon and the circulation, *Pharmacol Rev* 35:181, 1983.

Fuchs F: Mechanical modulation of the Ca^{2+} regulatory protein complex in cardiac muscle, *News Physiol Sci* 10:6, 1995.

Gwathmey JK, Hajjar RJ: Relation between steady-state force and intracellular $[Ca^{2+}]$ in intact human myocardium: index of myofibrillar responsiveness to Ca^{2+}, *Circulation* 82:1266, 1990.

Hakumäki MOK: Seventy years of the Bainbridge reflex, *Acta Physiol Scand* 130:177, 1987.

Kohmoto O, Spitzer KW, Movsesian MA, Barry WH: Effects of intracellular acidosis on (Ca^{2+}) transients, transsarcolemmal Ca^{2+} fluxes, and contraction in ventricular myocytes, *Circ Res* 66:622, 1990.

Koizumi K, Kollai M: Multiple modes of operation of cardiac autonomic control: development of the ideas from Cannon and Brooks to the present, *J Auton Nerv Syst* 41:19, 1992.

Kowallik P, Meesman M: Independent autonomic modulation of the human sinus and AV nodes: evidence from beat-to-beat measurements of PR and PP intervals during sleep, *J Cardiovasc Electrophysiol* 6:993, 1995.

Lakatta EG: Starling's law of the heart is explained by an intimate interaction of muscle length and myofilament calcium activation, *J Am Coll Cardiol* 10:1157, 1987.

Löffelholz K, Pappano AJ: The parasympathetic neuroeffector junction of the heart, *Pharmacol Rev* 37:1, 1985.

Marshall JM: Peripheral chemoreceptors and cardiovascular regulation, *Physiol Rev* 74:543, 1994.

Mayoux E, Coutry N, Lechêne P et al: Effects of acidosis and alkalosis on mechanical properties of hypertrophied rat heart fiber bundles, *Am J Physiol* 266:H2051, 1994.

Mohabir R, Lee H-C, Kurz RW, Clusin WT: Effects of ischemia and hypercarbic acidosis on myocyte calcium transient, contraction, and pH_i in perfused rabbit hearts, *Circ Res* 69:1525, 1991.

Morgan JP: Abnormal intracellular modulation of calcium as a major cause of cardiac contractile dysfunction, *N Engl J Med* 325:625, 1991.

Polikar R, Burger AG, Scherrer U et al: The thyroid and the heart, *Circulation* 87:1435, 1993.

Rea RF, Thames MD: Neural control mechanisms and vasovagal syncope, *J Cardiovasc Electrophysiol* 4:587, 1993.

Seals DR, Suwarno NO, Joyner MJ et al: Respiratory modulation of muscle sympathetic nerve activity in intact and lung denervated humans, *Circ Res* 72:440, 1993.

Seed WA, Walker JM: Relation between beat interval and force of the heartbeat and its clinical implications, *Cardiovasc Res* 22:303, 1988.

Spyer KM: Central nervous mechanisms contributing to cardiovascular control, *J Physiol (Lond), 474*:1, 1994.

Taha BH, Simon PM, Dempsey JA et al: Respiratory sinus arrhythmia in humans: an obligatory role for vagal feedback from the lungs, *J Appl Physiol* 78:638, 1995.

Walley KR, Ford LE, Wood LDH: Effects of hypoxia and hypercapnia on the force-velocity relation of rabbit myocardium, *Circ Res* 69:1616, 1991.

Yan G-X, Kleber AG: Changes in extracellular and intracellular pH in ischemic rabbit papillary muscle, *Circ Res* 71:460, 1992.

Books and monographs

Armour JA, Ardell JL, editors: *Neurocardiology,* New York, 1994, Oxford University Press.

Bishop VS, Malliani A, Thorén P: *Cardiac mechanoreceptors.* In *Handbook of physiology,* Section 2: *The cardiovascular system—peripheral circulation and organ blood flow,* vol III, Bethesda, Md, 1983, American Physiological Society.

Fowler NO: *Pericardium in health and disease,* Mount Kisco, NY, 1985, Futura.

Fozzard HA, Haber E, Jennings RB, Katz AM, Morgan HE, editors: *Heart and cardiovascular system: scientific foundations,* ed 2, 2 vols, New York, 1991, Raven Press.

Garfein OB, editor: *Current concepts in cardiovascular physiology,* San Diego, 1990, Academic Press.

Katz AM: *Physiology of the heart,* ed 2, New York, 1991, Raven Press.

Kulbertus HE, Franck G, editors: *Neurocardiology,* Armonk, NY, 1988, Futura.

Levy MN, Schwartz PJ, editors: *Vagal control of the heart: experimental basis and clinical implications,* Armonk, NY, 1994, Futura.

Opie LH: *The heart: physiology and metabolism,* ed 2, New York, 1991, Raven Press.

Randall WC, editor: *Nervous control of cardiovascular function,* New York, 1984, Oxford University Press.

Rowell LB: *Human cardiovascular control,* New York, 1993, Oxford University Press.

Sagawa K, Maughan L, Suga H, Sunagawa K: *Cardiac contraction and the pressure-volume relationship,* New York, 1988, Oxford University Press.

Sperelakis N, editor: *Physiology and pathophysiology of the heart,* ed 3, Boston, 1995, Kluwer Academic.

Zucker IH, Gilmore JP: *Reflex control of the circulation,* Boca Raton, FL, 1990, CRC Press.

Hemodynamics

The problem of treating the pulsatile flow of blood through the cardiovascular system in precise mathematical terms is insuperable. The heart is a complicated pump, and its behavior is affected by a variety of physical and chemical factors. The blood vessels are multibranched, elastic conduits of continuously varying dimensions. The blood itself is not a simple, homogeneous solution but instead is a complex suspension of red and white corpuscles, platelets, and lipid globules dispersed in a colloidal solution of proteins.

Despite these complicating factors, considerable insight may be gained from an understanding of the elementary principles of fluid mechanics as they pertain to simple physical systems. Such principles are expounded in this chapter to explain the interrelationships among velocity of blood flow, blood pressure, and the dimensions of the various components of the systemic circulation.

■ VELOCITY OF THE BLOODSTREAM

In describing the variations in blood flow in different vessels, it is first essential to distinguish between the terms **velocity** and **flow.** The former term, sometimes designated as **linear velocity,** refers to the rate of displacement with respect to

time and has the dimensions of distance per unit time, for example, cm/s. The flow is frequently designated as **volume flow** and has the dimensions of volume per unit time, for example, cm^3/s. In a conduit of varying cross-sectional dimensions, velocity, v, flow, Q, and cross-sectional area, A, are related by the equation:

$$v = Q/A \qquad (1)$$

The interrelationships among velocity, flow, and area are portrayed in Figure 5-1. The flow of an incompressible fluid past successive cross sections of a rigid tube must be constant. For a given constant flow, the velocity varies inversely as the cross-sectional area (see Figure 1-3). Thus, for the same volume of fluid per second passing from section a into section b, where the cross-sectional area is five times greater, the velocity diminishes to one fifth of its previous value. Conversely, when the fluid proceeds from section b to section c, where the cross-sectional area is one tenth as great, the velocity of each particle of fluid must increase tenfold.

The velocity at any point in the system depends not only on the cross-sectional area, but also on the flow, Q. This in turn depends on the pressure gradient, properties of the fluid, and di-

$A = 2\ cm^2$ $\quad$ $10\ cm^2$ $\quad$ $1\ cm^2$

$Q = 10\ ml/s$

$v = 5\ cm/s$ $\quad$ $1\ cm/s$ $\quad$ $10\ cm/s$

Figure 5-1 ■ As fluid flows through a tube of variable cross-sectional area, A, the linear velocity, v, varies inversely as the cross-sectional area.

mensions of the entire hydraulic system, as discussed in the following section. For any given flow, however, the ratio of the velocity past one cross section relative to that past a second cross section depends only on the inverse ratio of the respective area; that is,

$$v_1/v_2 = A_2/A_1 \qquad (2)$$

This rule pertains regardless of whether a given cross-sectional area applies to a system that consists of a single large tube or to a system made up of several smaller tubes in parallel.

As shown in Figure 1-3, velocity decreases progressively as the blood traverses the aorta, its larger primary branches, the smaller secondary branches, and the arterioles. Finally, a minimal value is reached in the capillaries. As the blood then passes through the venules and continues centrally toward the venae cavae, the velocity progressively increases again. The relative velocities in the various components of the circulatory system are related only to the cross-sectional area. Thus, each point on the cross-sectional area curve is inversely proportional to the corresponding point on the velocity curve (see Figure 1-3).

■ RELATIONSHIP BETWEEN VELOCITY AND PRESSURE

In that portion of a hydraulic system in which the total energy remains virtually constant, changes in velocity may be accompanied by appreciable alterations in the measured pressure.

$v = 100\ cm/s$ $\quad$ $200\ cm/s$ $\quad$ $100\ cm/s$

$^1/_2\,\rho v^2 = 3.8\ mm\ Hg$ $\quad$ $15\ mm\ Hg$ $\quad$ $3.8\ mm\ Hg$

Figure 5-2 ■ In a narrow section, B, of a tube, the linear velocity, v, and hence the dynamic component of pressure, $^1/_2\,\rho v^2$, are greater than in the wide sections, A and C, of the same tube. If the total energy is virtually constant throughout the tube (i.e., if the energy loss because of viscosity is negligible), the total pressures (P_1, P_3, and P_5) will not be detectably different, but the lateral pressure, P_4, in the narrow section will be less than the lateral pressures (P_2 and P_6) in the wide sections of the tube.

Consider three sections (**A, B,** and **C**) of such a hydraulic system, as depicted in Figure 5-2. Six pressure probes, or **Pitot tubes,** have been inserted. The openings of three of these (**2, 4,** and **6**) are tangential to the direction of flow and hence measure the **lateral,** or **static,** pressure within the tube. The openings of the remaining three Pitot tubes (**1, 3,** and **5**) face upstream. Therefore, they detect the **total pressure,** which is the lateral pressure plus a dynamic pressure component that reflects the kinetic energy of the flowing fluid. This dynamic component, P_d, of the total pressure may be calculated from the following equation:

$$P_d = \rho v^2/2 \qquad (3)$$

where ρ is the density of the fluid and v is the velocity. If the midpoints of segments A, B, and C are at the same hydrostatic level, the corresponding total pressure, P_1, P_3, and P_5, will be equal, provided that the energy loss from viscosity in these segments is negligible. However, because of the changes in cross-sectional area, the concomitant velocity changes alter the dynamic component.

In sections *A* and *C*, let $\rho = 1$ g/cm^3 and $v = 100$ cm/s. From equation 3

$$P_d = 5000 \text{ dynes/cm}^2$$
$$= 3.8 \text{ mm Hg}$$

because 1330 dynes/cm^2 = 1 mm Hg. In the narrow section, *B*, let the velocity be twice as great as in sections *A* and *C*. Therefore,

$$P_d = 20{,}000 \text{ dynes/cm}^2$$
$$= 15 \text{ mm Hg}$$

Hence, in the wide sections of the conduit the lateral pressures (P_2 and P_6) will be only 3.8 mm Hg less than the respective total pressures (P_1 and P_5), whereas in the narrow section the lateral pressure (P_4) is 15 mm Hg less than the total pressure (P_3).

The peak velocity of flow in the ascending aorta of normal dogs is about 150 cm/s. Therefore, the measured pressure at this site may vary significantly, depending on the orientation of the pressure probe. In the descending thoracic aorta the peak velocity is substantially less than that in the ascending aorta (Figure 5-3), and lesser velocities have been recorded in still more distal arterial sites. In most arterial locations the dynamic component is a negligible fraction of the total pressure, and the orientation of the pressure probe does not materially influence the pressure recorded. At the site of a constriction, however, the dynamic pressure component may attain substantial values. In **aortic stenosis,** for example, the entire output of the left ventricle is ejected through a narrow aortic valve orifice. The high flow velocity is associated with a large kinetic energy, and therefore the lateral pressure is correspondingly reduced.

Figure 5-3 ■ Velocity of the blood in the ascending and descending aorta of a dog. (Redrawn from Falsetti HL, Kiser KM, Francis GP, Belmore ER: *Circ Res* 31:328, 1972. By permission of the American Heart Association, Inc.)

The pressure tracings shown in Figure 5-4 were obtained from two pressure transducers inserted into the left ventricle of a patient with aortic stenosis. The transducers were located on the same catheter and were 5 cm apart. When both transducers were well within the left ventricular cavity (Figure 5-4, *A*), they both recorded the same pressures. However, when the proximal transducer was positioned in the aortic valve orifice (Figure 5-4, *B*), the lateral pressure recorded during ejection was much less than that recorded by the transducer in the ventricular cavity. This pressure difference was associated almost entirely with the much greater velocity of flow in the narrowed valve orifice than in the ventricular cavity. The pressure difference reflects mainly the conversion of some potential energy to kinetic energy. When the catheter was withdrawn still farther, so that the proximal transducer was in the aorta (Figure 5-4, *C*), the pressure difference was even more pronounced, because substantial energy was lost through friction (viscosity) as blood flowed rapidly through the narrow aortic valve.

The reduction of lateral pressure in the region of the stenotic valve orifice influences coronary blood flow in patients with aortic stenosis. The orifices of the right and left coronary arteries are located in the sinuses of Valsalva, just behind the valve leaflets. Hence, the initial segments of these

Figure 5-4 ■ Pressures *(P)* recorded by two transducers in a patient with aortic stenosis. **A, Both transducers were in the left ventricle** *(LV-LV)*. **B, One transducer was in the left ventricle and the other was in the aortic valve orifice** *(LV-AVO)*. **C, One transducer was in the left ventricle, and the other was in the ascending aorta** *(LV-AO)*. (Redrawn from Pasipoularides A, Murgo JP, Bird JJ, Craig WE: *Am J Physiol* 246:H542, 1984.)

Angiographc studies in patients with aortic stenosis have revealed that the direction of flow often reverses in the large coronary arteries toward the end of the ejection phase of systole; that is, blood flows toward the aorta rather than toward the myocardial capillaries. The decreased lateral pressure in the aorta in aortic stenosis is undoubtedly an important factor in causing this reversal of coronary blood flow.

An important aggravating feature in aortic stenosis is that the demands of the heart muscle for oxygen are greatly increased. Therefore, the pronounced drop in lateral pressure during cardiac ejection may contribute to the tendency for patients with severe aortic stenosis to experience **angina pectoris** (anterior chest pain associated with inadequate blood supply to the heart muscle) and to die suddenly.

vessels are oriented at right angles to the direction of blood flow through the aortic valves. Therefore, the lateral pressure is that component of total pressure that propels the blood through the two major coronary arteries. During the ejection phase of the cardiac cycle, the lateral pressure is diminished by the conversion of potential energy to kinetic energy. This process is grossly exaggerated in aortic stenosis, because of the high flow velocities.

■ RELATIONSHIP BETWEEN PRESSURE AND FLOW

The most fundamental law governing the flow of fluids through cylindric tubes was derived empirically by the French physiologist Poiseuille. He was primarily interested in the physical determinants of blood flow, but he substituted simpler

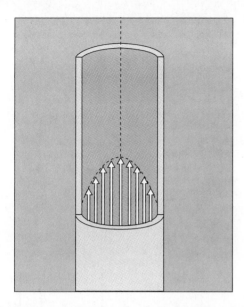

Figure 5-5 ■ In laminar flow, all elements of the fluid move in streamlines that are parallel to the axis of the tube; movement does not occur in a radial or circumferential direction. The layer of fluid in contact with the wall is motionless; the fluid that moves along the axis of the tube has the maximal velocity.

liquids for blood in his measurements of flow through glass capillary tubes. His work was so precise and important that his observations have been designated **Poiseuille's law.** Subsequently, this same law has been derived theoretically.

Poiseuille's law is applicable to the flow of fluids through cylindric tubes only under special conditions. It applies to the case of steady, laminar flow of newtonian fluids. The term **steady flow** signifies the absence of variations of flow in time, that is, a nonpulsatile flow. **Laminar flow** is the type of motion in which the fluid moves as a series of individual layers, with each stratum moving at a different velocity from its neighboring layers (Figure 5-5). In the case of flow through a tube, the fluid consists of a series of infinitesimally thin concentric tubes sliding past one another. Laminar flow is described in

greater detail below, where it is distinguished from turbulent flow. Also, a **newtonian fluid** is defined more precisely. For the present discussion, it may be considered to be a homogeneous fluid, such as water, in contradistinction to a suspension, such as blood.

Pressure is one of the principal determinants of the rate of flow. The pressure, P, in dynes/cm^2, at a distance h centimeters below the surface of a liquid is

$$P = h\rho g \qquad (4)$$

where ρ is the density of the liquid in g/cm^3 and g is the acceleration of gravity in cm/s^2. For convenience, however, pressure is frequently expressed simply in terms of height, h, of the column of liquid above some arbitrary reference point.

Consider the tube connecting reservoirs R_1 and R_2 in Figure 5-6, A. Let reservoir R_1 be filled with liquid to height h_1, and let reservoir R_2 be empty, as in section 1 of Figure 5-6. The outflow pressure, P_o, is therefore equal to the atmospheric pressure, which shall be designated as the zero, or reference, level. The inflow pressure, P_i, is then equal to the same reference level plus the height, h_1, of the column of liquid in reservoir R_1. Under these conditions, let the flow, Q, through the tube be 5 ml/s.

If reservoir R_1 is filled to height h_2, which is twice h_1, and reservoir R_2 is again empty (as in panel B), the flow will be twice as great, that is, 10 ml/s. Thus, with reservoir R_2 empty, the flow will be directly proportional to the inflow pressure, P_i.

If reservoir R_2 is now allowed to fill to height h_1, and the fluid level in R_1 is maintained at h_2 (as in panel C), the flow will again become 5 ml/s. Thus, flow is directly proportional to the difference between inflow and outflow pressures:

$$Q \propto P_i - P_o \qquad (5)$$

A, When R_2 is empty, fluid flows from R_1 to R_2 at a rate proportional to the pressure in R_1.

B, When the fluid level in R_1 is increased twofold, the flow increases proportionately.

C, Flow from R_1 to R_2 is proportional to the difference between the pressures in R_1 and R_2.

D, When pressure in R_2 rises to equal the pressure in R_1, flow ceases in the connecting tube.

Figure 5-6 ■ The flow, *Q,* of fluid through a tube connecting two reservoirs, R_1 and R_2, is proportional to the difference between the pressure, P_i, at the inflow end and the pressure, P_o, at the outflow end of the tube.

If the fluid level in R_2 attains the same height as in R_1, flow will cease (panel *D*).

For any given pressure difference between the two ends of a tube, the flow will depend on the dimensions of the tube. Consider the tube connected to the reservoir in Figure 5-7, *A*. With length l_1 and radius r_1, the flow Q_1 is observed to be 10 ml/s.

The tube connected to the reservoir in panel *B* has the same radius but is twice as long. Under those conditions the flow Q_2 is found to be 5 ml/s, or only half as great as Q_1. Conversely, for a tube half as long as l_1, the flow would be twice as great as Q_1. In other words, flow is inversely proportional to the length of the tube:

$$Q \propto l/l \qquad (6)$$

The tube connected to the reservoir in Figure 5-7, *C* is the same length as l_1, but the radius is twice as great. Under these conditions, the flow Q_3 is found to increase to a value of 160 ml/s, which is 16 times greater than Q_1. The precise measurements of Poiseuille revealed that flow varies directly as the fourth power of the radius:

$$Q \propto r^4 \qquad (7)$$

Thus, in the example above (Figure 5-7, *C*), because $r_3 = 2r_1$, Q_3 will be proportional to $(2r_1)^4$, or $16r_1^4$; therefore, Q_3 will equal $16Q_1$.

Finally, for a given pressure difference and for a cylindric tube of given dimensions, the flow will vary as a function of the nature of the fluid itself. This flow-determining property of fluids is termed **viscosity**, η, which has been defined by

A, Reference condition: for a given pressure, length, radius, and viscosity, let the flow (V_1) equal 10 ml/s.

B, If tube length doubles, flow decreases by 50%.

C, If tube radius doubles, flow increases 16-fold.

D, If viscosity doubles, flow decreases by 50%.

Figure 5-7 ■ **The flow, Q, of fluid through a tube is inversely proportional to the length, l, and the viscosity, η, and is directly proportional to the fourth power of the radius, r.**

Newton as the ratio of **shear stress** to the **shear rate** of the fluid. Those fluids for which the shear rate is proportional to the shear stress are known as **newtonian fluids.** If the shear rate is not proportional to the shear stress, the fluid is **nonnewtonian.**

These terms may be comprehended most clearly by considering the flow of a homogeneous fluid between parallel plates. In Figure 5-8, let the bottom plate (the bottom of a large basin) be stationary, and let the upper plate move at a constant velocity along the upper surface of the fluid. The **shear stress**, τ, is defined as the ratio of F:A, where F is the force applied to the upper plate in the direction of its motion along the up-

per surface of the fluid, and A is the area of the upper plate in contact with the fluid. The **shear rate** is du/dy, where u is the velocity of a minute element of the fluid in the direction parallel to the motion of the upper plate, and y is the distance of that fluid element above the bottom, stationary plate.

For a movable plate traveling with constant velocity across the surface of a homogeneous fluid, the velocity profile of the fluid will be linear. The fluid layer in contact with the upper plate will adhere to it and therefore will move at the same velocity, U, as the plate. Each minute element of fluid between the plates will move at a velocity, u, proportional to its distance, y, from the

$$\eta = \frac{\tau}{du/dy} = \frac{F/A}{U/Y}$$

Figure 5-8 ■ For a newtonian fluid, the viscosity, η, is defined as the ratio of shear stress, τ, to shear rate, *du/dy*. For a plate of contact area, *A*, moving across the surface of a liquid, τ equals the ratio of the force, *F*, applied in the direction of motion to the contact area, *A*, and *du/dy* equals the ratio of the velocity of the plate, *U*, to the depth of the liquid, *Y*.

lower plate. Therefore, the shear rate will be U/Y, where Y is the total distance between the two plates. Because viscosity, η, is defined as the ratio of shear stress, τ, to the shear rate, du/dy, in the example illustrated in Figure 5-8,

$$\eta = (F/A)/(U/Y) \qquad (8)$$

Thus, the dimensions of viscosity are dynes/cm^2 divided by (cm/s)/cm, or dyne-s/cm^2. In honor of Poiseuille, 1 dyne-s/cm^2 has been termed a **poise.** The viscosity of water at 20° C is approximately 0.01 poise, or 1 centipoise.

With regard to the flow of newtonian fluids through cylindric tubes, the flow varies inversely as the viscosity. Thus, in the example of flow from the reservoir in Figure 5-7, *D*, if the viscosity of the fluid in the reservoir were doubled, the flow would be halved (5 ml/s instead of 10 ml/s).

In summary, for the steady, laminar flow of a newtonian fluid through a cylindric tube, the flow, Q, varies directly as the pressure difference, $P_i - P_o$, and the fourth power of the radius, r, of the tube, and it varies inversely as the length, l, of the tube and the viscosity, η, of the fluid. The full statement of Poiseuille's law is

$$Q = \frac{\pi(P_i - P_o)r^4}{8\eta l} \qquad (9)$$

where $\pi/8$ is the constant of proportionality.

■ RESISTANCE TO FLOW

In electrical theory the resistance, R, is defined as the ratio of voltage drop, E, to current flow, I. Similarly, in fluid mechanics the hydraulic resistance, R, may be defined as the ratio of pressure drop, $P_i - P_o$, to flow, Q; P_i and P_o are the pressures at the inflow and outflow ends, respectively, of the hydraulic system. For the steady, laminar flow of a newtonian fluid through a cylindric tube, the physical components of hydraulic resistance may be appreciated by rearranging Poiseuille's law to give the **hydraulic resistance equation**

$$R = \frac{P_i - P_o}{Q} = \frac{8\eta l}{\pi r^4} \qquad (10)$$

Thus, when Poiseuille's law applies, the resistance to flow depends only on the dimensions of the tube and on the characteristics of the fluid.

The principal determinant of the resistance to blood flow through any individual vessel within the circulatory system is its caliber, because resistance varies with the fourth power of the tube radius. The resistance to flow through small blood vessels in cat mesentery has been measured, and the resistance per unit length of vessel (R/l) is plotted against the vessel diameter in Figure 5-9. The resistance is highest in the capillaries (diameter 7 μm), and it diminishes as the vessels increase in diameter on the arterial and venous sides of the capillaries. The values of R/l were found to be virtually proportional to the fourth power of the diameter (or radius) for the larger vessels on both sides of the capillaries.

Figures 1-2 and 1-3 show that the greatest upstream to downstream drop in internal pressure occurs in the arterioles and small arteries. Because the total flow is the same through the var-

Figure 5-9 ■ **The resistance per unit length** *(R/l)* **for individual small blood vessels in the cat mesentery. The capillaries, diameter 7 μm, are denoted by the vertical dashed line. Resistances of the arterioles are plotted to the left and resistances of the venules are plotted to the right of the vertical dashed line. The solid circles represent the actual data. The two curves through the data represent the following regression equations for the arteriole and venule data, respectively: (a) arterioles, R/l = 1.02 × 10⁶D⁻⁴·⁰⁴, and (b) venules, R/l = 1.07 × 10⁶D⁻³·⁹⁴. Note that for both types of vessels, the resistance per unit length is inversely proportional to the fourth power (within 1%) of the vessel diameter *(D)*.** (Redrawn from Lipowsky HH, Kovalcheck S, Zweifach BW: *Circ Res* 43:738, 1978. By permission of the American Heart Association, Inc.)

ious series components of the circulatory system, it follows that the greatest resistance to flow resides in the arterioles. For example, if R_a represents the resistance of the arterioles, and R_x represents the resistance of any other component of the vascular system in series with the arterioles, then by the definition of hydraulic resistance (equation 10),

$$R_a = (P_i - P_o)_a/Q_a \text{ for the arterioles, and}$$
$$R_x = (P_i - P_o)_x/Q_x \text{ for the other component.}$$

However, because the two components are in series, $Q_a = Q_x$, as stated above. Therefore,

$$R_a/R_x = (P_i - P_o)_a/(P_i - P_o)_x \qquad (11)$$

That is, the ratio of the pressure drop across the length of the arterioles to the pressure drop across the length of any other series component of the vascular system is equal to the ratio of the hydraulic resistances of these two vascular components.

The reason why the highest resistance does not reside in the capillaries (as might otherwise be suspected from Figure 5-9) is related to the relative numbers of parallel capillaries and parallel arterioles, as explained below (p 123). The arterioles are vested with a thick coat of circularly arranged smooth muscle fibers, by means of which the lumen radius may be varied. From the hydraulic resistance equation, wherein R varies inversely as r^4, it is clear that small changes in radius will alter resistance greatly.

Resistances in Series and in Parallel

In the cardiovascular system the various types of vessels listed along the horizontal axis in Figures 1-2 and 1-3 lie in series with one another. For two vessels arranged in series, a red blood cell that flows through the upstream vessel will also flow through the downstream vessel. Furthermore, the individual members of a given category of vessels are ordinarily arranged in parallel with one another (see Figure 1-4). For two vessels arranged in parallel, a red cell will pass through one of these vessels but not through the other during one circuit around the body. For example, the capillaries throughout the body are in most instances parallel elements. However, notable exceptions are the renal vasculature (wherein the peritubular capillaries are in series with the glomerular capillaries) and the splanchnic vasculature (wherein the intestinal and hepatic capillaries are aligned in series). Formulas for the total hydraulic resistance of tubes arranged in series and in parallel have been derived in the same manner as those for similar combinations of electrical resistances.

Three hydraulic resistances, R_1, R_2, and R_3, are arranged in series in the schema depicted in Figure 5-10. The pressure drop across the entire system—that is, the difference between inflow pressure, P_i, and outflow pressure, P_o—consists of the sum of the pressure drops across each of the individual resistances (equation *a*). Under steady-state conditions, the flow, Q, through any given cross section must equal the flow through any other cross section. By dividing each component in equation *a* by Q (equation *b*), it becomes evident from the definition of resistance (equation *c*) that *the total resistance, R_t, of the entire system of tubes in series equals the sum of the individual resistances,* that is,

$$R_t = R_1 + R_2 + R_3 \qquad (12)$$

For resistances in parallel, as illustrated in Figure 5-11, the inflow and outflow pressures are the same for all tubes. Under steady-state conditions, the total flow, Q_t, through the system equals the sum of the flows through the individual parallel elements (equation *a*). Because the pressure gradient ($P_i - P_o$) is identical for all parallel elements, each term in equation *a* may be divided by that pressure gradient to yield equation *b*. From the definition of resistance, equation *c* may be derived. This states that *the reciprocal*

of the total resistance, R_t, of tubes in parallel equals the sum of the reciprocals of the individual resistances, that is,

$$\frac{1}{R_t} = \frac{1}{R_1} + \frac{1}{R_2} + \frac{1}{R_3} \qquad (13)$$

Stated in another way, if we define hydraulic **conductance** as the reciprocal of resistance, it becomes evident that, *for tubes in parallel, the total conductance is the sum of the individual conductances.*

By considering a few simple illustrations, some of the fundamental properties of parallel hydraulic systems become apparent. For example, if the resistance of the three parallel elements in Figure 5-11 were all equal, then

$$R_1 = R_2 = R_3$$

Therefore,

$$1/R_t = 3/R_1$$

and

$$R_t = R_1/3$$

(a) $Q_t = Q_1 + Q_2 + Q_3$

(b) $\dfrac{Q_t}{P_i - P_o} = \dfrac{Q_1}{(P_i - P_o)} + \dfrac{Q_2}{(P_1 - P_o)} + \dfrac{Q_3}{(P_i - P_o)}$

(c) $\dfrac{1}{R_t} = \dfrac{1}{R_1} + \dfrac{1}{R_2} + \dfrac{1}{R_3}$

Figure 5-11 ■ For resistances (R_1, R_2, and R_3) arranged in parallel, the reciprocal of the total resistance, R_t, equals the sum of the reciprocals of the individual resistances.

(a) $P_i - P_o = (P_i - P_1) + (P_1 - P_2) + (P_2 - P_o)$

(b) $\dfrac{P_i - P_o}{Q} = \dfrac{(P_i - P_1)}{Q} + \dfrac{(P_1 - P_2)}{Q} + \dfrac{(P_2 - P_o)}{Q}$

(c) $R_t = R_1 + R_2 + R_3$

Figure 5-10 ■ For resistances (R_1, R_2, and R_3) arranged in series, the total resistance, R_t, equals the sum of the individual resistances.

Thus, the total resistance is less than any of the individual resistances. After further consideration, it becomes evident that for any parallel arrangement, the total resistance must be less than that of *any* individual component. For example, consider a system in which a very high-resistance tube is added in parallel to a low-resistance tube. The total resistance must be less than that of the low-resistance component by itself, because the high-resistance component affords an additional pathway, or conductance, for fluid flow.

As a physiologic illustration of these principles, consider the relationship between the **total peripheral resistance (TPR)** of the entire systemic vascular bed and the resistance of one of its components, such as the renal vasculature. In an individual with a cardiac output of 5000 ml/min and an arterial pressure of 100 mm Hg, the TPR would be 0.02 mm Hg/ml/min, or 0.02 peripheral resistance units (PRU). Blood flow through one kidney would be approximately 600 ml/min. Renal resistance would therefore be 100 mm Hg/600 ml/min, or 0.17 PRU, which is 8.5 times as great as the TPR.

From Figures 1-2 and 1-3 it seems paradoxical that the resistance to flow through the arterioles (as manifested by the pressure drop between the arterial and capillary ends of these vessels) is considerably greater than that through certain other vascular components, despite the fact that the total cross-sectional area of the arterioles exceeds that for these same vascular components. For example, the total cross-sectional area of the arterioles greatly exceeds that of the large arteries, yet the resistance to flow through the arterioles exceeds that through the large arteries.

Consideration of simple models of tubes in parallel will help resolve this apparent paradox. In Figure 5-12 the resistance to flow through one wide tube of cross-sectional area A_w is compared with that through four narrower tubes in parallel, each of area A_n. The total cross-sectional area of the parallel system of four narrow tubes equals the area of the wide tube; that is,

$$A_w = 4A_n \tag{14}$$

Because resistance, R, is inversely proportional to the fourth power of the radius, r, and because

$$A = \pi r^2 \tag{15}$$

for cylindric tubes, it follows that

$$R = k/A^2 \tag{16}$$

The proportionality constant, k, is related to tube length and fluid viscosity, both of which will be held constant in the example under consideration. From equation 16, the resistances of the wide tube, R_w, and a single narrow tube, R_n, are

$$R_w = k/A_2{}^2 \tag{17}$$
$$R_n = k/A_n{}^2 \tag{18}$$

From equation 13,

$$\frac{1}{R_r} = \frac{1}{R_n} + \frac{1}{R_n} + \frac{1}{R_n} + \frac{1}{R_n} = \frac{4}{R_n} \tag{19}$$

Substituting the value of R_n in equation 18,

$$1/R_t = 4A_n{}^2/k \tag{20}$$

Rearranging,

$$R_t = k/4A_n{}^2 \tag{21}$$

From equations 14 and 17,

$$R_t = 4k/A_w{}^2 = 4R_w \tag{22}$$

Hence, resistance of four such narrow tubes in parallel is four times as great as that of a single wide tube of equal total cross-sectional area.

If a similar calculation is made for eight such tubes in parallel, with each tube having one fourth the cross-sectional area of the single wide tube, it will be found that the total resistance will equal $2R_w$. In this circumstance the resistance to flow through eight such narrow tubes in parallel will still be twice as great as that through the single tube, despite the fact that the total cross-sectional area for the eight narrow tubes is twice as great as for the single wide tube. This is analogous to the relationship that exists between resistance and area in the circulatory system when the arterioles are com-

Figure 5-12 ■ When four narrow tubes, each of area A_n, are connected in parallel, the total cross-sectional area equals the area, A_w, of a wide tube of area such that $A_w = 4A_n$. Although the total areas are equal, the total resistance, R_t, to flow through the parallel narrow tubes is four times as great as the resistance, R_w, through the single wide tube.

pared with the large arteries. Despite the fact that the total cross-sectional area of all the arterioles greatly exceeds that of all the large arteries, the resistance to flow through the arterioles is considerably greater than that through the large arteries.

If the example is carried still further, it will be found that 16 such narrow tubes in parallel, now with four times the total cross-sectional area of the single wide tube, will exert a resistance to flow just equal to the resistance through the wide tube. Any number of these narrow tubes in excess of 16, then, will have a lower resistance than that of the single wide tube. This is analogous to the situation for the arterioles and capillaries. The resistance to flow through a single capillary is much greater than that through a single arteriole (Figure 5-9). Yet the number of capillaries so greatly exceeds the number of arterioles, as reflected by the relative difference in total cross-sectional areas, that the pressure drop across the arterioles is considerably greater than the pressure drop across the capillaries (see Figures 1-2 and 1-3).

■ LAMINAR AND TURBULENT FLOW

Under certain conditions, the flow of a fluid in a cylindric tube is **laminar** (sometimes called **streamlined**), as illustrated in Figure 5-5. The thin layer of fluid in contact with the wall of the tube adheres to the wall and thus is motionless. The layer of fluid just central to this external lamina must shear against this motionless layer and therefore moves slowly, but with a finite velocity. Similarly, the adjacent, more central layer travels still more rapidly. The longitudinal velocity profile is that of a paraboloid (Figure 5-5). The velocity of the fluid adjacent to the wall is zero, whereas the velocity at the center of the stream is maximum and equal to twice the mean velocity of flow across the entire cross section of the tube. In laminar flow, fluid elements remain in one lamina, or streamline, as the fluid progresses longitudinally along the tube.

Irregular motions of the fluid elements may develop in the flow of fluid through a tube; this flow is called **turbulent.** Under such conditions, fluid elements do not remain confined to definite

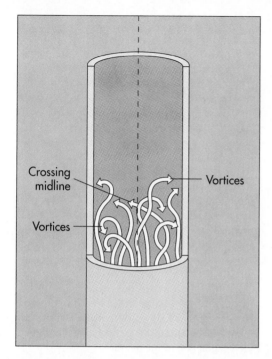

Crossing midline

Vortices

Vortices

Figure 5-13 ■ In turbulent flow the elements of the fluid move irregularly in axial, radial, and circumferential directions. Vortices frequently develop.

Turbulence is usually accompanied by audible vibrations. When turbulent flow exists within the cardiovascular system, it is usually detected as a **murmur.** The factors listed above that predispose to turbulence may account for murmurs heard clinically. In severe anemia, **functional cardiac murmurs** (murmurs not caused by structural abnormalities) are frequently detectable. The physical basis for such murmurs resides in (1) the reduced viscosity of blood in anemia and (2) the high flow velocities associated with the high cardiac output that usually prevails in anemic patients. Turbulence also occurs when the cross-sectional area of the bloodstream suddenly changes, as when the blood passes through a narrowed (stenotic) cardiac valve or when it passes through an abnormal widening (aneurysm) of a large artery. Such abrupt changes in dimensions of the bloodstream cause audible murmurs.

Blood clots, or **thrombi,** are much more likely to develop in turbulent than in laminar flow. One of the problems with the use of artificial valves in the surgical treatment of valvular heart disease is that thrombi may occur in association with the prosthetic valve. The thrombi may be dislodged and occlude a crucial artery. It is thus important to design such valves to avert turbulence.

laminae, but rapid, radial mixing occurs (Figure 5-13). A considerably greater pressure is required to force a given flow of fluid through the same tube when the flow is turbulent than when it is laminar. In turbulent flow the pressure drop is approximately proportional to the square of the flow rate, whereas in laminar flow the pressure drop is proportional to the first power of the flow rate. Hence, to produce a given flow, a pump such as the heart must do considerably more work to generate a given flow if turbulence develops.

Whether turbulent or laminar flow will exist in a tube under given conditions may be predicted on the basis of a dimensionless number called **Reynold's number,** N_R. This number represents the ratio of inertial to viscous forces. For a fluid flowing through a cylindric tube,

$$N_R = \rho D \, \bar{v} / \eta \qquad (23)$$

where D is the tube diameter, $\bar{v}$ is the mean velocity, ρ is the density, and η is the viscosity. For $N_R < 2000$, the flow usually is laminar; for $N_R > 3000$, the flow is turbulent. Various possible conditions may develop in the transition range of N_R between 2000 and 3000. Because flow tends to be laminar at low N_R and turbulent at high N_R, the definition of N_R indicates that large diameters, high velocities, and low viscosities predispose to turbulence. In addition to these factors, abrupt variations in tube dimensions or irregularities in the tube walls may produce turbulence.

■ SHEAR STRESS ON THE VESSEL WALL

In Figure 5-8 an external force is applied to a plate floating on the surface of a liquid in a large basin. This force, exerted parallel to the surface, caused a shearing stress on the liquid below and thereby produced a differential motion of each layer of liquid relative to the adjacent layers. At the bottom of the basin, the flowing liquid exerted a shearing stress on the surface of the basin in contact with the liquid. By rearranging the equation for viscosity stated in Figure 5-8, it is apparent that the shear stress, τ, equals η (du/dy); that is, the shear stress equals the product of the viscosity and the shear rate. Hence, *the greater the rate of flow, the greater the shear stress that the liquid exerts on the walls of the container in which it flows.*

For precisely the same reasons, the rapidly flowing blood in a large artery tends to pull the endothelial lining of the artery along with it. This force **(viscous drag)** is proportional to the shear rate (du/dy) of the layers of blood near the wall. For a flow regimen that obeys Poiseuille's law,

$$\tau = 4\eta Q/\pi r^3 \qquad (24)$$

The greater the rate of blood flow (Q) in the artery, the greater will be du/dy near the arterial wall, and the greater will be the viscous drag (τ).

■ RHEOLOGIC PROPERTIES OF BLOOD

The viscosity of a newtonian fluid, such as water, may be determined by measuring the rate of flow of the fluid at a given pressure gradient through a cylindric tube of known length and radius. As long as the fluid flow is laminar, the viscosity may be computed by substituting these values into Poiseuille's equation. The viscosity of a given new-

In certain types of arterial disease, particularly in patients with hypertension, the subendothelial layers tend to degenerate locally, and small regions of the endothelium may lose their normal support. The viscous drag on the arterial wall may cause a tear between a normally supported and an unsupported region of the endothelial lining. Blood may then flow from the vessel lumen through the rift in the lining and dissect between the various layers of the artery. Such a lesion is called a **dissecting aneurysm.** It occurs most commonly in the proximal portions of the aorta and is extremely serious. One reason for its predilection for this site is the high velocity of blood flow, with the associated large values of du/dy at the endothelial wall. The shear stress at the vessel wall also influences many other vascular functions, such as the permeability of the vascular walls to large molecules, the biosynthetic activity of the endothelial cells, the integrity of the formed elements in the blood, and the coagulation of the blood.

tonian fluid at a specified temperature will be constant over a wide range of tube dimensions and flows. However, for a nonnewtonian fluid, the viscosity calculated by substituting into Poiseuille's equation may vary considerably as a function of tube dimensions and flows. Therefore, in considering the rheologic properties of a suspension such as blood, the term **viscosity** does not have a unique meaning. The terms **anomalous viscosity** and **apparent viscosity** are frequently applied to the value of viscosity obtained for blood under the particular conditions of measurement.

Rheologically, blood is a suspension of formed elements, principally erythrocytes, in a relatively homogeneous liquid, the blood plasma. For this reason, the apparent viscosity of blood varies as a function of the **hematocrit ratio** (ratio of volume of red blood cells to volume of whole blood). In Figure 5-14 the upper curve represents

Figure 5-14 ■ **The viscosity of whole blood, relative to that of plasma, increases at a progressively greater rate as the hematocrit ratio increases. For any given hematocrit ratio, the apparent viscosity of blood is less when measured in a biological viscometer (such as the hind leg of a dog) than in a conventional capillary tube viscometer.** (Redrawn from Levy MN, Share L: *Circ Res* 1:247, 1953.)

Figure 5-15 ■ **The viscosity of blood, relative to that of water, increases as a function of tube diameter up to a diameter of about 0.3 mm.** (Redrawn from Fåhraeus R, Lindqvist T: *Am J Physiol* 96:562, 1931.)

the ratio of the apparent viscosity of whole blood to that of plasma over a range of hematocrit ratios from 0% to 80%, measured in a tube 1 mm in diameter. The viscosity of plasma is 1.2 to 1.3 times that of water. Figure 5-14 (upper curve) shows that blood, with a normal hematocrit ratio of 45%, has an apparent viscosity 2.4 times that of plasma.

For any given hematocrit ratio, the apparent viscosity of blood depends on the dimensions of the tube employed in estimating the viscosity. Figure 5-15 demonstrates that the apparent viscosity of blood diminishes progressively as tube diameter decreases below a value of about 0.3 mm. The diameters of the highest-resistance blood vessels, the arterioles, are considerably less than this critical value. This phenomenon there-

In severe anemia, blood viscosity is low. With increasing hematocrit ratios, the slope of the curve increases progressively; it is especially steep at the upper range of erythrocyte concentrations. A rise in hematocrit ratio from 45% to 70%, which occurs in **polycythemia,** increases the relative viscosity more than twofold, with a proportionate effect on the resistance to blood flow. The effect of such a change in hematocrit ratio on peripheral resistance may be appreciated when it is recognized that even in the most severe cases of essential hypertension, total peripheral resistance rarely increases by more than a factor of two. In hypertension, the increase in peripheral resistance is achieved by arteriolar vasoconstriction.

fore reduces the resistance to flow in the blood vessels that possess the greatest resistance.

The apparent viscosity of blood, when measured in living tissues, is considerably less than when measured in a conventional capillary tube viscometer with a diameter greater than 0.3 mm. In the lower curve of Figure 5-14, the apparent viscosity of blood was assessed by using the hind leg of an anesthetized dog as a biological viscometer. Over the entire range of hematocrit ratios, the apparent viscosity was less as measured in the living tissue than in the capillary tube viscometer (upper curve), and the disparity was greater the higher the hematocrit ratio.

The influence of tube diameter on apparent viscosity depends in part on the change in actual composition of the blood as it flows through small tubes. The composition changes because the red blood cells tend to accumulate in the faster axial stream in the blood vessels, whereas the blood component that flows in the slower marginal layers is mainly plasma. To illustrate this phenomenon, a reservoir such as R_1 in Figure 5-6, *C* has been filled with blood possessing a given hematocrit ratio. The blood in R_1 was constantly agitated to prevent settling and was permitted to flow through a narrow capillary tube into reservoir R_2. As long as the tube diameter was substantially greater than the diameter of the red blood cells, the hematocrit ratio of the blood in R_2 was not detectably different from that in R_1. Surprisingly, however, the hematocrit ratio of the blood contained within the tube was found to be considerably lower than the hematocrit ratio of the blood in either reservoir.

In Figure 5-16, the relative hematocrit is the ratio of the hematocrit in the tube to that in the reservoir at either end of the tube. For tubes of 500 μm diameter or greater, the relative hematocrit ratio was close to 1. However, as the tube diameter was reduced below 500 μm, the relative hematocrit ratio progressively diminished; for a tube diameter of 30 μm, the relative hematocrit ratio was only 0.65.

The fact that this situation results from a disparity in the relative velocities of the red cells and plasma can be appreciated on the basis of the following analogy. Consider the flow of auto-

Figure 5-16 ■ **The relative hematocrit ratio of blood flowing from a feed reservoir through capillary tubes of various calibers, as a function of the tube diameter. The relative hematocrit is the ratio of the hematocrit of the blood in the tubes to that of the blood in the feed reservoir.** (Redrawn from Barbee JH, Cokelet GR: *Microvasc Res* 3:6, 1971.)

mobile traffic across a bridge that is 3 miles long. Let the cars move in one lane at a speed of 60 miles per hour and the trucks in another lane at 20 miles per hour, as illustrated in Figure 5-17. If one car and one truck start out across the bridge each minute, then except for the initial few minutes of traffic flow across the bridge, one car and one truck will arrive at the other end each minute. Yet, if one counts the actual number of cars and trucks on the bridge at any moment, there will be three times more of the slower trucks than of the faster cars.

Because the axial portions of the bloodstream contain a greater proportion of red cells and move with a greater velocity, the red cells tend to traverse the tube in less time than does the plasma. Therefore, the red cells correspond to the fast cars in the analogy, and the plasma corresponds to the slow trucks. Measurement of transit times through various organs has shown that red cells do travel faster than the plasma. Furthermore, the hematocrit ratios of the blood contained in various tissues are lower than those

Figure 5-17 ■ When the car velocity is three times as great as the truck velocity, the ratio of the number of cars to trucks on a bridge will be 1:3, even though one of each type of vehicle enters and leaves the bridge each minute.

in blood samples withdrawn from large arteries or veins in the same animal (Figure 5-18).

The physical forces responsible for the drift of the erythrocytes toward the axial stream and away from the vessel walls are not fully understood. One factor is the great flexibility of the red blood cells. At low flow (or shear) rates, compa-rable with those in the microcirculation, rigid particles do not migrate toward the axis of a tube, whereas flexible particles do migrate. The concentration of flexible particles near the tube axis is enhanced by increasing the shear rate.

The apparent viscosity of blood diminishes as the shear rate is increased (Figure 5-19), a phe-

Figure 5-18 ■ **The hematocrit ratio (*H*_{*micro*}) of the blood in various-sized arterial and venous microvessels in the cat mesentery, relative to the hematocrit ratio (*H*_{*sys*}) in the large systemic vessels. The hematocrit ratio is least in the capillaries and tiny venules.** (Modified from Lipowsky HH, Usami S, Chien S: *Microvasc Res* 19:297, 1980.)

nomenon called **shear thinning.** The greater tendency of the erythrocytes to accumulate in the axial laminae at higher flow rates is partly responsible for this nonnewtonian behavior. However, a more important factor is that at very slow rates of shear, the suspended cells tend to form aggregates, which would increase viscosity. As the flow is increased, this aggregation would decrease and so also would the apparent viscosity (Figure 5-19).

The tendency for the erythrocytes to aggregate at low flows depends on the concentration in the plasma of the larger protein molecules, especially fibrinogen. For this reason, the changes in blood viscosity with shear rate are much more pronounced when the concentration of fibrinogen is high. Also, at low flow rates, the leukocytes tend to adhere to the endothelial cells of the microvessels and thereby increase the apparent viscosity.

The deformability of the erythrocytes is also a factor in shear thinning, especially at high hematocrit ratios. The mean diameter of human red blood cells is about 8 μm, yet they are able to pass through openings with a diameter of only 3 μm. As blood that is densely packed with erythrocytes is caused to flow at progressively greater rates, the erythrocytes become more and more deformed, which diminishes the apparent viscosity of the blood. The flexibility of human erythrocytes is enhanced as the concentration of fibrinogen in the plasma increases (Figure 5-20).

Figure 5-19 ■ Decrease in the viscosity of blood (centipoise) at increasing rates of shear. The shear rate refers to the velocity of one layer of fluid relative to that of the adjacent layers and is directionally related to the rate of flow. (Redrawn from Amin TM, Sirs JA: *Q J Exp Physiol* 70:37, 1985.)

Figure 5-20 ■ The effect of the plasma fibrinogen concentration on the flexibility of human erythrocytes. (Redrawn from Amin TM, Sirs JA: *Q J Exp Physiol* 70:37, 1985.)

If the red blood cells become hardened, as they are in certain **spherocytic anemias,** shear thinning may become much less prominent. When erythrocytes are extremely deformed, especially in **sickle cell anemia,** they tend to aggregate and completely block flow in small vessels; the tissues supplied by those vessels frequently become infarcted.

■ SUMMARY

1. The vascular system is composed of two major subdivisions in series with one another: the systemic circulation and the pulmonary circulation.

2. Each subdivision consists of several types of vessels (e.g., arteries, arterioles, capillaries) aligned in series with one another. In general, the vessels of a given type are arranged in parallel with each other.

3. The mean velocity (v) of blood flow in a given type of vessel is directly proportional to the total blood flow (Q_t) being pumped by the heart, and it is inversely proportional to the cross-sectional area (A) of all the parallel vessels of that type; i.e., $v = Q_t/A$.

4. The laterally directed pressure in the bloodstream decreases as the flow velocity increases; the decrement in lateral pressure is proportional to the square of the velocity. The changes are insignificant, however, except when flow is very large.

5. When blood flow is relatively steady and laminar in vessels larger than arterioles, the flow (Q) is proportional to the pressure drop down the vessel ($P_i - P_o$) and to the fourth power of the radius (r), and it is inversely proportional to the length (l) of the vessel and to the viscosity (η) of the fluid; i.e., $Q = \pi(P_i - P_o)r^4/8\eta l$ (Poiseuille's law).

6. For resistances aligned in series, the total resistance equals the sum of the individual resistances.

7. For resistances aligned in parallel, the reciprocal of the total resistance equals the sum of the reciprocals of the individual resistances.

8. Flow tends to become turbulent when flow velocity is high, when fluid viscosity is low, when tube diameter is large, or when the wall of the vessel is very irregular.

9. Blood flow is nonnewtonian in very small vessels; i.e., Poiseuille's law is not applicable. The apparent viscosity of blood diminishes as shear rate (flow) increases and as the tube dimensions decrease.

■ KEY WORDS AND CONCEPTS

- Velocity of the blood
- Blood flow
- Blood pressure
- Blood viscosity
- Aortic stenosis
- Poiseuille's law
- Steady flow
- Laminar flow
- Reynold's number
- Turbulent fluid
- Newtonian flow
- Shear stress
- Shear rate
- Hydraulic resistance
- Resistances in series
- Resistances in parallel
- Total peripheral resistance
- Functional cardiac murmur
- Viscous drag
- Dissecting aneurysm
- Blood rheology
- Anomalous viscosity
- Hematocrit ratio
- Shear thinning
- Sickle cell anemia

■ SELF-STUDY PROBLEMS

1. A renal physiologist found that the mean arterial pressure in an anesthetized animal was 100 mm Hg and the blood flow to each kidney was 200 ml/min. What was the resistance to blood flow through one kidney, and what was the resistance to blood flow through both kidneys? Explain the reason for the disparity in the resistances for one and two kidneys.

2. A patient is found to have a loud cardiac murmur, but the cardiac valves appear to function normally. Laboratory examinations revealed that the patient was severely anemic and that cardiac output was abnormally high. What factors operated in this patient to produce the "functional" murmur?

3. In a patient who has a small dissecting aneurysm of the thoracic aorta, what is the rationale for giving a drug that will reduce cardiac output?

4. Why is the hematocrit ratio of the blood in small blood vessels, such as the arterioles, consistently less than the hematocrit ratio in the large blood vessels?

■ BIBLIOGRAPHY

Journal articles

Alonso C, Pries AR, Kiesslich O et al: Transient rheological behavior of blood in low-shear tube flow: velocity profiles and effective viscosity, *Am J Physiol* 268:H25, 1995.

Amin TM, Sirs JA: The blood rheology of man and various animal species, *Q J Exp Physiol* 70:37, 1985.

Cokelet GR, Goldsmith HI: Decreased hydrodynamic resistance in the two-phase flow of blood through small vertical tubes at low flow rates, *Circ Res* 68:1, 1991.

Hoeks APG, Samijo SK, Brands PJ et al: Noninvasive determination of shear-rate distribution across the arterial wall, *Hypertension* 26:26, 1995.

Klanchar M, Tarbell JM, Wang D-M: In vitro study of the influence of radial wall motion on wall shear stress in an elastic tube model of the aorta, *Circ Res* 66:1624, 1990.

Lee RT, Kamm RD: Vascular mechanics for the cardiologist, *J Am Coll Cardiol* 23:1289, 1994.

Maeda N, Shiga T: Velocity of oxygen transfer and erythrocyte rheology, *News Physiol Sci* 9:22, 1994.

McKay CB, Meiselman HJ: Osmolality-mediated Fåhraeus and Fåhraeus-Lindqvist effects for human RBC suspensions, *Am J Physiol* 254:H238, 1988.

Melkumyants AM, Balashov SA, Khayutin VM: Control of arterial lumen by shear stress on endothelium, *News Physiol Sci* 10:204, 1995.

Morita T, Kurihara H, Maemura K et al: Role of Ca^{2+} and protein kinase C in shear stress–induced actin depolymerization and endothelin 1 gene expression, *Circ Res* 75:630, 1994.

Pries AR, Secomb TW, Gessner T et al: Resistance to blood flow in microvessels in vivo, *Circ Res* 75:904, 1994.

Pries AR, Secomb TW, Gaetgens P: Design principles of vascular beds, *Circ Res* 77:1017, 1995.

Reinhart WH, Boulanger CM, Lüscher TF et al: Influence of endothelial surface on flow velocity in vitro, *Am J Physiol* 265:H523, 1993.

Tangelder GJ, Slaaf DW, Arts T, Reneman RS: Wall shear rate in arterioles in vivo: least estimates from platelet velocity profiles, *Am J Physiol* 254:H1059, 1988.

White KC, Kavanaugh JF, Wang D-M et al: Hemodynamics and wall shear rate in the abdominal aorta of dogs: effects of vasoactive agents, *Circ Res* 75:637, 1994.

Books and monographs

Chien S, Usami S, Skalak R: *Blood flow in small tubes.* In Renkin EM, Michel CC, editors: *Handbook of physiology,* Section 2: *The cardiovascular system—Microcirculation,* vol IV, Bethesda, Md, 1984, American Physiological Society.

Cokelet GR, Meiselman HJ, Brooks DE, editors: *Erythrocyte mechanics and blood flow,* New York, 1980, Alan R Liss.

Fung YC: *Biodynamics: circulation,* New York, 1984, Springer-Verlag.

Lowe GDO: *Clinical blood rheology,* vol I, Boca Raton, FL, 1988, CRC Press.

Taylor DEM, Stevens AL, editors: *Blood flow: theory and practice,* New York, 1983, Academic Press.

The Arterial System

■ HYDRAULIC FILTER

The principal function of the systemic and pulmonary arterial systems is to distribute blood to the capillary beds throughout the body. The arterioles, the terminal components of the arterial system, regulate the distribution of flow to the various capillary beds. Between the heart and the arterioles, the aorta and pulmonary artery and their major branches constitute a system of conduits of considerable volume and distensibility. An arterial system composed of elastic conduits and high-resistance terminals constitutes a **hydraulic filter** analogous to the resistance-capacitance filters of electrical circuits.

Hydraulic filtering converts the intermittent output of the heart to a steady flow through the capillaries. This important function of the large elastic arteries has been likened to the **Windkessels** of antique fire engines. The Windkessel contained a large volume of trapped air. The compressibility of the trapped air converted the intermittent inflow of water to a steady outflow at the nozzle of the fire hose.

The analogous function of the large elastic arteries is illustrated in Figure 6-1. The heart is an intermittent pump. The entire stroke volume is discharged into the arterial system during sys-

tole, which usually occupies approximately one third of the duration of the cardiac cycle. In fact, as shown in Figure 3-10, most of the stroke volume is pumped during the rapid ejection phase, which constitutes about half of the systole. Part of the energy of cardiac contraction is dissipated as forward capillary flow during systole; the remainder is stored in the arteries as potential energy, in that much of the stroke volume is retained by stretching the distensible arteries (Figure 6-1, *A, B*). During diastole the elastic recoil of the arterial walls converts this potential energy into capillary blood flow. If the arterial walls were rigid, capillary flow would cease during diastole (Figure 6-1, *C, D*).

Hydraulic filtering minimizes the workload of the heart. More work is required to pump a given flow intermittently than steadily; the more effective the filtering, the less is the excess work. A simple example will illustrate this point.

Consider first the steady flow of a fluid at a rate of 100 ml/s through a hydraulic system with a resistance of 1 mm Hg/ml/s. This combination of flow and resistance would result in a constant pressure of 100 mm Hg, as shown in Figure 6-2, *A*.

Compliant arteries

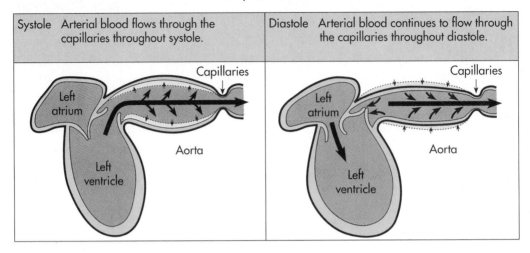

A, When the arteries are normally compliant, a substantial fraction of the stroke volume is stored in the arteries during ventricular systole. The arterial walls are stretched.

B, During ventricular diastole the previously stretched arteries recoil. The volume of blood that is displaced by the recoil furnishes continuous capillary flow throughout diastole.

Rigid arteries

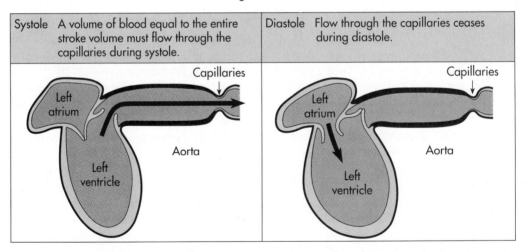

C, When the arteries are rigid, virtually none of the stroke volume can be stored in the arteries.

D, Rigid arteries cannot recoil appreciably during diastole.

Figure 6-1 ■ When the arteries are normally compliant, blood flows through the capillaries throughout the cardiac cycle. When the arteries are rigid, blood flows through the capillaries during systole, but flow ceases during diastole.

Neglecting any inertial effect, hydraulic work, W, may be defined as

$$W = \int_{t_1}^{t_2} PdV \qquad (1)$$

that is, each small increment of volume, dV, pumped is multiplied by the pressure, P, existing at the time, and the products are integrated over the time interval of interest, $t_2 - t_1$, to give the total work, W. For steady flow,

$$W = PV \qquad (2)$$

In the example in Figure 6-2, *A*, the work done in pumping the fluid for 1 s would be 10,000 mm Hg • ml (or 1.33×10^7 dyne-cm).

Next, consider an intermittent pump that puts out the same volume per second but pumps the entire volume at a steady rate over 0.5 s and then pumps nothing during the next 0.5 s. Hence, it pumps at the rate of 200 ml/s for 0.5 s, as shown in Figure 6-2, *B* and *C*. In *B* the conduit is rigid and the fluid is incompressible, but the system has the same resistance as in *A*. During the pumping phase of the cycle (systole) the flow of 200 ml/s through a resistance of 1 mm Hg/ml/s would produce a pressure of 200 mm Hg. During the filling phase of the pump (diastole) the pressure would be 0 mm Hg in this rigid system. The work done during systole would be 20,000 mm Hg • ml, which is twice that required in the example shown in Figure 6-2, *A*.

If the system were very distensible, hydraulic filtering would be very effective and the pressure would remain virtually constant throughout the entire cycle (Figure 6-2, *C*). Of the 100 ml of fluid pumped during the 0.5 s of systole, only 50 ml would be emitted through the high-resistance outflow end of the system during systole. The remaining 50 ml would be stored by the distensible conduit during systole and would flow out during diastole. Hence, the pressure would be virtually constant at 100 mm Hg throughout the cycle. The fluid pumped during systole would be ejected at only half the pressure that prevailed in Figure 6-2, *B*, and there-fore the work would be only half as great. With nearly perfect filtering, as in Figure 6-2, *C*, the work would be identical to that for steady flow (Figure 6-2, *A*).

Naturally, the filtering accomplished by the systemic and pulmonic arterial systems is intermediate between the examples in Figure 6-2, *B* and *C*. Ordinarily, the additional work imposed by intermittency of pumping, in excess of that for steady flow, is about 35% for the right ventricle and about 10% for the left ventricle. These fractions change, however, with variations in heart rate, peripheral resistance, and arterial distensibility.

The increased cardiac energy requirement imposed by a rigid arterial system is illustrated by the experimental results shown in Figure 6-3. In a group of anesthetized dogs, the cardiac output pumped by the left ventricle could be allowed to flow through the natural route (the aorta) or it could be diverted through a stiff plastic tube to the peripheral arteries. The total peripheral resistance (TPR) readings were virtually identical regardless of which pathway was selected. The data (Figure 6-3) from a representative animal show that for any given stroke volume, the myocardial oxygen consumption (MVO_2) was substantially greater when the blood was diverted through the plastic tubing than when it flowed through the aorta. This increase in MVO_2 indicates that the left ventricle had to expend more energy to pump blood through a less compliant conduit than through a more compliant conduit.

■ ARTERIAL ELASTICITY

The elastic properties of the arterial wall may be appreciated by considering first the **static pressure-volume relationship** for the aorta. To obtain the curves shown in Figure 6-4, aortas were obtained at autopsy from individuals in different age groups. All branches of the aorta were ligated and successive volumes of liquid were injected into this closed elastic system. After each

A, The flow is steady, and pressure will remain constant regardless of the distensibility of the conduit.

B, The flow *(Q)* produced by the pump is intermittent; it is steady for half the cycle and ceases for the remainder of the cycle. The conduit is rigid, and therefore the flow produced by the pump during its downstroke must exit through the resistance during the same 0.5 second that elapses during the downstroke. The pump must do twice as much work as the pump in **A**.

C, The pump operates as in **B**, but the conduit is infinitely distensible. This results in perfect filtering of the pressure; that is, the pressure is steady, and the flow through the resistance is also steady. The work equals that in **A**.

Figure 6-2 ■ The relationships between pressure and flow for three hydraulic systems. In each the overall flow is 100 ml/s and the resistance is 1 mm Hg/ml/s.

Figure 6-3 ■ The relationship between myocardial oxygen consumption *(ml/100 g/beat)* and
stroke volume *(ml)* in an anesthetized dog
whose cardiac output could be pumped by the
left ventricle either through the aorta or through
a stiff plastic tube to the peripheral arteries.
(Modified from Kelly RP, Tunin R, Kass DA: *Circ Res*
71:490, 1992. By permission of the American Heart Association, Inc.)

Figure 6-4 ■ Pressure-volume relationships for
aortas obtained at autopsy from humans in different age groups (denoted by the numbers at
the right end of each of the curves). (Redrawn
from Hallock P, Benson IC: *J Clin Invest* 16:595, 1937.)

increment of volume, the internal pressure was
measured. In Figure 6-4 the curve that relates
pressure to volume for the youngest age group
(curve *a*) is sigmoidal. Although the curve is
nearly linear over most of its extent, the slope decreases at the upper and lower ends. At any
point, the slope (dV/dP) represents the aortic
compliance. Thus, in young individuals the aortic compliance is least at very high and low pressures and greatest over the usual range of pressure variations. This sequence of compliance
changes resembles the familiar compliance
changes encountered in inflating a balloon. The
greatest difficulty in introducing air into the balloon is experienced at the beginning of inflation
and again at near-maximal volume, just before
rupture of the balloon. At intermediate volumes,
the balloon is relatively easy to inflate; that is, it is
more compliant.

The above effects of the subject's age on the

It is also apparent from Figure 6-4 that the
curves become displaced downward and the
slopes diminish as a function of advancing age.
Thus, for any pressure above about 80 mm Hg,
the compliance decreases with age, a manifestation of increased rigidity **(atherosclerosis)**
caused by progressive changes in the collagen
and elastin contents of the arterial walls.

elastic characteristics of the arterial system were
derived from aortas removed at autopsy (Figure
6-4). Such age-related changes have been confirmed in living subjects by ultrasound imaging
techniques. These studies have disclosed that the
increase in the diameter of the aorta produced
by each cardiac contraction is much less in el-

derly persons than in young persons (Figure 6-5). The effects of aging on the **elastic modulus** of the aorta in healthy subjects are shown in Figure 6-6. The elastic modulus, E_p, is defined as

$$E_p = \Delta P / (\Delta D / D) \qquad (3)$$

where ΔP is the aortic pulse pressure (Figure 6-7), D is the mean aortic diameter during the cardiac cycle, and ΔD is the maximal change in aortic diameter during the cardiac cycle.

Figure 6-5 ■ The pulsatile changes in diameter, measured ultrasonically, in a 22-year-old and in a 63-year-old man. (Modified from Imura T, Yamamoto K, Kanamori K, Mikawi T, Yasvda H: *Cardiovasc Res* 20:208, 1986.)

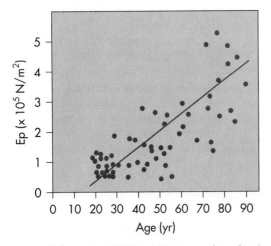

Figure 6-6 ■ The effects of age on the elastic modulus *(Ep)* of the abdominal aorta in a group of 61 human subjects. (Modified from Imura T, Yamamoto K, Kanamori K, Mikawi T, Yasvda H: *Cardiovasc Res* 20:208, 1986.)

The fractional change in diameter ($\Delta D/D$) of the aorta during the cardiac cycle reflects its change in volume as the left ventricle ejects its stroke volume into the aorta each systole. Thus, E_p is **inversely** related to compliance, which is the ratio of ΔV to ΔP. Consequently, the **increase** in elastic modulus with aging (Figure 6-6) and the **decrease** in compliance with aging (Figure 6-4) both reflect the stiffening of the arterial walls **(atherosclerosis)** as individuals age.

■ DETERMINANTS OF ARTERIAL BLOOD PRESSURE

The determinants of the pressure within the arterial system of intact subjects cannot be evaluated precisely. Nevertheless, arterial blood pressure is routinely measured in patients and provides a useful clue to cardiovascular status. We will therefore take a simplified approach to explain the principal determinants of arterial blood pressure. To accomplish this, the determinants of **mean arterial pressure** (defined in the next section) will first be analyzed. **Systolic** and **diastolic arterial pressures** will then be considered as the upper and lower limits of periodic oscillations about this mean pressure. Finally, the changes in arterial pressure as the pulse wave progresses from the origin of the aorta toward the capillaries will be discussed.

The determinants of arterial blood pressure may be arbitrarily subdivided into "physical" and "physiologic" factors (Figure 6-8). The arterial system is assumed to be a static, elastic system, and the only two "physical" factors considered are the **blood volume** within the arterial system and the **elastic characteristics** (compliance) of the system. Certain "physiologic" factors will be considered: **cardiac output,** which equals **heart rate × stroke volume,** and **peripheral resistance.** *Such physiologic factors will be shown to operate through one or both of the physical factors, however.*

Mean Arterial Pressure

Mean arterial pressure is the pressure in the arteries, averaged over time. It may be obtained from an arterial pressure tracing by measuring the area under the curve and dividing this area by the time interval involved, as shown in Figure 6-7. The mean arterial pressure, $\bar{P}_a$, can usually be approximated satisfactorily from the measured values of the systolic (P_s) and diastolic (P_d) pressures by means of the following empirical formula:

$$\bar{P}_a \cong P_d + \frac{1}{3}(P_s - P_d) \qquad (4)$$

The mean pressure will be considered to depend only on the mean blood volume in the arterial system and on the arterial compliance (Figure 6-8). The arterial volume, V_a, in turn depends on the rate of inflow, Q_h, from the heart into the arteries **(cardiac output)** and the rate of outflow, Q_r, from the arteries through the resistance vessels **(peripheral runoff)**; expressed mathematically,

$$dV_a/dt = Q_h - Q_r \qquad (5)$$

This equation is an expression of the law of conservation of mass. It states that the change in arterial blood volume per unit time (dV_a/dt) represents the difference between the rate at which blood is pumped into the arterial system by the heart (Q_h) and the rate at which it leaves the arterial system through the resistance vessels (Q_r).

If arterial inflow exceeds outflow, arterial volume increases, the arterial walls are stretched more, and pressure rises. The converse happens when arterial outflow exceeds inflow. When inflow equals outflow, arterial pressure remains constant.

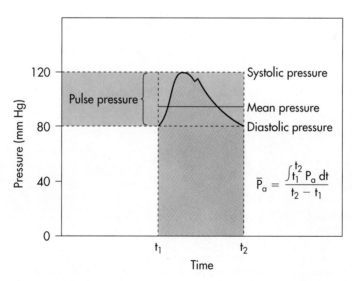

Figure 6-7 ■ **Arterial systolic, diastolic, pulse, and mean pressures. The mean arterial pressure ($\bar{P}_a$) represents the area under the arterial pressure curve *(shaded area)* divided by the cardiac cycle duration *($t_2 - t_1$)*.**

Cardiac Output

The change in pressure in response to an alteration of cardiac output can be better appreciated by considering some simple examples. Under control conditions, let cardiac output be 5 L/min and mean arterial pressure ($\bar{P}_a$) be 100 mm Hg (Figure 6-9, *A*). From the definition of total peripheral resistance,

$$R = (\bar{P}_a - \bar{P}_{ra})/Q_r \tag{6}$$

If $\bar{P}_{ra}$ (mean right atrial pressure) is negligible compared with $\bar{P}_a$,

$$R \cong \bar{P}_a/Q_r \tag{7}$$

Therefore, in the example, R is 100/5, or 20 mm Hg/L/min.

Now let cardiac output, Q_h, suddenly increase to 10 L/min (Figure 6-9, *B*). Instantaneously, $\bar{P}_a$ will be unchanged. Because the outflow, Q_r, from the arteries depends on $\bar{P}_a$ and R, Q_r will also remain unchanged at first. Therefore, Q_h, now 10 L/min, will exceed Q_r, still only

5 L/min. This will increase the mean arterial blood volume ($\bar{V}_a$). From equation 5, when $Q_h > Q_r$, $d\bar{V}_a/dt > 0$; that is, volume is increasing.

Because $\bar{P}_a$ depends on the mean arterial blood volume, $\bar{V}_a$, and the arterial compliance, C_a, an increase in $\bar{V}_a$ will raise the $\bar{P}_a$. By definition,

$$C_a = d\bar{V}_a/d\bar{P}_a \tag{8}$$

Therefore,

$$d\bar{V}_a = C_a d\bar{P}_a \tag{9}$$

and

$$\frac{d\bar{V}_a}{dt} = C_a \frac{d\bar{P}_a}{dt} \tag{10}$$

From equation 5,

$$\frac{d\bar{P}_a}{dt} = \frac{Q_h - Q_r}{C_a} \tag{11}$$

Hence, $\bar{P}_a$ will rise when $Q_h > Q_r$, will fall when $Q_h < Q_r$, and will remain constant when $Q_h = Q_r$.

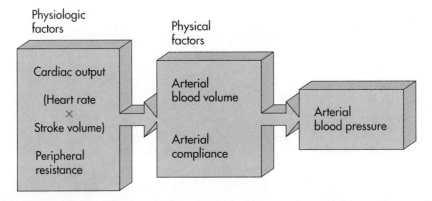

Figure 6-8 ■ Arterial blood pressure is determined directly by two major physical factors, the arterial blood volume and the arterial compliance. These physical factors are affected in turn by certain physiologic factors, primarily the heart rate, stroke volume, cardiac output (heart rate × stroke volume), and peripheral resistance.

2.5 L/min →
5 L/min →
10 L/min →

A

Control conditions

$\bar{P}_a = 100$ mm Hg

$Q_h = 5$ L/min

$Q_r = 5$ L/min

$R = \dfrac{20 \text{ mm Hg}}{\text{L/min}}$

$Q_r = \dfrac{\bar{P}_a}{R} = \dfrac{100}{20} = 5$

A, Under control conditions $Q_h = 5$ L/min, $\bar{P}_a = 100$ mm Hg, and $R = 20$ mm Hg/L/min. Q_r must equal Q_h, and therefore the mean blood volume ($\bar{V}_a$) in the arteries will remain constant from heartbeat to heartbeat.

B Instantaneous increase in cardiac output

$\bar{P}_a = 100$

$Q_h = 10$ L/min

$Q_r = 5$ L/min

$R = \dfrac{20 \text{ mm Hg}}{\text{L/min}}$

$Q_r = \dfrac{\bar{P}_a}{R} = \dfrac{100}{20} = 5$

B, If Q_h suddenly increases to 10 L/min, Q_h will initially exceed Q_r, and therefore $\bar{P}_a$ will begin to rise rapidly.

D Instantaneous increase in peripheral resistance

$\bar{P}_a = 100$

$Q_h = 5$ L/min

$Q_r = 2.5$ L/min

$R = \dfrac{40 \text{ mm Hg}}{\text{L/min}}$

$Q_r = \dfrac{\bar{P}_a}{R} = \dfrac{100}{40} = 2.5$

D, If R abruptly increases to 40 mm Hg/L/min, Q_r suddenly decreases and therefore Q_h exceeds Q_r. Thus $\bar{P}_a$ will rise progressively.

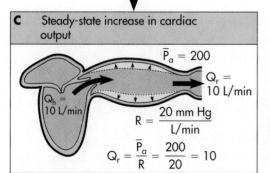

C Steady-state increase in cardiac output

$\bar{P}_a = 200$

$Q_h = 10$ L/min

$Q_r = 10$ L/min

$R = \dfrac{20 \text{ mm Hg}}{\text{L/min}}$

$Q_r = \dfrac{\bar{P}_a}{R} = \dfrac{200}{20} = 10$

C, The disparity between Q_h and Q_r progressively increases arterial blood volume. The volume continues to increase until $\bar{P}_a$ reaches a level of 200 mm Hg.

E Steady-state increase in peripheral resistance

$\bar{P}_a = 200$

$Q_h = 5$ L/min

$Q_r = 5$ L/min

$R = \dfrac{40 \text{ mm Hg}}{\text{L/min}}$

$Q_r = \dfrac{\bar{P}_a}{R} = \dfrac{200}{40} = 5$

E, The excess of Q_h over Q_r accumulates blood in the arteries. Blood continues to accumulate until $\bar{P}_a$ rises to a level of 200 mm Hg.

Figure 6-9 ■ **The relationship of mean arterial blood pressure ($\bar{P}_a$) to cardiac output (Q_h), peripheral runoff (Q_r), and peripheral resistance (R) under control conditions (A), in response to an increase in cardiac output (B and C) and in response to an increase in peripheral resistance (D and E).**

In this example, in which Q_h is suddenly increased to 10 L/min, $\bar{P}_a$ will continue to rise as long as Q_h exceeds Q_r. It is evident from equation 7 that Q_r will not attain a value of 10 L/min until $\bar{P}_a$ reaches a level of 200 mm Hg, as long as R remains constant at 20 mm Hg/L/min. Hence, as $\bar{P}_a$ approaches 200, Q_r will almost equal Q_h, and $\bar{P}_a$ will rise very slowly. When Q_h is first raised, however, Q_h is greatly in excess of Q_r, and therefore $\bar{P}_a$ will rise sharply. The pressure-time tracing in Figure 6-10 indicates that, regardless of the value of C_a, the slope gradually diminishes as pressure rises, to approach a final value asymptotically.

Furthermore, the **height** to which $\bar{P}_a$ will rise is independent of the elastic characteristics of the arterial walls. $\bar{P}_a$ must rise to a level such that peripheral runoff will equal cardiac output; that is, $Q_r = Q_h$. It is apparent from equation 6 that Q_r depends only on the pressure gradient and the resistance to flow. Hence, C_a determines only the rate at which the new equilibrium value of $\bar{P}_a$ will be approached, as illustrated in Figure 6-10. When C_a is small (rigid vessels), a relatively slight

increment in $\bar{V}_a$ (caused by a transient excess of Q_h over Q_r) increases $\bar{P}_a$ greatly. Hence, $\bar{P}_a$ attains its new equilibrium level quickly. Conversely, when C_a is large, considerable volumes can be accommodated with relatively small pressure changes. Therefore, the new equilibrium value of $\bar{P}_a$ is reached at a slower rate.

Peripheral Resistance Similar reasoning may now be applied to explain the changes in $\bar{P}_a$ that accompany alterations in peripheral resistance. Let the control conditions be identical with those of the preceding example, that is, $Q_h = 5$, $\bar{P}_a = 100$, and R = 20 (Figure 6-9, *A*). Then, let R suddenly be increased to 40 (Figure 6-9, *D*). Instantaneously, $\bar{P}_a$ will be unchanged. With $\bar{P}_a = 100$ and R = 40, $Q_r = \bar{P}_a/R = 2.5$ L/min. Thus, the peripheral runoff will momentarily be only 2.5 L/min, even though cardiac output equals 5 L/min. If Q_h remains constant at 5 L/min, $Q_h \geq Q_h$ and $\bar{V}_a$ will increase; hence, $\bar{P}_a$ will rise. $\bar{P}_a$ will continue to rise until it reaches 200 mm Hg (Figure 6-9, *E*). At this level, $Q_r = 200/40 = 5$ L/min, which equals Q_h. $\bar{P}_a$ will then remain at this new elevated equilibrium level as long as Q_h and R do not change.

It is clear, therefore that *the level of the mean arterial pressure depends on cardiac output and peripheral resistance.* It is immaterial whether any change in cardiac output is accomplished by an alteration of heart rate, of stroke volume, or of both. Any change in heart rate that is balanced by a concomitant, oppositely directed change in stroke volume will not alter Q_h. Hence, $\bar{P}_a$ will not be affected.

Pulse Pressure

If we assume (Figure 6-8) that the arterial pressure, P_a, at any moment depends on the two physical factors arterial blood volume, V_a, and arterial capacitance, C_a, it can be deduced that the arterial **pulse pressure** (difference between systolic and diastolic pressures) is principally a function of **stroke volume** and **arterial compliance**.

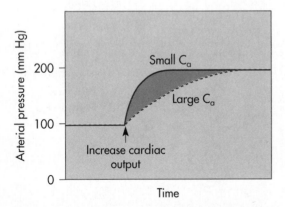

Figure 6-10 ■ **When cardiac output is suddenly increased, the arterial compliance (*C~a~*) determines the rate at which the mean arterial pressure will attain its new, elevated value but will not determine the magnitude of the new pressure.**

Stroke Volume The effect of a change in stroke volume on pulse pressure may be analyzed under conditions in which C_a remains virtually constant over a substantial range of pressures. C_a is constant over any linear region of the pressure-volume curve (Figure 6-11). Volume is plotted along the vertical axis, and pressure is plotted along the horizontal axis; the slope, dV/dP, equals the compliance, C_a.

In an individual with such a linear $P_a:V_a$ curve, the arterial pressure would oscillate about some mean value ($\bar{P}_A$ in Figure 6-11) that depends entirely on cardiac output and peripheral resistance, as explained previously. This mean pressure corresponds to some mean arterial blood volume, $\bar{V}_A$. The coordinates $\bar{P}_A, \bar{V}_A$ define point $\bar{A}$ on the graph. During diastole, peripheral runoff from the arterial system occurs in the absence of ventricular ejection of blood, and P_a and V_a diminish to minimal values, P_1 and V_1, just before the next ventricular ejection. P_1 is then, by definition, the **diastolic pressure.**

During the rapid ejection phase of systole, the volume of blood introduced into the arterial system exceeds the volume that exits through the arterioles. Arterial pressure and volume therefore rise from point A_1 toward point A_2 in Figure 6-11. The maximal arterial volume, V_2, is reached at the end of the rapid ejection phase (see Figure 3-10), and this volume corresponds to a peak pressure, P_2, which is the **systolic pressure.**

The **pulse pressure** is the difference between systolic and diastolic pressures ($P_2 - P_1$ in Figure 6-11), and it corresponds to some **arterial volume increment,** $V_2 - V_1$. *This increment equals the volume of blood discharged by the left ventricle during the rapid ejection phase minus the volume that has run off to the periphery during this same phase of the cardiac cycle.* When a normal heart beats at a normal frequency, the volume increment during the rapid ejection phase is a large fraction of the stroke volume (about 80%). It is this increment that will raise arterial volume rapidly from V_1 to V_2 and hence will cause the arterial pressure to rise from the diastolic to the systolic level (P_1 to P_2 in Figure 6-11). During the remainder of the cardiac cycle, peripheral runoff will exceed cardiac ejection. During diastole, of course, cardiac ejection equals zero. The resultant arterial blood volume decrement will cause volumes and pressures to fall from point A_2 back to point A_1.

If stroke volume is now doubled, while heart rate and peripheral resistance remain constant, the mean arterial pressure will be doubled, to $\bar{B}$ in Figure 6-11. Thus, the arterial pressure will now oscillate each heartbeat about this new value of the mean arterial pressure. A normal, vigorous heart will eject this greater stroke volume during a fraction of the cardiac cycle approximately equal to the fraction that prevailed at the lower stroke volume. Therefore, the arte-

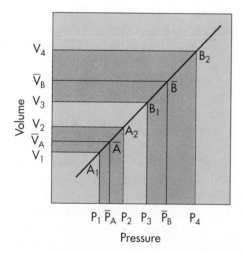

Figure 6-11 ■ **Effect of a change in stroke volume on pulse pressure in a system in which arterial compliance is constant over the range of pressures and volumes involved. A larger volume increment ($V_4 - V_3$ as compared with $V_2 - V_1$) results in a greater mean pressure ($\bar{P}_B$ as compared with $\bar{P}_A$) and a greater pulse pressure ($P_4 - P_3$ as compared with $P_2 - P_1$).**

Arterial pulse pressure affords valuable clues about a person's stroke volume, provided that the arterial compliance is essentially normal. Patients who have severe **congestive heart failure** or who have had a **severe hemorrhage** are likely to have very small arterial pulse pressures because their stroke volumes are abnormally small. Conversely, individuals with large stroke volumes, as in **aortic regurgitation,** are likely to have increased arterial pulse pressures. For example, **well-trained athletes** at rest tend to have low heart rates. The prolonged ventricular filling times in these subjects induce the ventricles to pump a large quantity of blood per heartbeat, and thus their pulse pressures are large.

Figure 6-12 ■ **For a given volume increment ($V_2 - V_1$), a reduced arterial compliance (curve B as compared with curve A) results in an increased pulse pressure ($P_4 - P_1$ as compared with $P_3 - P_2$).**

rial volume increment, $V_4 - V_3$, will be a large fraction of the new stroke volume, and hence it will be approximately twice as great as the previous volume increment ($V_2 - V_1$). If the P_a:V_a curve is linear, the greater volume increment will be reflected by a pulse pressure ($P_4 - P_3$) approximately *twice as great* as the original pulse pressure ($P_2 - P_1$). Inspection of Figure 6-11 reveals that with a rise in both mean and pulse pressures, the rise in systolic pressure (from P_2 to P_4) exceeds the rise in diastolic pressure (from P_1 to P_3). Thus, an increase in stroke volume raises systolic pressure more than it raises diastolic pressure.

Arterial Compliance To assess how arterial compliance affects pulse pressure, the relative effects of a given volume increment ($V_2 - V_1$ in Figure 6-12) in a young person (curve A) and in an elderly person (curve B) will be compared. Let cardiac output and TPR be the same in both people; therefore, $\bar{P}_a$ will be the same. It is apparent from Figure 6-12 that the same volume increment ($V_2 - V_1$) will cause a greater pulse pressure ($P_4 - P_1$) in the less distensible arteries of the elderly individual than in the more compliant arteries of the young person ($P_3 -$

P_2). For the reasons enunciated on page 137, this will impose a greater workload on the left ventricle of the elderly person than on that of the young person, even if the stroke volumes, TPR, and mean arterial pressures are equivalent.

Figure 6-13 displays the effects of changes in arterial compliance and in peripheral resistance, R_p, on arterial pressure in an isolated cat heart preparation. As the compliance was reduced from 43 to 14 to 3.6 units, the pulse pressure increased significantly. In this preparation, the stroke volume decreased as the arterial compliance was diminished. This accounts for the failure of the mean arterial pressure to remain constant at the different levels of arterial compliance. The effects of changes in peripheral resistance in this same preparation are described in the next section.

Total Peripheral Resistance and Arterial Diastolic Pressure It is often asserted that increased TPR affects the diastolic more than the

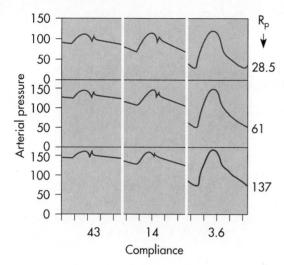

Figure 6-13 ■ The changes in aortic pressure induced by changes in arterial compliance and peripheral resistance (*R*ₚ) in an isolated cat heart preparation. (Modified from Elizinga G, Westerhof N: *Circ Res* 32:178, 1973. By permission of the American Heart Association, Inc.)

systolic arterial pressure. The validity of such an assertion deserves close scrutiny. First, let TPR be increased in an individual with a linear $P_a:V_a$ curve, as depicted in Figure 6-14, *A*. If the person's heart rate and stroke volume remain constant, an increase in TPR will increase $\bar{P}_a$ proportionately (from P_2 to P_5). If the volume increments ($V_2 - V_1$ and $V_4 - V_3$) are equal at both levels of TPR, the pulse pressures ($P_3 - P_1$ and $P_6 - P_4$) will also be equal. Hence, systolic (P_6) and diastolic (P_4) pressures will have been elevated by exactly the same amounts from their respective control levels (P_3 and P_1).

The combination of an increased resistance and diminished arterial compliance on arterial blood pressure would be represented in Figure 6-13 by a shift in direction from the top left panel to the bottom right panel; that is, both the mean pressure and the pulse pressure would be increased significantly. These results also coincide with the changes predicted by Figure 6-14, *B*.

Chronic **hypertension,** a condition characterized by a persistent elevation of TPR, occurs more commonly in older persons than in younger persons. The $P_a:V_a$ curve for a hypertensive patient would therefore resemble that shown in Figure 6-14, *B*, which is like the curves in Figure 6-4 for older individuals. In Figure 6-14, *B*, the slope of the $P_a:V_a$ curve diminishes as pressure and volume are increased. Hence, C_a is less at higher than at lower pressures. As before, if cardiac output remains constant, an increase in TPR would increase $\bar{P}_a$ proportionately (from P_2 to P_5). For equivalent increases in TPR, the elevation of pressure from P_2 to P_5 will be the same in panel *A* as in panel *B*, for reasons discussed on page 144. If the volume increment ($V_4 - V_3$ in Figure 6-14, *B*) at elevated TPR were equal to the control increment ($V_2 - V_1$), the pulse pressure ($P_6 - P_4$) in the hypertensive range would greatly exceed that ($P_3 - P_1$) at normal pressure levels. In other words, a given volume increment produces a greater pressure increment (i.e., pulse pressure) when the arteries are more rigid than when they are more compliant. Hence, the rise in systolic pressure ($P_6 - P_3$) will exceed the increase in diastolic pressure ($P_4 - P_1$). These hypothetical changes in arterial pressure closely resemble those actually seen in patients with **hypertension.** Diastolic pressure is indeed elevated in such individuals, but ordinarily not more than 10 to 40 mm Hg above the average normal level of 80 mm Hg, whereas it is not uncommon for systolic pressures to be elevated by 50 to 150 mm Hg above the average normal level of 120 mm Hg. *Thus, an increase in peripheral resistance will raise systolic pressure more than it will raise diastolic pressure.*

■ **PERIPHERAL ARTERIAL PRESSURE CURVES**

The radial stretch of the ascending aorta brought about by left ventricular ejection initiates a pressure wave that is propagated down the aorta and its branches. *The pressure wave travels much*

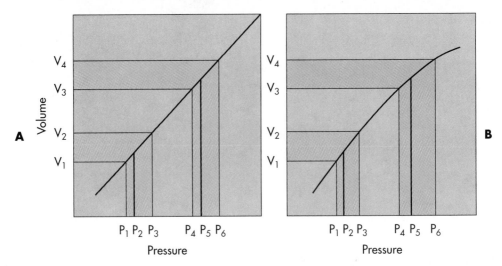

Figure 6-14 ■ **Effect of a change in total peripheral resistance (volume increment remaining constant) on pulse pressure when the pressure-volume curve for the arterial system is rectilinear (A) or curvilinear (B).**

faster than does the blood itself. It is this pressure wave that one perceives by palpating a peripheral artery.

The velocity of the pressure wave varies inversely with the vascular compliance. Accurate measurement of the transmission velocity has provided valuable information about the elastic characteristics of the arterial tree. In general, transmission velocity increases with age. This finding confirms the observation that the arteries become less compliant with advancing age (Figures 6-4 and 6-6). Also, velocity increases progressively as the pulse wave travels from the ascending aorta toward the periphery. This indicates that vascular compliance is less in the more distal than in the more proximal portions of the arterial system.

The arterial pressure contour becomes distorted as the wave is transmitted down the arterial system; the changes in configuration of the pulse with distance are shown in Figure 6-15. Aside from the increasing delay in the onset of the initial pressure rise, three major

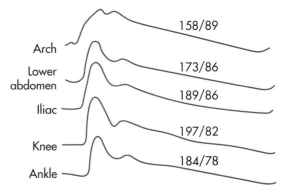

Figure 6-15 ■ **Arterial pressure curves recorded from various sites in an anesthetized dog.** (From Remington JW, O'Brien LJ: *Am J Physiol* 218:437, 1970.)

changes occur in the arterial pulse contour as the pressure wave travels distally. First, the high-frequency components of the pulse, such as the **incisura** (the notch that appears at the end of ventricular ejection), are damped out and soon disappear. Second, the systolic portions of the pressure wave become narrowed and elevated. In the curves shown in Figure 6-15, the systolic pressure at the level of the knee was 39 mm Hg greater than that recorded in the aortic arch. Third, a hump may appear on the diastolic portion of the pressure wave. These changes in contour are pronounced in young individuals but diminish with age. In elderly patients the pulse wave may be transmitted virtually unchanged from the ascending aorta to the periphery.

The damping of the high-frequency components of the arterial pulse is largely caused by the viscoelastic properties of the arterial walls. The precise mechanism for the peaking of the pressure wave is controversial. Probably several factors contribute, including reflection, tapering, resonance, and changes in transmission velocity with pressure level.

■ BLOOD PRESSURE MEASUREMENT IN HUMANS

In hospital intensive care units, arterial blood pressure can be measured **directly** by introducing a needle or catheter into a peripheral artery. Ordinarily, however, the blood pressure is estimated **indirectly** by means of a **sphygmomanometer.** This instrument consists of an inextensible cuff containing an inflatable bag. The cuff is wrapped around the extremity (usually the arm, occasionally the thigh) so that the inflatable bag lies between the cuff and the skin, directly over the artery to be compressed. The artery is occluded by inflating the bag, by means of a rubber squeeze bulb, to a pressure in excess of arterial systolic pressure. The pressure in the bag is measured by means of a mercury or an aneroid manometer. Pressure is released from the bag at a rate of 2 or 3 mm Hg per heartbeat by means of a needle valve in the inflating bulb (Figure 6-16).

When blood pressure readings are taken from the arm, the systolic pressure may be estimated by palpating the radial artery at the wrist **(palpatory method).** When pressure in the bag exceeds the systolic level, no pulse will be perceived. As the pressure falls just below the systolic level (Figure 6-16, *A*), a spurt of blood will pass through the brachial artery under the cuff during the peak of systole, and a slight pulse will be felt at the wrist.

The **auscultatory method** is a more sensitive and therefore a more precise method for measuring systolic pressure, and it also permits estimation of diastolic pressure. The practitioner listens with a stethoscope applied to the skin of the antecubital space over the brachial artery. While the pressure in the bag exceeds the systolic pressure, the brachial artery is occluded and no sounds are heard (Figure 6-16, *B*). When the inflation pressure falls just below the systolic level (120 mm Hg in Figure 6-16, *A*), small spurts of blood escape through the cuff and slight tapping sounds (called **Korotkoff sounds**) are heard with each heartbeat. The pressure at which the first sound is detected represents the **systolic pressure.** It usually corresponds closely with the directly measured systolic pressure.

As inflation pressure continues to fall, more blood escapes under the cuff per beat and the sounds become louder thuds. As the inflation pressure approaches the diastolic level, the Korotkoff sounds become muffled. As they fall just below the diastolic level (80 mm Hg in Figure 6-16, *A*), the sounds disappear; this indicates the **diastolic pressure.** The origin of the Korotkoff sounds is related to the spurt of blood passing under the cuff and meeting a static column of blood; the impact and turbulence generate audible vibrations. Once the inflation pressure is less than the diastolic pressure, flow is continuous in the brachial artery and sounds are no longer heard (Figure 6-16, *C*).

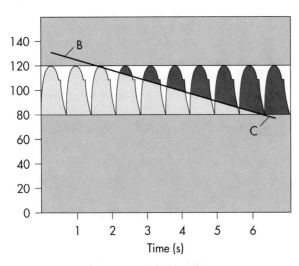

B, When the cuff pressure exceeds the systolic arterial pressure (120 mm Hg), no blood progresses through the arterial segment under the cuff, and no sounds can be detected by a stethoscope bell placed on the arm distal to the cuff.

A, Consider that the arterial blood pressure is being measured in a patient whose blood pressure is 120/80 mm Hg. The pressure (represented by the *oblique line*) in a cuff around the patient's arm is allowed to fall from greater than 120 mm Hg (point *B*) to below 80 mm Hg (point *C*) in about 6 seconds.

C, When the cuff pressure falls below the diastolic arterial pressure, arterial flow past the region of the cuff is continuous, and no sounds are audible. When the cuff pressure is between 120 and 80 mm Hg, spurts of blood traverse the artery segment under the cuff with each heartbeat, and the Korotkoff sounds are heard through the stethoscope.

Figure 6-16 ■ **Measurement of arterial blood pressure with a sphygmomanometer.**

■ **SUMMARY**

1. The arteries serve not only to conduct blood from the heart to the capillaries, but also to store some of the ejected blood during each cardiac systole so that flow can continue through the capillaries during cardiac diastole.

2. The aging process diminishes the compliance of the arteries.

3. The less compliant the arteries, the more work the heart must do to pump a given cardiac output.

4. The mean arterial pressure varies directly with the cardiac output and total peripheral resistance.

5. The arterial pulse pressure varies directly with the stroke volume but inversely with the arterial compliance.

6. The contour of the systemic arterial pressure wave is distorted as it travels from the as-

cending aorta to the periphery. The high-frequency components of the wave are damped, the systolic components are narrowed and elevated, and a hump may appear in the diastolic component of the wave.

7. When blood pressure is measured by a sphygmomanometer in humans, (a) systolic pressure is manifested by the occurrence of a tapping sound that originates in the artery distal to the cuff as the cuff pressure falls below peak arterial pressure, which permits spurts of blood to pass through the compressed artery; and (b) diastolic pressure is manifested by disappearance of the sound as the cuff pressure falls below minimal arterial pressure, which permits flow through the artery to become continuous.

■ KEY WORDS AND CONCEPTS

- Hydraulic filter
- Windkessels
- Hydraulic work
- Arterial compliance
- Atherosclerosis
- Elastic modulus
- Mean arterial pressure
- Systolic arterial pressure
- Diastolic arterial pressure
- Arterial pulse pressure
- Cardiac output
- Peripheral runoff
- Arterial volume increment per heartbeat
- Essential hypertension
- Peripheral arterial pulse
- Sphygmomanometer
- Korotkoff sounds

■ SELF-STUDY PROBLEMS

1. Why would a patient with normal cardiac output and normal total peripheral resistance (TPR), but with generalized atherosclerosis, re-

quire greater coronary blood flow than would a patient with a normal arterial system?

2. How would the systolic, diastolic, and mean arterial pressures in a well-trained athlete with a heart rate of 45 beats/min differ from the systolic, diastolic, and mean arterial pressures in a nonathletic person of the same age, and with the same cardiac output and TPR, but with a heart rate of 75 beats/min?

3. A 20-year-old person and a 70-year-old person each had the same cardiac output, heart rate, and TPR under basal conditions. Assume that a vasoconstrictor drug was given to each person, and that it increased their TPR identically by 50% but did not affect their cardiac output or heart rate. What changes in systolic, diastolic, and mean arterial pressures would you expect in each of these subjects?

4. The left ventricle of a patient with aortic valve insufficiency ejects 100 ml of blood during systole, but 30 ml leak back into the ventricle during diastole. Thus, the patient's net stroke volume (i.e., the quantity of blood pumped through the peripheral vasculature each heartbeat) is 70 ml. If the patient's heart rate is 70 beats/min, cardiac output would be 4.9 L/min. How would the systolic, diastolic, and mean arterial pressures in this patient compare with those pressures in a normal person without aortic valve disease but with the same cardiac output, heart rate, and TPR as the patient with aortic valve insufficiency?

■ BIBLIOGRAPHY

Journal articles

Alexander J Jr, Burkhoff D, Schipke J, Sagawa K: Influence of mean pressure on aortic impedance and reflections in the systemic arterial system, *Am J Physiol* 257:H969, 1989.

Armentano RL, Barra JG, Levenson J et al: Arterial wall mechanics in conscious dogs: assessment of viscous, inertial, and elastic moduli to characterize aortic wall behavior, *Circ Res* 76:468, 1995.

Burattini R, Campbell KB: Effective distributed compliance of the canine descending aorta estimated by modified T-tube model, *Am J Physiol* 264:H1977, 1993.

Campbell KB, Lee LC, Frasch HF, Noordergraaf A: Pulse reflection sites and effective length of the arterial system, *Am J Physiol* 256:H1684, 1989.

Farrar DJ, Bond MG, Riley WA et al: Anatomic correlates of aortic pulse wave velocity and carotid artery elasticity during atherosclerosis progression and regression in monkeys, *Circulation* 83:1754, 1991.

Folkow B, Svanborg A: Physiology of cardiovascular aging, *Physiol Rev* 73:725, 1993.

Imura T, Yamamoto K, Kanamori K, Mikami T, Yasvda H: Noninvasive ultrasonic measurement of the elastic properties of the human abdominal aorta, *Cardiovasc Res* 20:208, 1986.

Kelly RP, Ting C-T, Yang T-M et al: Effective arterial elastance as index of arterial vascular load in humans, *Circulation* 86:513, 1992.

Kelly RP, Tunin R, Kass DA: Effects of reduced aortic compliance on cardiac efficiency and contractile function of in situ canine left ventricle, *Circ Res* 71:490, 1992.

Kingwell BA, Cameron JD, Gillies KJ et al: Arterial compliance may influence baroreflex function in athletes and hypertensives, *Am J Physiol* 268:H411, 1995.

Laskey WK, Parker HG, Ferrari VA, Kussmaul WG, Noordergraaf A: Estimation of total systemic arterial compliance in humans, *J Appl Physiol* 69:112, 1990.

Lee RT, Kamm RD: Vascular mechanics for the cardiologist, *J Am Coll Cardiol* 23:1289, 1994.

Mulvany MJ, Aalkjaer C: Structure and function of small arteries, *Physiol Rev* 70:921, 1990.

O'Rourke M: Mechanical principles in arterial disease, *Hypertension* 26:2, 1995.

Perloff D, Grim C, Flack J et al: Human blood pressure determination by sphygmomanometry, *Circulation* 88:2460, 1993.

Piene H: Pulmonary arterial impedance and right ventricular function, *Physiol Rev* 66:606, 1986.

Rabbany SY, Drzewiecke GM, Noordergraaf A: Peripheral vascular effects on auscultatory blood pressure measurement, *J Clin Monit* 9:9, 1993.

Stergiopulos N, Meister JJ, Westerhof N: Evaluation of methods for estimation of total arterial compliance, *Am J Physiol* 268:H1540, 1995.

Zuckerman BD, Weisman HF, Yin FCP: Arterial hemodynamics in a rabbit model of atherosclerosis, *Am J Physiol* 257:H891, 1989.

Books and monographs

Fung YC: *Biodynamics: circulation,* Heidelberg, 1984, Springer-Verlag.

Li JK-J: *Arterial system dynamics: hemodynamics of arteries,* New York, 1987, New York University Press.

Milnor WR: *Hemodynamics,* Baltimore, 1982, Williams & Wilkins.

O'Rourke M, Kelly R, Avolio A: *Arterial pulse,* Baltimore, 1992, Williams & Wilkins.

Taylor DEM, Stevens AL, editors: *Blood flow: theory and practice,* New York, 1983, Academic Press.

Westerhof N, Gross DR: *Vascular dynamics,* New York, 1989, Plenum Press.

The Microcirculation and Lymphatics

The entire circulatory system is geared to supply the body tissues with blood in amounts commensurate with their requirements for oxygen and nutrients. The capillaries, consisting of a single layer of endothelial cells, permit rapid exchange of gases, water, and solutes with interstitial fluid. The muscular arterioles, which are the major **resistance vessels,** regulate regional blood flow to the capillary beds, and the venules and veins serve primarily as collecting channels and storage, or **capacitance, vessels.**

The arterioles, which range in diameter from about 5 to 100 μm, have a thick smooth muscle layer, a thin adventitial layer, and an endothelial lining (see Figure 1-1). The arterioles give rise directly to the capillaries (5 to 10 μm in diameter) or in some tissues to **metarterioles** (10 to 20 μm in diameter), which then give rise to capillaries (Figure 7-1). The metarterioles can serve either as thoroughfare channels to the venules, bypassing the capillary bed, or as conduits to supply the capillary bed. There are often cross connections between arterioles and between venules, as well as in the capillary network. Arterioles that give rise directly to capillaries regulate flow through their cognate capillaries by constriction or dilation. The capillaries form an interconnecting network of tubes of different lengths with an average length of 0.5 to 1 mm.

Capillary distribution varies from tissue to tissue. In metabolically active tissues, such as cardiac and skeletal muscle and glandular structures, capillaries are numerous, whereas in less active tissues, such as subcutaneous tissue or cartilage, **capillary density** is low. Also, all capillaries are not of the same diameter, and because some capillaries have diameters less than that of the erythrocytes, it is necessary for the cells to become temporarily deformed in their passage through these capillaries. Fortunately, the normal red cells are quite flexible and readily change their shape to conform with that of the small capillaries.

Blood flow in the capillaries is not uniform and depends chiefly on the contractile state of the arterioles. The average velocity of blood flow in the capillaries is approximately 1 mm/s; however, it can vary from zero to several millimeters per second in the same vessel within a brief period. These changes in capillary blood flow may be of random type or may show rhythmical oscillatory behavior of different frequencies that are caused by contraction and relaxation **(vasomotion)** of the precapillary vessels. This vasomotion is to some extent

153

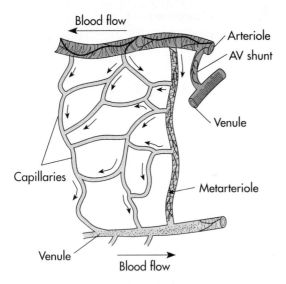

Figure 7-1 ■ **Composite schematic drawing of the microcirculation. The circular structures on the arteriole and venule represent smooth muscle fibers, and the branching solid lines represent sympathetic nerve fibers. The arrows indicate the direction of blood flow.**

an intrinsic contractile behavior of the vascular smooth muscle and is independent of external input. Furthermore, changes in **transmural pressure** (intravascular minus extravascular pressure) influence the contractile state of the precapillary vessels. An increase in transmural pressure, whether produced by an increase in venous pressure or by dilation of arterioles, results in contraction of the terminal arterioles at the points of origin of the capillaries, whereas a decrease in transmural pressure elicits precapillary vessel relaxation (see myogenic response, p 175). In addition, humoral and possibly neural factors also affect vasomotion. For example, when the precapillary vessels contract in response to increased transmural pressure, the contractile response can be overridden and vasomotion abolished. This effect is accomplished by metabolic (humoral) factors (p 177) when the oxygen supply becomes too low for the requirements of the parenchymal tissue, as occurs in muscle during exercise.

Although reduction of transmural pressure induces relaxation of the terminal arterioles, blood flow through the capillaries obviously cannot increase if the reduction in intravascular pressure is caused by severe constriction of the parent arterioles, metarterioles, or small arteries. Large arterioles and metarterioles also exhibit vasomotion, but in the contraction phase they usually do not completely occlude the lumen of the vessel and arrest blood flow, as may occur with contraction of the terminal arterioles (Figure 7-2). Thus, *flow rate may be altered by contraction and relaxation of small arteries, arterioles, and metarterioles.*

Because blood flow through the capillaries provides for exchange of gases and solutes between blood and tissue, it has been termed **nutritional flow,** whereas blood flow that bypasses the capillaries in traveling from the arterial to the venous side of the circulation has been termed **nonnutritional,** or **shunt, flow** (Figure 7-1). In some areas of the body (e.g., fingertips, ears), true **arteriovenous shunts** exist (p 239). However, in many tissues, such as muscle, evidence of anatomic shunts is lacking. Nevertheless, nonnutritional flow can occur and has been termed physiologic shunting of blood flow. It is the result of a greater flow of blood through previously open capillaries with either no change or an increase in the number of closed capillaries. In tissues that have metarterioles, shunt flow may be continuous from arteriole to venule during low metabolic activity when many precapillary vessels are closed. When metabolic activity increases in such tissues and more precapillary vessels open, blood passing through the metarterioles is readily available for capillary perfusion.

The true capillaries are devoid of smooth muscle and are therefore incapable of active constriction. Nevertheless, the endothelial cells that form the capillary wall contain actin and myosin and can alter their shape in response to certain chemical stimuli. There is no evidence, however, that changes in endothelial cell shape regulate

Figure 7-2 ■ **A, Arterioles of a hamster cheek pouch before microinjection of norepinephrine. B, After injection of norepinephrine. Note the complete closure of the arteriole between the arrows, and the narrowing of a branch arteriole at the upper right. *Insert*: Capillary with red cells during a period of complete closure of the feeding arteriole. Scale in A and B, 30 μm; in insert, 5 μm.** (Courtesy David N. Damon.)

blood flow through the capillaries. Hence, *changes in capillary diameter are passive and are caused by alterations in precapillary and postcapillary resistance.*

The thin-walled capillaries can withstand high internal pressures without bursting because of their narrow lumen. This can be explained in terms of the **law of Laplace** and is illustrated in the following comparison of wall tension of a capillary with that of the aorta (Table 7-1). The Laplace equation is

$$T = Pr$$

where
T = Tension in the vessel wall
P = Transmural pressure
r = Radius of the vessel

Wall tension is the force per unit length tangential to the vessel wall that opposes the distending force (Pr) that tends to pull apart a theoretical longitudinal slit in the vessel (Figure 7-3). Transmural pressure is essentially equal to intraluminal pressure, because extravascular pressure is negligible. The Laplace equation applies to very thin-walled vessels, such as capillaries. Wall thickness must be taken into consideration when the equation is applied to thick-walled vessels, such as the aorta. This is done by dividing Pr (pressure × radius) by wall thickness (w). The equation now becomes

$$\sigma \text{ (wall stress)} = Pr/w$$

Pressure in mm Hg (height of Hg column) is converted to dynes per square centimeter ac-

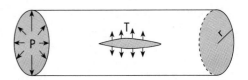

Figure 7-3 ■ Diagram of a small blood vessel to illustrate the law of Laplace—$T = Pr$, where P = intraluminal pressure, r = radius of the vessel, and T = wall tension as the force per unit length tangential to the vessel wall, tending to pull apart a theoretical longitudinal slit in the vessel.

TABLE 7-1

Vessel wall tension in the aorta and a capillary

	Aorta	Capillary
Radius (r)	1.5 cm	5×10^{-4} cm
Height of Hg column (h)	10 cm Hg	2.5 cm Hg
ρ	13.6 g/cm^3	13.6 g/cm^3
g	980 cm/s^2	980 cm/s^2
P	$10 \times 13.6 \times 980 = 1.33 \times 10^5$ dyne/cm^2	$2.5 \times 13.6 \times 980 = 3.33 \times 10^4$ dyne/cm^2
w	0.2 cm	1×10^{-4} cm
T = Pr	$(1.33 \times 10^5)(1.5) = 2 \times 10^5$ dyne/cm	$(3.33 \times 10^4)(5 \times 10^{-4}) = 16.7$ dyne/cm
$\sigma = \dfrac{Pr}{w}$	$\dfrac{2 \times 10^5}{0.2} = 1 \times 10^6$ dyne/cm^2	$\dfrac{16.7}{1 \times 10^{-4}} = 1.67 \times 10^5$ dyne/cm^2

cording to the equation $P = h\rho g$, where h = the height of a Hg column in centimeters, ρ = the density of Hg in g/cm^3, g = gravitational acceleration in cm/s^2, and wall stress (σ) = force per unit area.

Thus, at normal aortic and capillary pressures the wall tension of the aorta is about 12,000 times greater than that of the capillary (Table 7-1). In a person standing quietly, capillary pressure in the feet may reach 100 mm Hg. Under such conditions, capillary wall tension increases to 66.5 dynes/cm, a value that is still only one three-thousandth that of the wall tension in the aorta at the same internal pressure. However, σ (wall stress), which takes wall thickness into consideration, is only about tenfold greater in the aorta than in the capillary.

In addition to providing an explanation for the ability of capillaries to withstand large internal pressures, the above calculations also point out that in dilated vessels, wall stress increases even when internal pressure remains constant.

The diameter of the resistance vessels is determined by the balance between the contractile force of the vascular smooth muscle and the distending force produced by the intraluminal pressure. The greater the contractile activity of the vascular smooth muscle of an arteriole, the smaller is its diameter, until a point is reached, in the case of small arterioles, when complete occlusion of the vessel occurs. This is caused by infolding of the endothelium and by trapping of the cells in the vessel. With progressive reduction in the intravascular pressure, vessel diameter decreases (as does tension in the vessel wall—law of Laplace).

With a progressive decrease in perfusion pressure, a point is reached where blood flow ceases even though pressure within the arteriole or small artery is still positive relative to tissue pressure. This phenomenon has been referred to as the **critical closing pressure,** and its mechanism is still controversial. This critical closing pressure is low when vasomotor activity is reduced by inhibition of sympathetic nerve activity to the vessel, and is increased when vasomotor tone is enhanced by activation of the vascular sympathetic nerve fibers.

■ VASOACTIVE ROLE OF ENDOTHELIUM

For many years, it was thought that the endothelium was an inert single layer of cells that served solely as a passive filter to permit passage of water and small molecules across the blood vessel wall and to retain blood cells and large molecules (proteins) within the vascular compartment. However, it is now recognized that the endothelium is a source of substances that elicit contraction or relaxation of the vascular smooth muscle.

As shown in Figure 7-4, prostacyclin can relax vascular smooth muscle via an increase in the cyclic adenosine monophosphate (cAMP) concentration. **Prostacyclin** is formed in the endothelium from arachidonic acid, and the process is catalyzed by prostacyclin synthase. To what extent this occurs in vivo is not known, but the prostacyclin may be released by shear stress caused by the pulsatile blood flow. The primary function of prostacyclin is to inhibit platelet adherence to the endothelium and platelet aggregation, thus preventing intravascular clot formation.

Of far greater importance in endothelial-mediated vascular dilation is the formation and release of the **endothelium-derived relaxing factor (EDRF)** (Figure 7-4), which has been identified as **nitric oxide (NO).** Stimulation of the endothelial cells in vivo, in isolated arteries, or in culture by acetylcholine or several other agents (adenosine triphosphate [ATP], brady-

Figure 7-4 ■ Endothelial- and nonendothelial-mediated vasodilation. Prostacyclin *(PI$_2$)* is formed from arachidonic acid *(AA)* by the action of cyclooxygenase *(Cyc Ox)* and prostacyclin synthase *(Pr Syn)* in the endothelium, and elicits relaxation of the adjacent vascular smooth muscle via increases in cyclic adenosine monophosphate *(cAMP)*. Stimulation of the endothelial cells with acetylcholine *(ACh)* or other agents (see text) results in the formation and release of an endothelium-derived relaxing factor *(EDRF)*, identified as nitric oxide *(NO)*. The NO stimulates guanylyl cyclase *(G Cyc)* to increase cyclic guanosine monophosphate *(cGMP)* in the vascular smooth muscle to produce relaxation. The vasodilator agent nitroprusside *(NP)* acts directly on the vascular smooth muscle. Substances such as adenosine, hydrogen ions *(H$^+$)*, CO$_2$, and potassium ions *(K$^+$)* can arise in the parenchymal tissue and elicit vasodilation by direct action on the vascular smooth muscle (see p 178).

kinin, serotonin, substance P, histamine) causes the production and release of NO. In blood vessels from which the endothelium has been mechanically removed, these agents do not elicit vasodilation. The NO (synthesized from L-arginine) activates guanylyl cyclase in the vascular smooth muscle to increase the cyclic guanosine monophosphate (cGMP) concentration, which produces relaxation by decreasing cytosolic free Ca^{++}. NO release can be stimulated by the shear stress of blood flow on the endothelium, but the physiologic role of NO in the local regulation of blood flow remains to be elucidated. The drug nitroprusside also increases cGMP, which produces vasodilation, but it acts directly on the vascular smooth muscle and is not endothelial-mediated (Figure 7-4). Vasodilator agents such as adenosine, hydrogen ions, CO_2, and potassium may be released from parenchymal tissue and act locally on the resistance vessels (Figure 7-4).

The endothelium can also synthesize **endothelin,** a very potent vasoconstrictor peptide. Endothelin can affect vascular tone and blood pressure in humans and may be involved in pathologic states such as atherosclerosis, pulmonary hypertension, congestive heart failure, and renal failure.

■ PASSIVE ROLE OF ENDOTHELIUM
Transcapillary Exchange

Solvent and solute move across the capillary endothelial wall by three processes: diffusion, filtration, and endothelial vesicles (pinocytosis).

The permeability of the capillary endothelial membrane is not the same in all body tissues. For example, the liver capillaries are quite permeable, and albumin escapes at a rate several times greater than that from the less permeable muscle capillaries. Also, there is not uniform permeability along the whole capillary; the venous ends are more permeable than the arterial ends, and permeability is greatest in the venules. The greater permeability at the venous end of the capillaries and in the venules is attributed to the greater number of pores in these regions of the microvessels.

The sites where filtration occurs have been a controversial subject for a number of years. Some water flows through the capillary endothelial cell membranes, but most flows through apertures **(pores)** in the endothelial wall of the capillaries (Figures 7-5 and 7-6). Calculations based on the transcapillary movement of solutes of small molecular size led to the prediction of capillary pores with diameters of about 4 nm in skeletal and cardiac muscle. In agreement with this prediction, electron microscopy revealed clefts between adjacent endothelial cells with a gap at the narrowest point of about 4 nm (Figures 7-5 and 7-6). The clefts (pores) are sparse and represent only about 0.02% of the capillary surface area. In cerebral capillaries, where a blood-brain barrier to many small molecules exists, pores are absent.

Figure 7-5 ■ A, Cross-sectioned capillary in a mouse ventricular wall. The luminal diameter is approximately 4 μm. In this thin section, the capillary wall is formed by a single endothelial cell (*Nu,* endothelial nucleus), which forms a functional complex *(arrow)* with itself. The thin pericapillary space is occupied by a pericyte *(PC)* and a connective tissue *(CT)* cell ("fibroblast"). Note the numerous endothelial vesicles *(V).* B, Detail of the endothelial cell in panel A, showing plasmalemmal vesicles *(V)* attached to the endothelial cell surface. These vesicles are especially prominent in vascular endothelium and are involved in transport of substances across the blood vessel wall. Note the complex alveolar vesicle (*). *BM,* Basement membrane. C, Junctional complex in a capillary of mouse heart. "Tight" junctions *(TJ)* typically form in these small blood vessels and appear to consist of fusions between apposed endothelial cell surface membranes. D, Interendothelial junction in a muscular artery of monkey papillary muscle. Although tight junctions similar to those of capillaries are found in these large blood vessels, extensive junctions that resemble gap junctions in the intercalated disks between myocardial cells often appear in arterial endothelium (example shown at *GJ*).

Figure 7-5 ■ For legend see opposite page.

Figure 7-6 ■ Diagrammatic sketch of an electron micrograph of a composite capillary in cross section.

In addition to clefts, some of the more porous capillaries (e.g., in kidney, intestine) contain **fenestrations** (Figure 7-6) 20 to 100 nm wide, whereas others (e.g., in the liver) have a **discontinuous endothelium** (Figure 7-6). Fenestrations and discontinuous endothelium permit passage of molecules that are too large to pass through the intercellular clefts of the endothelium.

Diffusion Under normal conditions, only about 0.06 ml of water per minute moves back and forth across the capillary wall per 100 g of tissue as a result of filtration and absorption, whereas 300 ml of water per minute per 100 g of tissue does so by diffusion, a 5000-fold difference.

When filtration and diffusion are related to blood flow, about 2% of the plasma passing through the capillaries is filtered. In contrast, the diffusion of water is 40 times greater than the rate by which it is brought to the capillaries by blood flow. The transcapillary exchange of solutes is also primarily governed by diffusion. Thus, *diffusion is the key factor in providing exchange of gases, substrates, and waste products between the capillaries and the tissue cells.*

The process of diffusion is described by Fick's law:

$$J = -DA\frac{dc}{dx} \tag{1}$$

where

J = Quantity of a substance moved per unit time (t)

D = Free diffusion coefficient for a particular molecule (the value is inversely related to the square root of the molecular weight)

A = Cross-sectional area of the diffusion pathway

$\dfrac{dc}{dx}$ = Concentration gradient of the solute

Fick's law is also expressed as

$$J = -PS(C_o - C_i) \tag{2}$$

where

P = Capillary permeability of the substance

S = Capillary surface area

C_i = Concentration of the substance inside the capillary

C_o = Concentration of the substance outside the capillary

Hence, the PS product provides a convenient expression of available capillary surface, because permeability is rarely altered under physiologic conditions.

In the capillaries, diffusion of lipid-insoluble molecules is not free but is restricted to the pores, whose mean size can be calculated by measurement of the diffusion rate of an uncharged molecule whose free diffusion coefficient is known. Movement of solutes across the endothelium is complex and involves corrections for attractions between solute and solvent molecules, interactions between solute molecules, pore configuration, and charge on the molecules relative to charge on the endothelial cells. It is not simply a question of random thermal movements of molecules down a concentration gradient.

For small molecules, such as water, NaCl, urea, and glucose, the capillary pores offer little restriction to diffusion (low **reflection coefficient,** see p 164), and diffusion is so rapid that the mean concentration gradient across the capillary endothelium is extremely small. With lipid-insoluble molecules of increasing size, diffusion through muscle capillaries becomes progressively more restricted, until diffusion becomes minimal with molecules of a molecular weight above about 60,000. With small molecules, the only limitation to net movement across the capillary wall is the rate at which blood flow transports the molecules to the capillary **(flow limited).**

When transport across the capillary is flow limited, the concentration of a small molecule solute in the blood reaches equilibrium with its concentration in the interstitial fluid near the origin of the capillary from the cognate arteriole. If an inert small molecule tracer is infused intraarterially, its concentration falls to negligible levels near the arterial end of the capillary (Figure 7-7, A). If the flow is large, the small molecule tracer will be detectable farther downstream in the capillary. A somewhat larger molecule moves farther along the capillary before reaching an insignificant concentration in the blood, and the number of still larger molecules that enter the arterial end of the capillary and cannot pass through the capillary pores is the same as the number leaving the venous end of the capillary (Figure 7-7, A).

With large molecules, diffusion across the capillaries becomes the limiting factor **(diffusion limited).** In other words, capillary permeability to a large molecule solute limits its transport across the capillary wall (Figure 7-7, A). The diffusion of small lipid-insoluble molecules is so rapid that diffusion becomes limiting in blood-tissue exchange only when the distances between capillaries and parenchymal cells are large (e.g., tissue edema or very low capillary density) (Figure 7-7, B).

Movement of lipid-soluble molecules across the capillary wall is not limited to capillary pores (only about 0.02% of the capillary surface), because such molecules can pass directly through the lipid membranes of the entire capillary endothelium. Consequently, *lipid-soluble molecules move with great rapidity between blood and tissue. The degree of lipid solubility (oil-to-water partition coefficient) provides a good index of the ease of transfer of lipid molecules through the capillary endothelium.*

Oxygen and carbon dioxide are both lipid soluble and readily pass through the endothelial cells. Calculations based on (1) the diffusion coefficient for O_2, (2) capillary density and diffusion distances, (3) blood flow, and (4) tissue O_2 consumption indicate that the O_2 supply of normal tissue at rest and during activity is not limited by diffusion or the number of open capillaries.

Measurements of Po_2 and saturation of blood in the microvessels indicate that, in many tissues, O_2 saturation at the entrance of the capillaries has already decreased to a saturation of about 80% as a result of diffusion of O_2 from arterioles and small arteries. Also, CO_2 loading and the re-

Figure 7-7 ■ **Flow and diffusion-limited transport from capillaries *(Cap)* to tissue. A, Flow-limited transport. The smallest water-soluble inert tracer particles *(black dots)* reach negligible concentrations after passing only a short distance down the capillary. Larger particles *(colored circles)* with similar properties travel farther along the capillary before reaching insignificant intracapillary concentrations. Both substances cross the interstitial fluid *(ISF)* and reach the parenchymal tissue *(cell)*. Because of their size, more of the smaller particles are taken up by the tissue cells. The largest particles *(black circles)* cannot penetrate the capillary pores and hence do not escape from the capillary lumen except by pinocytotic vesicle transport. An increase in the volume of blood flow or an increase in capillary density increases tissue supply for the diffusible solutes. Note that capillary permeability is greater at the venous end of the capillary (also in the venule, not shown) because of the larger number of pores in this region. B, Diffusion-limited transport. When the distance between the capillaries and the parenchymal tissue is large, as a result of edema or low capillary density, diffusion becomes a limiting factor in the transport of solutes from capillary to tissue even at high rates of capillary blood flow.**

sultant intravascular shifts in the oxyhemoglobin dissociation curve occur in the precapillary vessels. Hence, direct flux of O_2 and CO_2 occurs between adjacent arterioles, venules, and possibly arteries and veins **(countercurrent exchange)**, in addition to gas exchange at the level of the capillaries. This countercurrent exchange of gas represents a diffusional shunt of gas around the capillaries, and, at low blood flow rates, it may limit the supply of O_2 to the tissue.

Capillary Filtration *The direction and magnitude of the movement of water across the capillary wall are determined by the algebraic sum of the hydrostatic and osmotic pressures that exist across the membrane.* An increase in intracapillary hydrostatic pressure favors movement of fluid from the vessel to the interstitial space, whereas an increase in the concentration of osmotically active particles within the vessels favors movement of fluid into the vessels from the interstitial space.

Hydrostatic Forces The hydrostatic pressure (blood pressure) within the capillaries is not constant and depends on arterial pressure, venous pressure, and precapillary (arterioles) and postcapillary (venules and small veins) resistances. An increase in arterial or venous pressure elevates capillary hydrostatic pressure, whereas a reduction in each has the opposite effect. An increase in arteriolar resistance or closure of arteries reduces capillary pressure, whereas greater venous resistance (venules and veins) increases capillary pressure.

Hydrostatic pressure is the principal force in

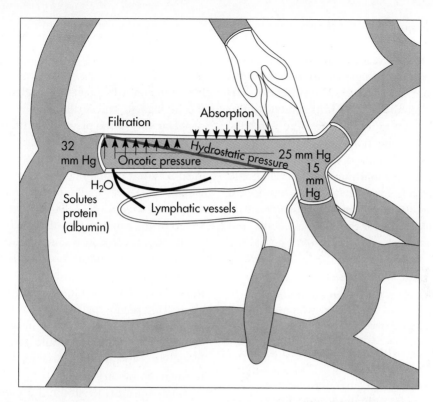

Figure 7-8 ■ Schematic representation of the factors responsible for filtration and absorption across the capillary wall and the formation of lymph.

capillary filtration. However, changes in the venous resistance affect capillary hydrostatic pressure more than do changes in arteriolar resistance. A given change in venous pressure produces a greater effect on capillary hydrostatic pressure than the same change in arterial pressure, and about 80% of an increase in venous pressure is transmitted back to the capillaries.

Despite the fact that capillary hydrostatic pressure (P_c) is variable from tissue to tissue (even within the same tissue), average values, obtained from many direct measurements in human skin, are about 32 mm Hg at the arterial end of the capillaries and 15 mm Hg at the venous end of the capillaries at the level of the heart (Figure 7-8). When a person stands, the hydrostatic pressure is higher in the legs and lower in the head.

Tissue pressure, or more specifically intersti-

tial fluid pressure (P_i) outside the capillaries, opposes capillary filtration, and it is $P_c - P_i$ that constitutes the driving force for filtration. In the normal (nonedematous) state, P_i is close to zero, so that P_c essentially represents the hydrostatic driving force.

Osmotic Forces The key factor that restrains fluid loss from the capillaries is the osmotic pressure of the plasma proteins—usually termed **colloid osmotic pressure** or **oncotic pressure** (π_p). The total osmotic pressure of plasma is about 6000 mm Hg, whereas the oncotic pressure is only about 25 mm Hg. However, this small oncotic pressure plays an important role in fluid exchange across the capillary wall, because the plasma proteins are essentially confined to the intravascular space, whereas the electrolytes that are responsible for the major fraction of plasma osmotic pressure are practically equal in concentration on both sides of the capillary endothelium. The relative permeability of solute to water influences the actual magnitude of the osmotic pressure. The **reflection coefficient** (σ) is the relative impediment to the passage of a substance through the capillary membrane. The reflection coefficient of water is zero and that of albumin (to which the endothelium is essentially impermeable) is 1. Filterable solutes have reflection coefficients between 0 and 1. Also, different tissues have different reflection coefficients for the same molecule, and therefore movement of a given solute across the endothelial wall varies with the tissue. The true oncotic pressure (π) is defined by

$$\pi = \sigma RT (C_i - C_o) \qquad (3)$$

where

σ = Reflection coefficient
R = Gas constant
T = Absolute temperature
C_i and C_o = Solute (albumin) concentration, respectively, inside and outside the capillary

Of the plasma proteins, albumin is preponderate in determining oncotic pressure. The average albumin molecule (molecular weight 69,000) is approximately half the size of the average globulin molecule (molecular weight 150,000) and is present in almost twice the concentration as the globulins (4.5 vs. 2.5 g/dl of plasma). Albumin also exerts a greater osmotic force than can be accounted for solely on the basis of the number of molecules dissolved in the plasma. Therefore, it cannot be completely replaced by inert substances of appropriate molecular size such as dextran. This additional osmotic force becomes disproportionately greater at high concentrations of albumin (as in plasma) and is weak to absent in dilute solutions of albumin (as in interstitial fluid). The reason for this behavior of albumin is its negative charge at the normal blood pH and the attraction and retention

of cations (principally Na^+) in the vascular compartment (the **Gibbs-Donnan effect**). Furthermore, albumin binds a small number of chloride ions, which increases its negative charge and, hence, its ability to retain more sodium ions inside the capillaries. The small increase in electrolyte concentration of the plasma over that of the interstitial fluid produced by the negatively charged albumin enhances its osmotic force to that of an ideal solution containing a solute of molecular weight of 37,000. If albumin did indeed have a molecular weight of 37,000, it would not be retained by the capillary endothelium because of its small size, and obviously could not function as a counterforce to capillary hydrostatic pressure. If, however, albumin did not have an enhanced osmotic force, it would require a concentration of about 12 g of albumin/dl of plasma to achieve a plasma oncotic pressure of 25mm Hg. Such a high albumin concentration would greatly increase blood viscosity and the resistance to blood flow through the vascular system.

Small amounts of albumin escape from the capillaries and enter the interstitial fluid, where they exert a very small osmotic force (0.1 to 5 mm Hg). This force, π_i, is small because of the low concentration of albumin in the interstitial fluid, and because at low concentrations the osmotic force of albumin is not enhanced as it is at high albumin concentrations.

Balance of Hydrostatic and Osmotic Forces
The relationship between hydrostatic pressure and oncotic pressure, and the role of these forces in regulating fluid passage across the capillary endothelium, were expounded by Starling in 1896 and constitute the **Starling hypothesis.** It can be expressed by the equation

$$Q_f = k[(P_c + \pi_i) - (P_i + \pi_p)] \qquad (4)$$

where

Q_f = Fluid movement
P_c = Capillary hydrostatic pressure
P_i = Interstitial fluid hydrostatic pressure
π_p = Plasma oncotic pressure

π_i = Interstitial fluid oncotic pressure

k = Filtration constant for capillary membrane

Filtration occurs when the algebraic sum is positive; absorption occurs when it is negative.

Classically, it has been thought that filtration occurs at the arterial end of the capillary and absorption at its venous end because of the gradient of hydrostatic pressure along the capillary. This is true for the idealized capillary, as depicted in Figure 7-8, but direct observations have revealed that many capillaries show only filtration, whereas others show only absorption. In some vascular beds (e.g., the renal glomerulus) hydrostatic pressure in the capillary is high enough to result in filtration along the entire length of the capillary. In other vascular beds, (e.g., the intestinal mucosa), the hydrostatic and oncotic forces are such that absorption occurs along the whole capillary.

As discussed earlier in this chapter, capillary pressure is variable and depends on several factors, the principal one being the contractile state of the precapillary vessel. In the normal steady state, arterial pressure, venous pressure, postcapillary resistance, interstitial fluid hydrostatic and oncotic pressures, and plasma oncotic pressure are relatively constant, and a change in precapillary resistance is the determining factor with respect to fluid movement across the wall for any given capillary. Because water moves so quickly across the capillary endothelium, the hydrostatic and osmotic forces are nearly in equilibrium along the entire capillary. Hence, filtration and absorption in the normal state occur at very small degrees of imbalance of pressure across the capillary wall. Only a small percentage (2%) of the plasma flowing through the vascular system is filtered, and of this about 85% is absorbed in the capillaries and venules. The remainder returns to the vascular system as lymph fluid along with the albumin that escapes from the capillaries.

In the lungs the mean capillary hydrostatic pressure is only about 8 mm Hg. Because the

---

In pathologic conditions, such as left ventricular failure or stenosis of the mitral valve, pulmonary capillary hydrostatic pressure may exceed plasma oncotic pressure. When this occurs, it may cause pulmonary edema, a condition that seriously interferes with gas exchange in the lungs.

---

plasma oncotic pressure is 25 mm Hg and the lung interstitial fluid pressure is approximately 15 mm Hg, the net force slightly favors reabsorption. Nevertheless, pulmonary lymph is formed and consists of fluid that is osmotically drawn out of the capillaries by the small amount of plasma protein that escapes through the capillary endothelium.

Capillary Filtration Coefficient The rate of movement of fluid across the capillary membrane (Q_f) depends not only on the algebraic sum of the hydrostatic and osmotic forces across the endothelium (ΔP), but also on the area of the capillary wall available for filtration (A_m), the distance across the capillary wall (Δx), the viscosity of the filtrate (η), and the filtration constant of the membrane (k). These factors may be expressed by the equation

$$Q_f = \frac{kA_m\Delta P}{\eta\Delta x} \tag{5}$$

The dimensions are units of flow per unit of pressure gradient across the capillary wall per unit of capillary surface area. This expression, which describes the flow of fluid through a membrane (pores), is essentially Poiseuille's law for flow through tubes (p 120).

Because the thickness of the capillary wall and the viscosity of the filtrate are relatively constant, they can be included in the filtration constant, k, and if the area of the capillary membrane is not known, the rate of filtration can be expressed per unit weight of tissue. Hence, the equation can be simplified to

$$Q_f = k_t \Delta P \qquad (6)$$

where k_t is the capillary filtration coefficient for a given tissue, and the units for Q_f are milliliters per minute per 100 g of tissue per millimeter of mercury pressure.

In any given tissue the filtration coefficient per unit area of capillary surface, and hence capillary permeability, is not changed by different physiologic conditions, such as arteriolar dilation and capillary distention, or by such adverse conditions as hypoxia, hypercapnia, or reduced pH. With capillary injury (toxins, severe burns), capillary permeability increases, as indicated by the filtration coefficient, and significant amounts of fluid and protein leak out of the capillaries into the interstitial space.

Because capillary permeability is constant under normal conditions, the filtration coefficient can be used to determine the relative number of open capillaries (total capillary surface area available for filtration in tissue). For example, increased metabolic activity of contracting skeletal muscle induces relaxation of precapillary resistance vessels with opening of more capillaries (**capillary recruitment,** resulting in an increased filtering surface area).

Disturbances in Hydrostatic-Osmotic Balance Changes in arterial pressure per se may have little effect on filtration, because the change in pressure may be countered by adjustments of the precapillary resistance vessels (autoregulation, p 175), so that hydrostatic pressure in the open capillaries remains the same. However, with severe reduction in arterial pressure, as may occur in hemorrhage, there may be arteriolar constriction mediated by the sympathetic nervous system and a fall in venous pressure resulting from the blood loss. These changes will lead to a decrease in capillary hydrostatic pressure. Furthermore, the low blood pressure in hemorrhage causes a decrease in blood flow (and hence O_2 supply) to the tissue,

with the result that vasodilator metabolites accumulate and induce relaxation of arterioles. Precapillary vessel relaxation is also engendered by the reduced transmural pressure (autoregulation, p 175). As a consequence of these several factors, absorption predominates over filtration and occurs at a larger capillary surface area. This is one of the compensatory mechanisms employed by the body to restore blood volume (p 278).

An increase in venous pressure alone, as occurs in the feet when one changes from the lying to the standing position, would elevate capillary pressure and enhance filtration. However, the increase in transmural pressure causes precapillary vessel closure (myogenic mechanism, p 175), so that the capillary filtration coefficient actually decreases. This reduction in capillary surface available for filtration protects against the extravasation of large amounts of fluid into the interstitial space (edema).

A large amount of fluid can move across the capillary wall in a relatively short time. In a normal individual the filtration coefficient (k_t) for the whole body is about 0.0061 ml/min/100 g of tissue/mm Hg. For a 70-kg man, elevation of venous pressure of 10 mm Hg for 10 minutes would increase filtration from capillaries by 342 ml. This would not lead to edema formation, because the fluid is returned to the vascular compartment by the lymphatic vessels. When edema does develop, it usually appears in the dependent

---

With prolonged standing, particularly when associated with some elevation of venous pressure in the legs (such as that caused by pregnancy) or with sustained increases in venous pressure (as seen in congestive heart failure), filtration is greatly enhanced and exceeds the capacity of the lymphatic system to remove the capillary filtrate from the interstitial space (see also Figure 9-19).

parts of the body, where the hydrostatic pressure is greatest, but its location and magnitude are also determined by the type of tissue. Loose tissues, such as the subcutaneous tissue around the eyes or in the scrotum, are more prone to collect larger quantities of interstitial fluid than are firm tissues, such as muscle, or encapsulated structures, such as the kidney.

The concentration of the plasma proteins may also change in different pathologic states and thus alter the osmotic force and movement of fluid across the capillary membrane. The plasma protein concentration is increased in dehydration (e.g., water deprivation, prolonged sweating, severe vomiting, and diarrhea), and water moves by osmotic forces from the tissues to the vascular compartment. In contrast, the plasma protein concentration is reduced in nephrosis (a renal disease in which there is loss of protein in the urine), and edema may occur.

Pinocytosis Some transfer of substances across the capillary wall can occur in tiny pinocytotic vesicles (pinocytosis). These vesicles (Figures 7-5 and 7-6), formed by a pinching off of the surface membrane, can take up substances on one side of the capillary wall, move by thermal kinetic energy across the cell, and deposit their contents at the other side. The amount of material that can be transported in this way is very small relative to that moved by diffusion. However, pinocytosis may be responsible for the movement of large lipid-insoluble molecules (30 nm) between blood and interstitial fluid. The number of pinocytotic vesicles in endothelium varies with the tissue (muscle > lung > brain) and increases from the arterial to the venous end of the capillary.

■ LYMPHATICS

The terminal vessels of the lymphatic system consist of a widely distributed closed-end network of highly permeable lymph capillaries similar in appearance to blood capillaries. However, they are generally lacking in tight junctions between endothelial cells, and possess fine filaments that anchor them to the surrounding connective tissue. With muscular contraction, these fine strands distort the lymphatic vessel to open spaces between the endothelial cells, and permit the entrance of protein and large particles and cells present in the interstitial fluid. The lymph capillaries drain into larger vessels that finally enter the right and left subclavian veins at their junctions with the respective internal jugular veins. Only cartilage, bone, epithelium, and tissues of the central nervous system are devoid of lymphatic vessels. The plasma capillary filtrate is returned to the circulation by virtue of tissue pressure, facilitated by intermittent skeletal muscle activity, contractions of the lymphatic vessels, and an extensive system of one-way valves. In this respect, they resemble the veins, although even the larger lymphatic vessels have thinner walls than the corresponding veins and contain only a small amount of elastic tissue and smooth muscle.

The volume of fluid transported through the lymphatics in 24 hours is about equal to an animal's total plasma volume, and the protein returned by the lymphatics to the blood in a day is about one fourth to one half of the circulating plasma proteins. This is the only means whereby protein (albumin) that leaves the vascular compartment can be returned to the blood, because back diffusion into the capillaries cannot occur against the large albumin concentration gradient.

> When capillary injury is extensive, as in burns, intravascular fluid *and* plasma protein leak into the interstitial space. The protein that escapes from the vessel lumen increases the oncotic pressure of the interstitial fluid. This greater osmotic force outside the capillaries leads to additional fluid loss and possibly to severe dehydration of the patient.

Were the protein not removed by the lymph vessels, it would accumulate in the interstitial fluid and act as an oncotic force to draw fluid from the blood capillaries to produce edema. In addition to returning fluid and protein to the vascular bed, the lymphatic system filters the lymph at the lymph nodes and removes foreign particles, such as bacteria. The largest lymphatic vessel, the **thoracic duct,** in addition to draining the lower extremities, returns protein lost through the permeable liver capillaries and carries substances absorbed from the gastrointestinal tract, principally fat in the form of chylomicrons, to the circulating blood.

Lymph flow varies considerably, being almost nil from resting skeletal muscle and increasing during exercise in proportion to the degree of muscular activity. It is increased by any mechanism that enhances the rate of blood capillary filtration: for example, increased capillary pressure or permeability or decreased plasma oncotic pressure. When either the volume of interstitial fluid exceeds the drainage capacity of the lymphatics or the lymphatic vessels become blocked, as may occur in certain disease states, interstitial fluid accumulates, chiefly in the more compliant tissues (e.g., subcutaneous tissue), and gives rise to clinical edema.

■ SUMMARY

1. Blood flow through the capillaries is chiefly regulated by contraction and relaxation of the arterioles (resistance vessels).
2. The capillaries, which consist of a single layer of endothelial cells, can withstand high transmural pressure by virtue of their small diameter. According to the law of Laplace, T (wall tension) = P (transmural pressure) $\times$ r (radius of the capillary).
3. The endothelium is the source of an endothelium-derived relaxing factor (EDRF—identified as nitric oxide) and prostacyclin, which relax vascular smooth muscles.

4. Movement of water and small solutes between the vascular and interstitial fluid compartments occurs through capillary pores mainly by diffusion but also by filtration and absorption.
5. Because the rate of diffusion is about 40 times greater than the blood flow in the tissue, exchange of small lipid-insoluble molecules is flow limited. The larger the molecules, the slower is the diffusion, until with large molecules the lipid-insoluble molecules become diffusion limited. Molecules larger than about 60,000 kd are essentially confined to the vascular compartment.
6. Lipid-soluble substances such as CO_2 and O_2 pass directly through the lipid membranes of the capillary, and the ease of transfer is directly proportional to the degree of lipid solubility of the substance.
7. Capillary filtration and absorption are described by the Starling equation: Fluid movement = k[($P_c + \pi_i$) − ($P_i + \pi_p$)] where P_c = capillary hydrostatic pressure; P_i = interstitial fluid hydrostatic pressure; π_i = interstitial fluid oncotic pressure; π_p = plasma oncotic pressure. Filtration occurs when the algebraic sum is positive; absorption occurs when it is negative.
8. Large molecules can move across the capillary wall in vesicles formed from the lipid membrane of the capillaries by a process called pinocytosis.
9. Fluid and protein that have escaped from the blood capillaries enter the lymphatic capillaries and are transported via the lymphatic system back to the blood vascular compartment.

■ KEY WORDS AND CONCEPTS

- Resistance vessels
- Capacitance vessels
- Metarterioles

- Vasomotion
- Transmural pressure
- Nutritional flow
- Shunt flow
- Law of Laplace
- Endothelium
- Prostacyclin
- Nitric oxide (NO)
- Adenosine
- Guanylyl cyclase
- Transcapillary exchange
- Capillary pores and fenestrations
- Discontinuous endothelium
- Diffusion
- Flow-limited transport
- Diffusion-limited transport
- Reflexion coefficient
- Lipid-soluble molecules
- Countercurrent exchange
- Capillary filtration
- Hydrostatic pressure
- Oncotic pressure
- Tissue pressure
- Gibbs-Donnan effect
- Starling hypothesis
- Capillary filtration coefficient
- Capillary recruitment
- Pinocytosis
- Lymphatic system

■ SELF-STUDY PROBLEMS

1. What physiologic factors influence capillary blood flow?
2. When a person is standing quietly, the pressure in the capillaries of the feet can reach as high as 100 mm Hg. Why do the thin-walled capillaries not rupture when subjected to such a high pressure?
3. If mean capillary hydrostatic pressure is 20 mm Hg, tissue pressure 4 mm Hg, plasma oncotic pressure 25 mm Hg, and tissue oncotic pressure 2 mm Hg, is there absorption or filtration in this capillary? Why? In the passage of solute across the capillary wall, how do filtration and absorption compare with diffusion?
4. In the movement of lipid-insoluble solutes from the capillary lumen to the interstitial fluid, what is meant by flow limited and diffusion limited?
5. By what mechanisms do lipid-soluble and lipid-insoluble solutes pass from the capillary lumen to the interstitial space?
6. How is albumin that has escaped from the capillaries returned to the systemic circulation?

■ BIBLIOGRAPHY

Journal articles

Aukland K: Why don't our feet swell in the upright position?, *News Physiol Sci* 9:214, 1994.

Aukland K, Reed RK: Interstitial-lymphatic mechanisms in the control of extracellular fluid volume, *Physiol Rev* 73:1, 1993.

Curry FRE: Regulation of water and solute exchange in microvessel endothelium: studies in single perfused capillaries, *Microcirculation* 1:11, 1994.

Davies PF: Flow-mediated endothelial mechanotransduction, *Physiol Rev* 75:519, 1995.

Duling BR, Klitzman B: Local control of microvascular function: role in tissue oxygen supply, *Annu Rev Physiol* 42:373, 1980.

Feng Q, Hedner T: Endothelium-derived relaxing factor (EDRF) and nitric oxide. II. Physiology, pharmacology, and pathophysiological implications, *Clin Physiol* 10:503, 1990.

Furchgott RF, Vanhoutte PM: Endothelium-derived relaxing and contracting factors, *FASEB J* 3:2007, 1989.

Krogh A: The number and distribution of capillaries in muscles with calculation of the oxygen pressure head necessary for supplying the tissue, *J Physiol* 52:409, 1919.

Lewis DH, editor: Symposium on lymph circulation, *Acta Phyiol Scand Suppl* 463:9, 1979.

Pries AR, Secomb TW, Gessner T, Sperandio MB, Gross JF, Gaehtgens P: Resistance to blood flow in microvessels in vivo, *Circ Res* 75:904, 1994.

Rippe B, Haraldsson B: Transport of macromolecules across microvascular walls: the two-pore theory, *Physiol Rev* 74:163, 1994.

Rosell S: Neuronal control of microvessels, *Annu Rev Physiol* 42:359, 1980.

Starling EH: On the absorption of fluids from the connective tissue spaces, *J Physiol* 19:312, 1896.

Books and monographs

Bert JL, Pearce RH: *The interstitium and microvascular exchange*. In *Handbook of physiology*, Section 2: *The cardiovascular system—microcirculation*, vol IV, Bethesda, Md., 1984, American Physiological Society.

Crone C, Levitt DG: *Capillary permeability to small solutes*. In *Handbook of physiology*, Section 2: *The cardiovascular system—microcirculation*, vol IV, Bethesda, Md., 1984, American Physiological Society.

Hudlicka O: *Development of microcirculation: capillary growth and adaptation*. In *Handbook of physiology*, Section 2: *The cardiovascular system—microcirculation*, vol IV, Bethesda, Md., 1984, American Physiological Society.

Krogh A: *The anatomy and physiology of capillaries*, New York, 1959, Hafner.

Luscher TF, Vanhoutte PM: *The endothelium: modulator of cardiovascular function*, Boca Raton, Fla., 1990, CRC Press.

Michel CC: *Fluid movements through capillary walls*. In *Handbook of physiology*, Section 2: *The cardiovascular system—microcirculation*, vol IV, Bethesda, Md., 1984, American Physiological Society.

Mortillaro NA: *Physiology and pharmacology of the microcirculation*, vol 1, New York, 1983, Academic Press.

Renkin EM: *Control microcirculation and blood-tissue exchange*. In *Handbook of physiology*, Section 2: *The cardiovascular system—microcirculation*, vol IV, Bethesda, Md., 1984, American Physiological Society.

Shepro D, D'Amore PA: *Physiology and biochemistry of the vascular wall endothelium*. In *Handbook of physiology*, Section 2: *The cardiovascular system—microcirculation*, vol IV, Bethesda, Md., 1984, American Physiological Society.

Simionescu M, Simionescu N: *Ultrastructure of the microvascular wall: functional correlations*. In *Handbook of physiology*, Section 2: *The cardiovascular system—microcirculation*, vol IV, Bethesda, Md., 1984, American Physiological Society.

Taylor AE, Granger DN: *Exchange of macromolecules across the microcirculation*. In *Handbook of physiology*, Section 2: *The cardiovascular system—microcirculation*, vol IV, Bethesda, Md., 1984, American Physiological Society.

Wiedeman MP: *Architecture*. In *Handbook of physiology*, Section 2: *The cardiovascular system—microcirculation*, vol IV, Bethesda, Md., 1984, American Physiological Society.

Zweifach BW, Lipowsky HH: *Pressure-flow relations in blood and lymph microcirculation*. In *Handbook of physiology*, Section 2: *The cardiovascular system—microcirculation*, vol IV, Bethesda, Md., 1984, American Physiological Society.

The Peripheral Circulation and Its Control

The peripheral circulation is essentially under dual control, centrally through the nervous system and locally in the tissues by the environmental conditions in the immediate vicinity of the blood vessels. The relative importance of these two control mechanisms is not the same in all tissues. In some areas of the body, such as the skin and splanchnic regions, neural regulation of blood flow predominates, whereas in others, such as the heart and brain, this mechanism plays a minor role.

The vessels chiefly involved in regulating the rate of blood flow throughout the body are called the **resistance vessels** (arterioles). These vessels offer the greatest resistance to the flow of blood pumped to the tissues by the heart and thus are important in the maintenance of arterial blood pressure. Smooth muscle fibers constitute a large percentage of the composition of the walls of the resistance vessels (see Figure 1-1). Therefore, the vessel lumen can be varied from one that is completely obliterated by strong contraction of the smooth muscle, with infolding of the endothelial lining, to one that is maximally dilated as a result of full relaxation of the vascular smooth muscle. Some resistance vessels are closed at any given moment in time, and partial contraction **(tone)** of the vascular smooth muscle exists in the arterioles. Were all the resistance vessels in the body to dilate simultaneously, blood pressure would fall precipitously to very low levels.

■ VASCULAR SMOOTH MUSCLE

Vascular smooth muscle is the tissue responsible for the control of total peripheral resistance, arterial and venous tone, and the distribution of blood flow throughout the body. The smooth muscle cells are small, mononucleate, and spindle shaped. They are generally arranged in helical or circular layers around the larger blood vessels and in a single circular layer around arterioles (Figure 8-1, A and B). Also, parts of endothelial cells project into the vascular smooth muscle layer **(myoendothelial junctions)** at various points along the arterioles (Figure 8-1, C). These projections suggest a functional interaction between endothelium and adjacent vascular smooth muscle. In general, the close association between action potentials and contraction observed in skeletal and cardiac muscle cells cannot be demonstrated in vascular smooth muscle. Also, vascular smooth muscle lacks transverse tubules.

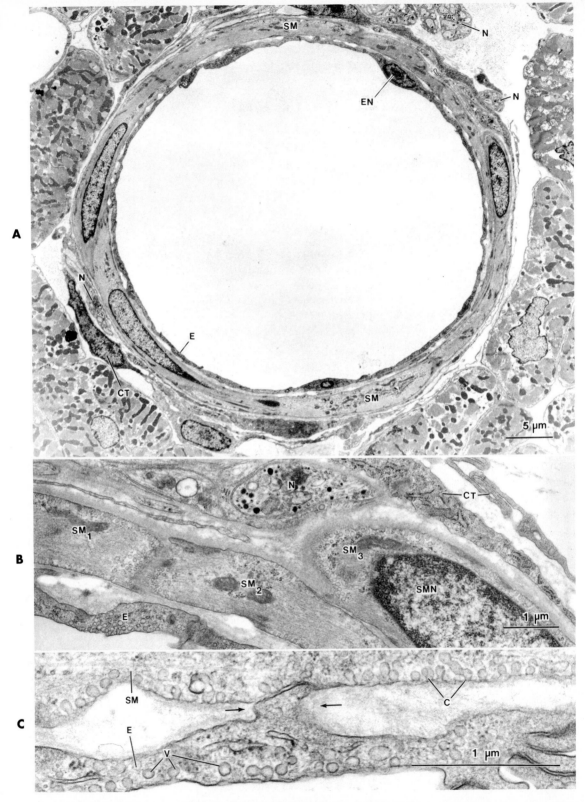

Figure 8-1 ■ For legend see opposite page.

Graded changes in membrane potential are often associated with increases or decreases in force. Contractile activity is generally elicited by neural or humoral stimuli. The behavior of smooth muscle in different vessels varies. For example, some vessels, particularly in the portal or mesenteric circulation, contain longitudinally oriented smooth muscle that is spontaneously active and shows action potentials that are correlated with the contractions and the electrical coupling between cells.

The vascular smooth muscle cells contain large numbers of thin, actin filaments and comparatively small numbers of thick, myosin filaments. These filaments are aligned in the long axis of the cell but do not form visible sarcomeres with striations. Nevertheless, the sliding filament mechanism is believed to operate in this tissue, and phosphorylation of crossbridges regulates their rate of cycling. Compared with skeletal muscle, the smooth muscle contracts very slowly, develops high forces, maintains force for long periods with low adenosine triphosphate (ATP) utilization, and operates over a considerable range of lengths under physiologic conditions. Cell-to-cell conduction is via gap junctions as occurs in cardiac muscle (see p 57).

The interaction between myosin and actin, leading to contraction, is controlled by the myoplasmic Ca^{++} concentration as in other muscles, but the molecular mechanism whereby Ca^{++} regulates contraction differs. For example, smooth muscle lacks troponin and fast sodium channels. The increased myoplasmic Ca^{++} that elicits contraction can come through voltage-gated calcium channels (**electromechanical coupling**) and through receptor-mediated calcium channels (**pharmacomechanical coupling**) in the sarcolemma, and by release from the sarcoplasmic reticulum (Figure 8-2). The cells relax when intracellular free Ca^{++} is pumped back into the sarcoplasmic reticulum and is extruded from the cell by the calcium pump in the cell membrane and by the Na-Ca exchanger.

The response to humoral stimuli, which is termed pharmacomechanical coupling, occurs without evidence of electrical excitation and is the predominant mechanism for eliciting contraction of vascular smooth muscle. In the category of pharmacologic stimuli that cause contraction or relaxation are such substances as catecholamines, histamine, acetylcholine, serotonin, angiotensin, adenosine, nitric oxide, CO_2, K^+, H^+, and prostaglandins (see Figure 7-4).

As illustrated in Figure 8-2, an agonist activates receptors in the vascular smooth muscle membrane. These receptors in turn activate phospholipase C in a reaction coupled to guanine nu-

---

Figure 8-1 ■ A, Low-magnification electron micrograph of an arteriole in cross section (inner diameter of approximately 40 μm) in cat ventricle. The wall of the blood vessel is composed largely of vascular smooth muscle cells *(SM)* whose long axes are directed approximately circularly around the vessel. A single layer of endothelial cells *(E)* forms the innermost portion of the blood vessel. Connective tissue elements *(CT)* such as fibroblasts and collagen make up the adventitial layer at the periphery of the vessel; nerve bundles also appear in this layer *(N)*. *EN,* Endothelial cell nucleus. B, Detail of the wall of the blood vessel in A. This field contains a single endothelial layer *(E),* the medial smooth muscle layer (three smooth muscle cell profiles: SM_1, SM_2, SM_3), and the adventitial layer (containing nerves *[N]* and connective tissue *[CT]*). *SMN,* Smooth muscle nucleus. C, Another region of the arteriole, showing the area in which the endothelial *(E)* and smooth muscle *(SM)* layers are apposed. A projection of an endothelial cell *(between arrows)* is closely applied to the surface of the overlying smooth muscle, forming a "myoendothelial junction." Plasmalemmal vesicles are prominent in both the endothelium *(V)* and the smooth muscle cell (where such vesicles are known as "caveolae," *C*).

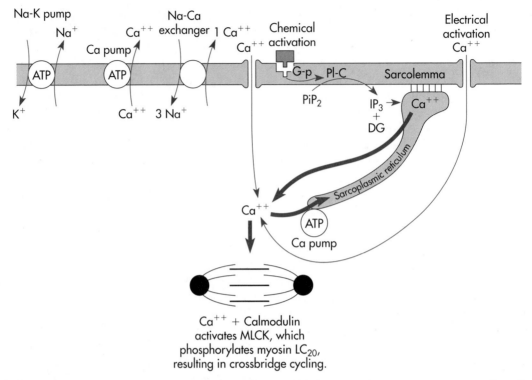

Figure 8-2 ■ **Excitation-contraction coupling in vascular smooth muscle. Calcium can enter the cell via electrically activated channels (electromechanical coupling) or via receptor-operated channels (chemical activation, termed pharmacomechanical coupling) in the sarcolemma. Calcium is also released from the sarcoplasmic reticulum in response to inositol trisphosphate *(IP$_3$)* stimulation and is taken back into the sarcoplasmic reticulum by a calcium pump. Calcium is extruded from the cell by a calcium pump and by the Na-Ca exchanger. *G-p,* Guanine nucleotide binding protein; *Pl-C,* phospholipase C; *PiP$_2$,* phosphatidyl inositol bisphosphate; *DG,* diacylglycerol; *MLCK,* myosin light chain kinase.**

cleotide binding proteins (G proteins). The phospholipase C hydrolyzes phosphatidyl inositol bisphosphate in the membrane to yield diacylglycerol and inositol trisphosphate; the latter causes the release of Ca^{++} from the sarcoplasmic reticulum. The Ca^{++} binds to calmodulin, which in turn binds to myosin light chain kinase. This activated Ca^{++}-calmodulin-myosin kinase complex phosphorylates the light chains (20,000 daltons) of myosin. The phosphorylated myosin ATPase is then activated by actin, and the resulting crossbridge cycling initiates contraction.

Finally, the sensitivity of the contractile regulatory apparatus to Ca^{++} is increased by agonists. The mechanism for this enhanced sensitivity is still unclear but appears to involve G proteins. Relaxation occurs when the myosin light chain kinase is inactivated by dephosphorylation and the cytosolic Ca^{++} is lowered by sarcoplasmic reticulum uptake and by Ca^{++} extrusion by the Ca pump and the Na-Ca exchanger. Local environmental changes alter the contractile state of vascular smooth muscle, and alterations such as increased temperature or increased carbon dioxide levels induce relaxation of this tissue.

Most of the arteries and veins of the body are supplied to different degrees solely by fibers of the sympathetic nervous system. These nerve fibers exert a tonic effect on the blood vessels, as evidenced by the fact that cutting or freezing the sympathetic nerves to a vascular bed (such as muscle) results in an increase in blood flow. Activation of the sympathetic nerves either directly or reflexly (pp 180 and 183) enhances vascular resistance. In contrast to the sympathetic nerves, the parasympathetic nerves tend to decrease vascular resistance, but they innervate only a small fraction of the blood vessels in the body, mainly in certain viscera and pelvic organs.

■ INTRINSIC OR LOCAL CONTROL OF PERIPHERAL BLOOD FLOW

Autoregulation and Myogenic Regulation

In a number of different tissues the blood flow appears to be adjusted to the existing metabolic activity of the tissue. Furthermore, imposed changes in perfusion pressure (arterial blood pressure) at constant levels of tissue metabolism, as measured by oxygen consumption, are met with vascular resistance changes that tend to maintain a constant blood flow. This mechanism is commonly referred to as **autoregulation** of blood flow and is illustrated graphically in Figure 8-3. In the skeletal muscle preparation from which these data were gathered, the muscle was completely isolated from the rest of the animal and was in a resting state. From a control pressure of 100 mm Hg, the pressure was abruptly increased or decreased, and the blood flows observed immediately after changing the perfusion pressure are represented by the closed circles. Maintenance of the altered pressure at each new level was followed within 30 to 60 seconds by a return of flow to or toward the control levels; the open circles represent these steady-state flows. Over the pressure range of 20 to 120 mm Hg, the

Figure 8-3 ■ Pressure-flow relationship in the skeletal muscle vascular bed of the dog. Closed circles represent the flows obtained immediately after abrupt changes in perfusion pressure from the control level *(point where lines cross).* **Open circles represent the steady-state flows obtained at the new perfusion pressure.** (Redrawn from Jones RD, Berne RM: *Circ Res* 14:126, 1964.)

steady-state flow is relatively constant. Calculation of resistance across the vascular bed (pressure-flow) during steady-state conditions indicates that with elevation of perfusion pressure the resistance vessels constricted, whereas with reduction of perfusion pressure, they dilated.

The reason for this constancy of blood flow in the presence of an altered perfusion pressure is not known, but it appears to be explained best by the **myogenic mechanism**.

According to the myogenic mechanism, the vascular smooth muscle contracts in response to an increase in transmural pressure and relaxes in response to a decrease in transmural pressure. Therefore, the initial flow increment produced by an abrupt increase in perfusion pressure that passively distends the blood vessels would be followed by a return of flow to the previous control level by contraction of the smooth muscles of the resistance vessels.

An example of a myogenic response is shown in Figure 8-4. Arterioles isolated from the hearts of young pigs were cannulated at each end, and the transmural pressure (intravascular pressure minus extravascular pressure) and flow through the arteriole could be adjusted to desired levels. With no flow through the arteriole, successive increases of transmural pressure elicited progressive decreases in the vessel diameter (Figure 8-4, *A*). This response was independent of the endothelium because it was identical in intact vessels and in vessels denuded of endothelium (Figure 8-4, *B*). Arterioles that were relaxed by direct action of nitroprusside on the vascular smooth muscle showed only a passive increase in diameter when transmural pressure was increased.

How vessel distension elicits contraction is unsettled, but because stretch of vascular smooth muscle elevates intracellular Ca^{++}, it has been proposed that an increase in transmural pressure activates membrane calcium channels.

Because blood pressure is reflexly maintained at a fairly constant level under normal conditions, it would be expected that operation of a myogenic mechanism would be minimized. However, when one changes position (from lying to standing), a large change in transmural pressure occurs in the lower extremities. The precapillary vessels constrict in response to this imposed stretch, which results in cessation of flow in most capillaries. After flow stops, capillary filtration diminishes until the increase in

Figure 8-4 ■ A, Constriction of an isolated cardiac arteriole in response to increases in transmural pressure without flow through the blood vessel. B, Constrictor response of the arteriole to an increase in transmural pressure is unaffected by removal of its endothelium. C, Diagram of cannulated arteriole. When the smooth muscle is relaxed by nitroprusside, the arteriole is passively distended by the increase in transmural pressure. (Redrawn from Kuo L, Davis MJ, Chilian WM: *Am J Physiol* 259:H1063, 1990.)

plasma oncotic pressure and the increase in interstitial fluid pressure balance the elevated capillary hydrostatic pressure produced by changing from a horizontal to a vertical position.

Endothelium-Mediated Regulation

As discussed on page 157, stimulation of the endothelium can elicit a vasoactive response of the vascular smooth muscle. To demonstrate this response, transmural pressure is kept constant in an isolated arteriole, and intravascular pressure is increased by raising the perfusion fluid reservoir connected to one end of the arteriole and simultaneously lowering the reservoir connected to the other end of the arteriole by an equal dis-

> If arteriolar resistance did not increase with standing, the hydrostatic pressure in the lower parts of the legs would reach such high levels that large volumes of fluid would pass from the capillaries into the interstitial fluid compartment and produce edema.

tance. This maneuver increases the longitudinal pressure gradient along the vessel, and vasodilation occurs (Figure 8-5, *A*). The vasodilation is presumably caused by the endothelium-derived relaxing factor (nitric oxide) (see p 157), which is released from the endothelium in response to the shear stress consequent to the increase in velocity of flow. If the arteriole is denuded of endothelium, the dilation of the vessel in response to increased flow is abolished (Figure 8-5, *B*).

Metabolic Regulation

According to the metabolic mechanism, blood flow is governed by the metabolic activity of the tissue. Any intervention that results in an O_2 supply that is inadequate for the requirements of the tissue gives rise to the formation of vasodilator metabolites. These metabolites are released from the tissue and act locally to dilate the resistance vessels. When the metabolic rate of the tissue increases or the O_2 delivery to the tissue decreases, more vasodilator substance is released and the metabolite concentration in the tissue increases.

Figure 8-5 ■ **A, Flow-induced vasodilation in an isolated cardiac arteriole at constant transmural pressure. Flow was increased progressively by increasing the pressure gradient in the long axis of the arteriole (longitudinal pressure gradient). B, Flow-induced vasodilation is abolished by removal of the endothelium of the arteriole.** (Redrawn from Kuo L, Davis MJ, Chilian WM: *Am J Physiol* 259:H1063, 1990.)

Many substances have been proposed as mediators of metabolic vasodilation. Some of the earliest ones suggested are lactic acid, CO_2, and hydrogen ions. However, the decrease in vascular resistance induced by supernormal concentrations of these dilator agents falls considerably short of the dilation observed under physiologic conditions of increased metabolic activity.

Changes in O_2 tension can evoke changes in the contractile state of vascular smooth muscle; an increase in Po_2 elicits contraction, and a decrease in Po_2, relaxation. If significant reductions in the intravascular Po_2 occur before the arterial blood reaches the resistance vessels (diffusion through the arterial and arteriolar walls, p 162), small changes in O_2 supply or consumption could elicit contraction or relaxation of the resistance vessels. However, direct measurements of Po_2 at the resistance vessels indicate that over a wide range of Po_2 (11 to 343 mm Hg), there is no correlation between O_2 tension and arteriolar diameter. Furthermore, if Po_2 were directly responsible for vascular smooth muscle tension, one would not expect to find a parallelism between the duration of arterial occlusion and the duration of the reactive hyperemia (flow above control level upon release of an arterial occlusion) (Figure 8-6). With either short occlusions (5 to 10 seconds) or long occlusions (1 to 3 minutes) the venous blood becomes bright red (well oxygenated) within 1 or 2 seconds after release of the arterial occlusion, and hence the smooth muscle of the resistance vessels must be exposed to a high Po_2 in each instance. Nevertheless, the longer occlusions result in longer periods of reactive hyperemia. These observations are more compatible with the release of a vasodilator metabolite from the tissue than with a direct effect of Po_2 on the vascular smooth muscle.

Potassium ions, inorganic phosphate, and interstitial fluid osmolarity can also induce vasodilation. Because K^+ and phosphate are released and osmolarity is increased during skeletal muscle contraction, it has been proposed that these factors contribute to **active hyperemia** (increased blood flow caused by enhanced tissue activity). However, significant increases of phosphate concentration and osmolarity are not consistently observed during muscle contraction, and they may produce only transient increases in blood flow. Therefore, they are not likely candidates as mediators of the vasodilation observed with muscular activity. Potassium release occurs with the onset of skeletal muscle contraction or an increase in cardiac activity, and could be responsible for the initial decrease in vascular resistance observed with exercise or increased cardiac work. However, K^+ release is not sustained, despite continued arteriolar dilation throughout the period of enhanced muscle activity. Therefore, some other agent must serve as mediator of the vasodilation associated with the greater metabolic activity of the tissue. Reoxygenated venous blood obtained from active cardiac and skeletal muscles under steady-state conditions of exercise does not elicit vasodilation when infused into a test vascular bed. It is difficult to see how oxygenation of the venous blood could alter its K^+ or phosphate content or its osmolarity and thereby destroy its vasodilator effect.

Adenosine, which is involved in the regulation of coronary blood flow, may also participate in the control of the resistance vessels in skeletal muscle; also, some of the prostaglandins have been proposed as important vasodilator mediators in certain vascular beds.

Thus, there are a number of candidates for the role of mediator of metabolic vasodilation, and the relative contribution of each of the various factors remains the subject for future investigation. Several factors may be involved in any given vascular bed, and different factors preponderate in different tissues.

Metabolic control of vascular resistance by the release of a vasodilator substance is predicated on the existence of basal vessel tone. This tonic activity, or **basal tone,** of the vascular smooth muscle is readily demonstrable, but, in contrast to tone in skeletal muscle, it is independent of the nervous system. The factor responsible for basal tone in blood vessels is not known, but one or more of the following factors may be involved: (1) an expression of myogenic activity in response to the stretch imposed by the blood pressure, (2) the high O_2 tension of arterial blood, (3) the presence of calcium ions, or (4) some unknown factor in plasma, because addition of plasma to the bathing solution of isolated vessel segments evokes partial contraction of the smooth muscle.

If arterial inflow to a vascular bed is stopped for a few seconds to several minutes, the blood flow, on release of the occlusion, immediately exceeds the flow before occlusion and only gradually returns to the control level **(reactive hyperemia).** This is illustrated in Figure 8-6: blood flow to the leg was stopped by clamping the femoral artery for 15, 30, and 60 seconds. Release of the 60-second occlusion resulted in a peak

blood flow 70% greater than the control flow, with a return to control flow within about 110 seconds. When this same experiment is performed in humans by inflating a blood pressure cuff on the upper arm, dilation of the resistance vessels of the hand and forearm, immediately after release of the cuff, is evident from the bright red color of the skin and the fullness of the veins. Within limits the peak flow, and particularly the duration of the reactive hyperemia, are proportional to the duration of the occlusion (Figure 8-6). If the extremity is exercised during the occlusion period, reactive hyperemia is increased. These observations, and the close relationship that exists between metabolic activity and blood flow in the unoccluded limb, are consonant with a metabolic mechanism in the local regulation of tissue blood flow.

When the vascular smooth muscle of the arterioles relaxes in response to vasodilator metabolites released by a decrease in the oxygen supply/oxygen demand ratio of the tissue, resistance may diminish in the arteries that feed these

Figure 8-6 ■ **Reactive hyperemia in the hind limb of the dog after 15-, 30-, and 60-s occlusions of the femoral artery.** (Berne RM: Unpublished observations.)

arterioles. This results in a greater blood flow than that produced by arteriolar dilation alone. Two possible mechanisms can account for this coordination of arterial and arteriolar dilation. First, vasodilation in the microvessels is propagated, and when initiated in the arterioles, it can propagate from arterioles back to arteries. Second, the metabolite-mediated dilation of the arterioles accelerates blood flow in the feeder arteries. This increases the shear stress on the arterial endothelium and can induce vasodilation by release of nitric oxide.

■ EXTRINSIC CONTROL OF PERIPHERAL BLOOD FLOW
Neural Sympathetic Vasoconstriction

A number of regions in the medulla influence cardiovascular activity. Some of the effects of stimulation of the dorsal lateral medulla (**pressor region**) are vasoconstriction, cardiac acceleration, and enhanced myocardial contractility. Caudal and ventromedial to the pressor region is a zone that produces a decrease in blood pressure on stimulation. This **depressor** area exerts its effect by direct spinal inhibition and by inhibition of the medullary pressor region. These areas constitute a center, not in an anatomic sense in that a dis-

crete group of cells is discernible, but in a physiologic sense in that stimulation of the pressor region produces the responses mentioned previously. From the vasoconstrictor regions, fibers descend in the spinal cord and synapse at different levels of the thoracolumbar region (T1 to L2 or L3). Fibers from the intermediolateral gray matter of the cord emerge with the ventral roots but leave the motor fibers to join the paravertebral sympathetic chains through the white communicating branches. These preganglionic white (myelinated) fibers may pass up or down the sympathetic chains to synapse in the various ganglia within the chains or in certain outlying ganglia. Postganglionic gray branches (unmyelinated) then join the corresponding segmental spinal nerves and accompany them to the periphery to innervate the arteries and veins. Postganglionic sympathetic fibers from the various ganglia join the large arteries and accompany them as an investing network of fibers to the resistance and capacitance vessels (veins).

The vasoconstrictor regions are tonically active, and reflexes or humoral stimuli that enhance this activity result in an increase in frequency of impulses reaching the terminal branches to the vessels, where a constrictor neurohumor (**norepinephrine**) is released and elicits constriction (alpha-adrenergic effect) of the resistance vessels. Inhibition of the vasoconstrictor areas reduces their tonic activity and hence diminishes the frequency of impulses in the efferent nerve fibers, resulting in vasodilation. In this manner, neural regulation of the peripheral circulation is accomplished primarily by alteration of the number of impulses passing down the vasoconstrictor fibers of the sympathetic nerves to the blood vessels. The vasomotor regions may show rhythmic changes in tonic activity manifested as oscillations of arterial pressure. Some occur at the frequency of respiration (**Traube-Hering waves**) and are caused by an increase in sympathetic impulses to the resis-

---

Disease of the arterial walls can lead to obstruction of the arteries and symptoms, called **intermittent claudication,** when it occurs in the legs. The symptoms consist of leg pain when walking or climbing stairs, which is relieved by rest. The disease is called **thromboangiitis obliterans** and is seen most frequently in men who are smokers. With minimal walking, the resistance vessels become maximally dilated by local metabolite release; when the oxygen demand of the muscles increases with further walking, blood flow cannot increase sufficiently to meet the muscle needs for oxygen, and pain caused by muscle ischemia results.

tance vessels coincident with inspiration. Others are independent of, and at a lower frequency than, respiration **(Mayer waves).**

Sympathetic Constrictor Influence on Resistance and Capacitance Vessels

The vasoconstrictor fibers of the sympathetic nervous system supply the arteries, arterioles, and veins, but neural influence on the larger vessels is of far less functional importance that it is on the arterioles and small arteries. Capacitance vessels are more responsive to sympathetic nerve stimulation than are resistance vessels; they reach maximal constriction at a lower frequency of stimulation than do the resistance vessels. However, capacitance vessels do not possess beta-adrenergic receptors, nor do they respond to vasodilator metabolites. Norepinephrine is the neurotransmitter released at the sympathetic nerve terminals in the blood vessels, and many factors, such as circulating hormones and particularly locally released substances, modify the liberation of norepinephrine from the vesicles of the nerve terminals.

The response of the resistance and capacitance vessels to stimulation of the sympathetic fibers is illustrated in Figure 8-7. At constant arterial pressure, sympathetic fiber stimulation evoked a reduction of blood flow (constriction of the resistance vessels) and a decrease in blood volume of the tissue (constriction of the capacitance vessels). The abrupt decrease in tissue volume is caused by movement of blood out of the capacitance vessels and out of the

hindquarters of the cat, whereas the late, slow, progressive decline in volume (to the right of the arrow) is caused by movement of extravascular fluid into the capillaries and hence away from the tissue. The loss of tissue fluid is a consequence of the lowered capillary hydrostatic pressure brought about by constriction of the resistance vessels, with establishment of a new equilibrium of the forces responsible for filtration and absorption across the capillary wall (see p 164).

In addition to active changes (contraction and relaxation of the vascular smooth muscle) in vessel caliber, there are passive changes caused

Figure 8-7 ■ **Effect of sympathetic nerve stimulation (2 Hz) on blood flow and tissue volume in the hindquarters of the cat. The arrow denotes the change in slope of the tissue volume curve where the volume decrease caused by emptying of capacitance vessels ceases and loss of extravascular fluid becomes evident.** (Redrawn from Mellander S: *Acta Physiol Scand* 50[suppl 176]:1-86, 1960.)

Section of the sympathetic nerves to an extremity, as might occur during peripheral arterial surgery, abolishes sympathetic vascular tone, thereby increasing limb blood flow. With time, vascular tone is regained by an increase in basal (intrinsic) tone.

solely by alteration in intraluminal pressure; an increase in intraluminal pressure produces distension of the vessels, and a decrease produces a reduction in caliber by recoil of the elastic components of the vessel walls.

At basal tone, approximately one third of the blood volume of a tissue can be mobilized on stimulation of the sympathetic nerves at physiologic frequencies. The basal tone is very low in capacitance vessels; with veins denervated, only small increases in volume are obtained with maximal doses of acetylcholine. Therefore, the blood volume at basal tone is close to the maximal blood volume of the tissue. More blood can be mobilized from the skin than from the muscle capacitance vessels, in part because of greater sensitivity of the skin vessels to sympathetic stimulation, but also because basal tone is lower in skin vessels than in muscle vessels. Therefore, in the absence of neural influence, the skin capacitance vessels contain more blood than do the muscle capacitance vessels.

Blood is mobilized from capacitance vessels in response to physiologic stimuli. In exercise, activation of the sympathetic nerve fibers produces constriction of veins and hence augments the cardiac filling pressure. Also, in arterial hypotension (as in hemorrhage), the capacitance vessels constrict to aid in overcoming the decreased central venous pressure associated with this condition.

In hemorrhagic shock the resistance vessels constrict, thereby assisting in the maintenance or restoration of arterial pressure. With arterial hypotension the enhanced arteriolar constriction also leads to a small mobilization of blood from the tissue by virtue of recoil of the postarteriolar vessels when intraluminal pressure is reduced. Furthermore, there is mobilization of extravascular fluid because of greater absorption into the capillaries in response to the lowered capillary hydrostatic pressure.

In brief, neural and humoral stimuli can exert similar or dissimilar effects on different segments of the vascular tree, and in so doing can alter blood flow, tissue blood volume, and extravascular volume to meet the physiologic requirements of the organism.

Parasympathetic Neural Influence

The efferent fibers of the cranial division of the parasympathetic nervous system supply blood vessels of the head and viscera, whereas fibers of the sacral division supply blood vessels of the genitalia, bladder, and large bowel. Skeletal muscle and skin do not receive parasympathetic innervation. Because only a small proportion of the resistance vessels of the body receive parasympathetic fibers, the effect of these cholinergic fibers on total vascular resistance is small.

Stimulation of the parasympathetic fibers to the salivary glands induces marked vasodilation. A vasodilator polypeptide, **bradykinin,** formed locally from the action of an enzyme on a plasma protein substrate present in the glandular lymphatics has been considered to be the metabolic mediator of the vasodilation produced by chorda tympani stimulation. Bradykinin is formed in other exocrine glands, such as the lacrimal glands and sweat glands. Its presence in sweat is thought to be partly responsible for the dilation of cutaneous blood vessels that occurs with sweating.

Humoral Factors

Epinephrine and norepinephrine exert a profound effect on the peripheral blood vessels. In skeletal muscle, epinephrine in low concentrations dilates resistance vessels **(beta-adrenergic effect)** and in high concentrations produces constriction **(alpha-adrenergic effect).** In skin only vasoconstriction is obtained with epinephrine, whereas in all vascular beds the primary effect of norepinephrine is vasoconstriction. When stimulated, the adrenal gland can release epinephrine and norepinephrine into the systemic circulation. However, under physiologic conditions, the effect of catecholamine release from the adrenal medulla is of lesser importance than norepinephrine release produced by sympathetic nerve activation.

Vascular Reflexes

Areas of the medulla that mediate sympathetic and vagal effects are under the influence of neural impulses arising in the baroreceptors, chemoreceptors, hypothalamus, cerebral cortex, and skin. These areas of the medulla are also affected by changes in the blood concentrations of CO_2 and O_2.

Arterial Baroreceptors The **baroreceptors** (or **pressoreceptors**) are stretch receptors located in the carotid sinuses (slightly widened areas of the internal carotid arteries at their points of origin from the common carotid arteries) and in the aortic arch (Figures 8-8 and 8-9). Impulses arising in the carotid sinus travel up the sinus nerve (nerve of Hering) to the glossopharyngeal nerve and, via the latter, to the nucleus of the **tractus solitarius (NTS)** in the medulla. The NTS is the site of central projection of the chemoreceptors and baroreceptors. Stimulation of the NTS inhibits sympathetic nerve impulses to the peripheral blood vessels (depressor), whereas lesions of the NTS produce vasoconstriction (pressor). Impulses arising in the pressoreceptors of the aortic arch reach the NTS via afferent fibers in the vagus nerves. The pres-

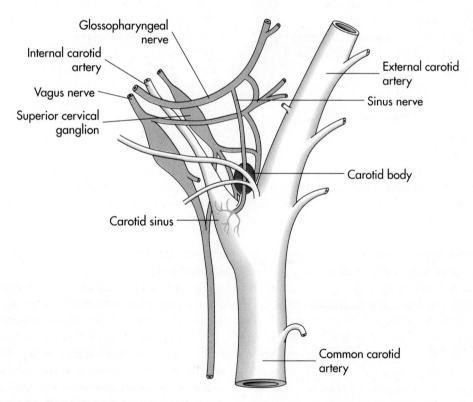

Figure 8-8 ■ **Diagrammatic representation of the carotid sinus and carotid body and their innervation in the dog.** (Redrawn from Adams WE: *The comparative morphology of the carotid body and carotid sinus,* Springfield, Ill, 1958, Charles C Thomas.)

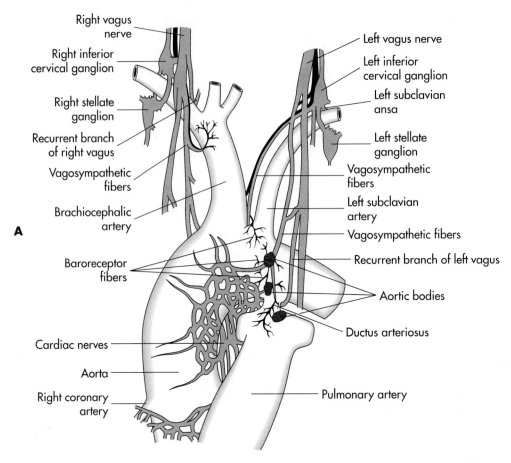

Figure 8-9 ■ A, Anterior view of the aortic arch showing the innervation of the aortic bodies and pressoreceptors in the dog. (Modified from Nonidez JF: *Anat Rec* 69:299, 1937.)

soreceptor nerve terminals in the walls of the carotid sinus and aortic arch respond to the stretch and deformation of the vessel induced by the arterial pressure. The frequency of firing is enhanced by an increase in blood pressure and diminished by a reduction in blood pressure. An increase in impulse frequency, as occurs with a rise in arterial pressure, inhibits the vasoconstrictor regions, resulting in peripheral vasodilation and a lowering of blood pressure. Contributing to a lowering of the blood pressure is a

bradycardia brought about by stimulation of the vagal regions.

The carotid sinus and aortic baroreceptors are not equipotent in their effects on peripheral resistance in response to nonpulsatile alterations in blood pressure. The carotid sinus baroreceptors are more sensitive than those in the aortic arch. Changes in pressure in the carotid sinus evoke greater alterations in systemic arterial pressure than do equivalent changes in aortic arch pressure. However, with pulsatile changes

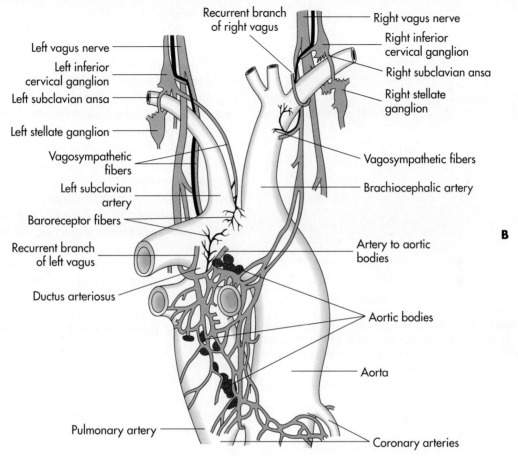

Figure 8-9, cont'd ▪ B, Posterior view of the aortic arch showing the innervation of the aortic bodies and pressoreceptors in the dog. (Modified from Nonidez JF: *Anat Rec* 69:299, 1937.)

in blood pressure, the two sets of baroreceptors respond similarly.

The carotid sinus with the sinus nerve intact can be isolated from the rest of the circulation and perfused by either a donor animal or an artificial perfusion system. Under these conditions, changes in the pressure within the carotid sinus are associated with reciprocal changes in the blood pressure of the experimental animal. The receptors in the walls of the carotid sinus show some adaptation and therefore are more respon-

sive to constantly changing pressures than to sustained constant pressures. This is illustrated in Figure 8-10, which shows that at normal levels of mean blood pressure (about 100 mm Hg) a barrage of impulses from a single fiber of the sinus nerve is initiated in early systole by the pressure rise, and only a few spikes are observed during late systole and early diastole. At lower pressures these phasic changes are even more evident, but the overall frequency of discharge is reduced. The blood pressure threshold for eliciting sinus

Figure 8-10 ■ **Relationship of phasic aortic blood pressure in the firing of a single afferent nerve fiber from the carotid sinus at different levels of mean arterial pressure.**

nerve impulses is about 50 mm Hg, and a maximal sustained firing is reached at around 200 mm Hg. Because the pressoreceptors show some degree of adaptation, their response at any level of mean arterial pressure is greater with a large than with a small pulse pressure. This is illustrated in Figure 8-11, which shows the effects of damping pulsations in the carotid sinus on the frequency of firing in a fiber of the sinus nerve and on the systemic arterial pressure. When the pulse pressure in the carotid sinuses is reduced with an air chamber, but mean pressure remains constant, the rate of electrical impulses recorded from a sinus nerve fiber decreases and the systemic arterial pressure increases. Restoration of the pulse pressure in the carotid sinus restores the frequency of sinus nerve discharge and systemic arterial pressure to control levels (Figure 8-11).

The resistance increases that occur in the peripheral vascular beds in response to reduced pressure in the carotid sinus vary from one vascular bed to another and thereby produce a redistribution of blood flow. For example, in the dog the resistance changes elicited by altering carotid sinus pressure around the normal operating sinus pressure are greatest in the femoral vessels, less in the renal, and least in the mesenteric and celiac vessels. Furthermore, the sensitivity of the carotid sinus reflex can be altered. Local application of norepinephrine or stimulation of sympathetic nerve fibers to the carotid sinuses enhances the sensitivity of the receptors in the sinus so that a given increase in intrasinus pressure produces a greater depressor response. A decrease in baroreceptor sensitivity occurs in hypertension when the carotid sinus becomes stiffer and less deformable as a result of the high intraarterial pressure. Under these conditions a given increase in carotid sinus pressure elicits a smaller decrement in systemic arterial pressure than it does at normal levels of blood pressure. In other words, the set point of the baroreceptors is raised in hypertension so that the threshold is increased and the receptors are less sensitive to change in transmural pressure.

As would be expected, denervation of the carotid sinus can produce temporary, and in some instances prolonged, hypertension.

The arterial baroreceptors play a key role in short-term adjustments of blood pressure when relatively abrupt changes in blood volume, cardiac output, or peripheral resistance (as in ex-

In some individuals the carotid sinus is quite sensitive to pressure. Hence, tight collars or other forms of external pressure over the region of the carotid sinus may elicit marked hypotension and fainting.

Figure 8-11 ■ **Effect of reducing pulse pressure in the vascularly isolated perfused carotid sinuses** *(top record)* **on impulses recorded from a fiber of a sinus nerve** *(middle record)* **and on mean systemic arterial pressure** *(bottom record)*. **Mean pressure in the carotid sinuses** *(horizontal line, top record)* **is held constant when pulse pressure is damped.**

ercise) *occur. However, long-term control of blood pressure—that is, over days, weeks, and longer—is determined by the fluid balance of the individual, namely, the balance between fluid intake and fluid output.* By far the single most important organ in the control of body fluid volume, and hence of blood pressure, is the kidney. With overhydration excessive fluid intake is excreted, whereas with dehydration there is a marked reduction in urine output.

Cardiopulmonary Baroreceptors In addition to the carotid sinus and aortic baroreceptors, there are cardiopulmonary receptors with vagal and sympathetic afferent and efferent nerves. These cardiopulmonary reflexes are tonically active and can alter peripheral resistance with changes in intracardiac, venous, or pulmonary vas-

cular pressures. The receptors are located in the atria, ventricles, and pulmonary vessels.

The atria contain two types of receptors: those activated by the tension developed during atrial contraction (**A receptors**) and those activated by the stretch of the atria during atrial filling (**B receptors**). Stimulation of these atrial receptors sends impulses up vagal fibers to the vagal center in the medulla. Consequently, the sympathetic activity is decreased to the kidney and increased to the sinus node. These changes in sympathetic activity increase renal blood flow, urine flow, and heart rate.

Activation of the cardiopulmonary receptors can also lower blood pressure reflexly by inhibiting the vasoconstrictor center in the medulla. Stimulation of the receptors inhibits angiotensin, aldosterone, and vasopressin (antidiuretic hormone) release; interruption of the reflex pathway has the opposite effects. Changes in urine volume elicited by changes in cardiopulmonary baroreceptor activation are important in the regulation of blood volume. For example, a decrease in blood volume (hypovolemia), as occurs in hemorrhage, enhances sympathetic vasoconstriction in the kidney and increases secretion of renin, angiotensin, aldosterone, and antidiuretic hormone. The renal vasoconstriction (primarily afferent arteriolar) reduces glomerular filtration and increases renin release from the kidney. Renin acts on a plasma substrate to form angiotensin, which increases aldosterone release from the adrenal cortex. The enhanced release of antidiuretic hormone increases water reabsorption. The net result is retention of salt and water by the kidney and a sensation of thirst. Angiotensin II (formed from angiotensin I by converting enzyme) also raises systemic arteriolar tone.

Peripheral Chemoreceptors The chemoreceptors consist of small, highly vascular bodies in the region of the aortic arch (aortic bodies—Figure 8-9) and just medial to the carotid sinuses (carotid bodies—Figure 8-8). They are sensitive to changes in the Po_2, Pco_2, and pH of the blood. Although they are primarily concerned with the regulation of respiration, they reflexly influence the vasomotor regions to a minor degree. A reduction in arterial blood O_2 tension (Pao_2) stimulates the chemoreceptors, and the increase in the number of impulses in the afferent nerve fibers from the carotid and aortic bodies stimulates the vasoconstrictor regions, resulting in increased tone of the resistance and capacitance vessels.

The chemoreceptors are also stimulated by increased arterial blood CO_2 tension ($Paco_2$) and reduced pH, but the reflex effect induced is quite small compared with the direct effect of hypercapnia (high $Paco_2$) and hydrogen ions on the va-

somotor regions in the medulla. When hypoxia and hypercapnia occur at the same time, the stimulation of the chemoreceptors is greater than the sum of the two stimuli when they act alone. The effects of hypoxia plus hypercapnia on blood pressure, heart rate, and respiration are shown in Figure 8-12 (see also Figures 4-14 and 4-15).

When the chemoreceptors are stimulated simultaneously with a reduction in pressure in the baroreceptors, the chemoreceptors potentiate the vasoconstriction observed in the peripheral vessels. However, when the baroreceptors and chemoreceptors are both stimulated (e.g., high carotid sinus pressure and low Pao_2), the effects of the baroreceptors predominate.

There are also chemoreceptors with sympathetic afferent fibers in the heart. These cardiac chemoreceptors are activated by ischemia and transmit the precordial pain (**angina pectoris**) associated with an inadequate blood supply to the myocardium.

Hypothalamus Optimal function of the cardiovascular reflexes requires the integrity of the pontine and hypothalamic structures. Furthermore, these structures are responsible for behavioral and emotional control of the cardiovascular system. Stimulation of the anterior hypothalamus produces a fall in blood pressure and bradycardia, whereas stimulation of the posterolateral region of the hypothalamus produces a rise in blood pressure and tachycardia. The hypothalamus also contains a temperature-regulating center that affects the skin vessels. Stimulation by cold applications to the skin or by cooling of the

---

At high altitudes the low Pao_2 stimulates the peripheral chemoreceptors to increase the rate and depth of respiration. This is the main mechanism involved in an attempt to restore the oxygen supply to the body.

Figure 8-12 ■ Effects of stimulation of the isolated perfused carotid body chemoreceptors at constant carotid sinus perfusion pressure, by substituting hypoxic hypercapnic blood (PO_2, 31.1 mm Hg; PCO_2, 84.9 mm Hg; pH, 7.242) for arterial blood (PO_2, 140.4 mm Hg; PCO_2, 42.1 mm Hg; pH, 7.33) between arrows. Note that the bradycardia was transient. The enhanced respiratory response abolishes bradycardia and can produce tachycardia, especially with sustained stimulation of the carotid body receptors (see Figures 4-14 and 4-15). The increase in pulse interval *(PI)* indicates a decrease in heart rate. $\overline{BP}$, Mean arterial blood pressure; V_T, tidal volume. (Redrawn from Daly MdeB, Kouner PI, Angell-James JE, Oliver JA: *Clin Exp Pharmacol Physiol* 5:511, 1978.)

blood perfusing the hypothalamus results in constriction of the skin vessels and heat conservation, whereas warm stimuli result in cutaneous vasodilation and enhanced heat loss (see p 241).

Cerebrum The cerebral cortex can also exert a significant effect on blood flow distribution in the body. Stimulation of the motor and premotor areas can affect blood pressure; usually a pressor response is obtained. However, vasodilation and depressor responses may be evoked, as in blushing or fainting, in response to an emotional stimulus.

Skin and Viscera Painful stimuli can elicit either pressor or depressor responses, depending on the magnitude and location of the stimu-

lus. Distension of the viscera often evokes a depressor response, whereas painful stimuli on the body surface usually evoke a pressor response.

Pulmonary Reflexes Inflation of the lungs reflexly induces systemic vasodilation and a decrease in arterial blood pressure. Conversely, collapse of the lungs evokes systemic vasoconstriction. Afferent fibers mediating this reflex run in the vagus nerves and possibly to a limited extent in the sympathetic nerves. Their stimulation by stretch of the lungs inhibits the vasomotor areas. The magnitude of the depressor response to lung inflation is directly related to the degree of inflation and to the existing level of vasoconstrictor tone.

Central Chemoreceptors Increases of Pa_{CO_2} stimulate chemosensitive regions of the medulla and elicit vasoconstriction and increased peripheral resistance. Reduction in Pa_{CO_2} below normal levels (as with hyperventilation) decreases the degree of tonic activity of these areas in the medulla, thereby decreasing peripheral resistance. The chemosensitive regions are also affected by changes in pH. A lowering of blood pH stimulates, and a rise in blood pH inhibits, these areas. These effects of changes in Pa_{CO_2} and blood pH possibly operate through changes in cerebrospinal fluid pH, as appears to be the case for the respiratory center.

Oxygen tension has relatively little direct effect on the medullary vasomotor region. The primary effect of hypoxia is reflexly mediated via the carotid and aortic chemoreceptors. Moderate reduction of Pa_{O_2} stimulates the vasomotor region, but severe reduction depresses vasomotor activity in the same manner that other areas of the brain are depressed by very low O_2 tensions.

■ BALANCE BETWEEN EXTRINSIC AND INTRINSIC FACTORS IN REGULATION OF PERIPHERAL BLOOD FLOW

Dual control of the peripheral vessels by intrinsic and extrinsic mechanisms makes possible a number of vascular adjustments that enable the body to direct blood flow to areas where it is needed in greater supply and away from areas whose immediate requirements are fewer. In some tissues a more or less fixed relative potency of extrinsic and intrinsic mechanisms exists; in other tissues the ratio is changeable, depending on the state of activity of that tissue.

In the brain and the heart, both vital structures with very limited tolerance for a reduced blood supply, intrinsic flow-regulating mechanisms are dominant. For instance, massive discharge of the vasoconstrictor region over the sympathetic nerves, which might occur in severe, acute hemorrhage, has negligible effects on the cerebral and cardiac resistance vessels, whereas skin, renal, and splanchnic blood vessels become greatly constricted.

In the skin the extrinsic vascular control is dominant. Not only do the cutaneous vessels participate strongly in a general vasoconstrictor discharge, but they also respond selectively through hypothalamic pathways to subserve the heat loss and heat conservation function required in body temperature regulation. However, intrinsic control can be demonstrated by local changes of temperature that can modify or override the central influence on resistance and capacitance vessels.

In skeletal muscle the interplay and changing balance between extrinsic and intrinsic mechanisms can be clearly seen. In resting skeletal muscle, neural control (vasoconstrictor tone) is dominant, as can be demonstrated by the large increment in blood flow that occurs immediately after section of the sympathetic nerves to the tissue. In anticipation of and at the start of exercise, such as running, blood flow increases in the leg muscles. After the onset of exercise the intrinsic flow-regulating mechanism assumes control, and because of the local increase in metabolites, vasodilation occurs in the active muscles. Vasoconstriction occurs in the inactive tissues as a manifestation of the general sympathetic discharge, but constrictor impulses reaching the resistance vessels of the active muscles

---

Cerebral ischemia, which may occur because of excessive pressure exerted by an expanding intracranial tumor, results in a marked increase in peripheral vasoconstriction. The stimulation is probably caused by a local accumulation of CO_2 and reduction of O_2, and possibly by excitation of intracranial baroreceptors. With prolonged, severe ischemia, central depression eventually supervenes and blood pressure falls.

are overridden by the local metabolic effect. Operation of this dual control mechanism thus provides increased blood where it is required and shunts it away from relatively inactive areas. Similar effects may be achieved with an increase in Pa_{CO_2}. Normally the hyperventilation associated with exercise keeps Pa_{CO_2} at normal levels. However, were Pa_{CO_2} to increase, a generalized vasoconstriction would occur because of stimulation of the medullary vasoconstrictor region by CO_2. In the active muscles, where the CO_2 concentration is highest, the smooth muscle of the arterioles would relax in response to the local P_{CO_2}. Factors affecting and affected by the vasomotor region are summarized in Figure 8-13.

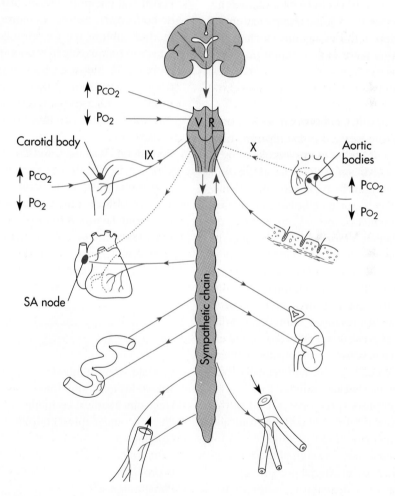

Figure 8-13 ■ **Schematic diagram illustrating the neural input and output of the vasomotor region** *(VR). IX,* **Glossopharyngeal nerve;** *X,* **vagus nerve.**

■ SUMMARY

1. The arterioles, often referred to as the resistance vessels, are important in the regulation of blood flow through their cognate capillaries. The smooth muscle, which makes up a major fraction of the walls of the arterioles, contracts and relaxes in response to neural and humoral stimuli.

2. Most tissues show autoregulation of blood flow, a phenomenon characterized by a constant blood flow in the face of a change in perfusion pressure. A logical explanation of autoregulation is the myogenic mechanism whereby an increase in transmural pressure elicits a contractile response, whereas a decrease in transmural pressure elicits relaxation.

3. The striking parallelism between tissue blood flow and tissue oxygen consumption indicates that blood flow is largely regulated by a metabolic mechanism. A decrease in the oxygen supply/oxygen demand ratio of a tissue releases a vasodilator metabolite that dilates arterioles to enhance the oxygen supply.

4. Neural regulation of blood flow is almost completely accomplished by the sympathetic nervous system. Sympathetic nerves to blood vessels are tonically active; inhibition of the vasoconstrictor center in the medulla reduces peripheral vascular resistance. Stimulation of the sympathetic nerves constricts resistance and capacitance (veins) vessels. Parasympathetic fibers innervate the head, viscera, and genitalia; they do not innervate skin and muscle.

5. The baroreceptors (pressoreceptors) in the internal carotid arteries and aorta are tonically active and regulate blood pressure on a moment-to-moment basis. Stretch of these receptors by an increase in arterial pressure reflexly inhibits the vasoconstrictor center in the medulla and induces vasodilation, whereas a decrease in arterial pressure disinhibits the vasoconstrictor center and induces vasoconstriction. The carotid baroreceptors predominate over those in the aorta and respond more vigorously to changes in pressure (stretch) than they do to elevated or reduced constant pressures; they adapt to an imposed constant pressure. Baroreceptors are also present in the cardiac chambers and large pulmonary vessels (cardiopulmonary baroreceptors); they have less influence on blood pressure but participate in blood volume regulation.

6. Peripheral chemoreceptors (carotid and aortic bodies) and central chemoreceptors in the medulla oblongata are stimulated by a decrease in blood oxygen tension (Pa_{O_2}) and an increase in blood carbon dioxide tension (Pa_{CO_2}). Stimulation of these chemoreceptors primarily increases the rate and depth of respiration but also produces peripheral vasoconstriction.

7. Peripheral resistance, and hence blood pressure, can be affected by stimuli arising in the skin, viscera, lungs, and brain.

8. The combined effect of neural and local metabolic factors is to distribute blood to active tissues and divert it from inactive tissues. In vital structures, such as the heart and brain and in contracting skeletal muscle, the metabolic factors predominate.

■ KEY WORDS AND CONCEPTS

- Vascular smooth muscle
- Myoendothelial junctions
- Electromechanical coupling
- Pharmacomechanical coupling
- Calcium
- Calmodulin
- G proteins
- Phospholipase C
- Inositol trisphosphate
- Na-Ca exchange
- Autoregulation of blood flow
- Myogenic mechanism

- Transmural pressure
- Shear stress vasodilation
- Metabolic mechanism
- Active hyperemia
- Reactive hyperemia
- Basal tone
- Neural vasoconstriction
- Norepinephrine
- Resistance vessels
- Capacitance vessels
- Parasympathetic nerves
- Bradykinin
- Beta-adrenergic effect
- Alpha-adrenergic effect
- Vascular reflexes
- Baroreceptors (pressoreceptors)
- Carotid sinus receptors
- Aortic arch receptors
- Pulse pressure
- Cardiopulmonary receptors
- Peripheral chemoreceptors
- Central chemoreceptors
- Aortic bodies
- Carotid bodies
- Peripheral vascular reflexes

■ SELF-STUDY PROBLEMS

1. What is meant by autoregulation of blood flow and what is the mechanism involved?
2. How can the endothelium affect the contractile state of vascular smooth muscle?
3. What is vascular tone?
4. Briefly describe the local and neural effects on vascular resistance in resting and contracting skeletal muscle.
5. How is blood pressure regulated by the carotid baroreceptors?

■ BIBLIOGRAPHY

Journal articles

Berne RM, Knabb RM, Ely SW, Rubio R: Adenosine in the local regulation of blood flow: a brief overview, *Fed Proc* 42:3136, 1983.

Brown AM: Receptors under pressure—an update on baroreceptors, *Circ Res* 46:1, 1980.

Cowley AW Jr: Long-term control of blood pressure, *Physiol Rev* 72:231, 1992.

Donald DE, Shepherd JT: Autonomic regulation of the peripheral circulation, *Annu Rev Physiol* 42:429, 1980.

Ellsworth ML, Forrester T, Ellis CG, Dietrich HH: The erythrocyte as a regulator of vascular tone, *Am J Physiol* 269:H2155, 1995.

Hainsworth R: Reflexes from the heart, *Physiol Rev* 71:617, 1991.

Hilton SM, Spyer KM: Central nervous regulation of vascular resistance, *Annu Rev Physiol* 42:399, 1980.

Hirst GDS, Edwards FR: Sympathetic neuroeffector transmission in arteries and arterioles, *Physiol Rev* 69:546, 1989.

Kuo L, Davis JJ, Chilian WM: Endothelium-dependent flow-induced dilation of isolated coronary arterioles, *Am J Physiol* 259:H1063, 1990.

Marshall JM: Peripheral chemoreceptors and cardiovascular regulation, *Physiol Rev* 74:543, 1994.

Monos E, Berczi V, Nadasy G: Local control of veins: biomechanical, metabolic, and humoral aspects, *Physiol Rev* 75:611, 1995.

Shen Y-T, Knight DR, Thomas JX Jr, Vatner SF: Relative roles of cardiac receptors and arterial baroreceptors during hemorrhage in conscious dogs, *Circ Res* 66:397, 1990.

Shepherd JT: Reflex control of arterial blood pressure, *Cardiovasc Res* 16:357, 1982.

Books and monographs

Abboud FM, Thames MD: *Interaction of cardiovascular reflexes in circulatory control.* In *Handbook of physiology,* Section 2: *The cardiovascular system—peripheral circulation and organ blood flow,* vol III, Bethesda, Md., 1983, American Physiological Society.

Bishop VS, Malliani A, Thoren P: *Cardiac mechanoreceptors.* In *Handbook of physiology,* Section 2: *The cardiovascular system—peripheral circulation and organ blood flow,* vol III, Bethesda, Md., 1983, American Physiological Society.

Eyzaguirre C, Fitzgerald RS, Lahiri S, Zapata P: *Arterial chemoreceptors.* In *Handbook of physiology,* Section 2: *The cardiovascular system—peripheral circulation and organ blood flow,* vol III, Bethesda, Md., 1983, American Physiological Society.

Johnson PC: *The myogenic response.* In *Handbook of physiology,* Section 2: *The cardiovascular system—vascular smooth muscle,* vol II, Bethesda, Md., 1980, American Physiological Society.

Kovach AGB, Sandos P, Kollii, M, editors: *Cardiovascular physiology: neural control mechanisms,* New York, 1981, Academic Press.

Mancia G, Mark AL: *Arterial baroreflexes in humans.* In *Handbook of physiology,* Section 2: *The cardiovascular system—peripheral circulation and organ blood flow,* vol III, Bethesda, Md., 1983, American Physiological Society.

Mark AL, Mancia G: *Cardiopulmonary baroreflexes in humans.* In *Handbook of physiology,* Section 2: *The cardiovascular system—peripheral circulation and organ blood flow,* vol III, Bethesda, Md., 1983, American Physiological Society.

Mulvany MJ, Strandgaard S, Hammersen F, editors: *Resistance vessels: physiology, pharmacology and hypertensive pathology,* Basel, Switzerland, 1985, S Karger.

Persson PB, Kirchheim HR, editors: *Baroreceptor reflexes,* Berlin, 1991, Springer-Verlag.

Rothe CF: *Venous system: physiology of the capacitance vessels.* In *Handbook of physiology,* Section 2: *The cardiovascular system—peripheral circulation and organ blood flow,* vol III, Bethesda, Md., 1983, American Physiological Society.

Sagawa K: *Baroreflex control of systemic arterial pressure and vascular bed.* In *Handbook of physiology,* Section 2:

The cardiovascular system—peripheral circulation and organ blood flow, vol III, Bethesda, Md., 1983, American Physiological Society.

Shepherd JT: *Cardiac mechanoreceptors.* In Fozzard HA, et al, editors: *The heart and cardiovascular system, scientific foundations,* ed 2, New York, 1991, Raven Press.

Somlyo AP, Somlyo AV: *Smooth muscle structure and function.* In Fozzard HA, et al, editors: *The heart and cardiovascular system, scientific foundations,* ed 2, New York, 1991, Raven Press.

Sparks HV Jr: *Effect of local metabolic factors on vascular smooth muscle.* In *Handbook of physiology,* Section 2: *The cardiovascular system—vascular smooth muscle,* vol II, Bethesda, Md., 1980, American Physiological Society.

Zucker IH, Gilmore JP, editors: *Reflex control of the circulation,* Boca Raton, Fla., 1991, CRC Press.

Control of Cardiac Output: Coupling of Heart and Blood Vessels

F our factors control cardiac output: heart rate, myocardial contractility, preload, and afterload (Figure 9-1). Heart rate and myocardial contractility are strictly **cardiac factors.** They are characteristics of the cardiac tissues, although they are modulated by various neural and humoral mechanisms. Preload and afterload, however, depend on the characteristics of both the heart and the vascular system. On the one hand, preload and afterload are important **determinants** of cardiac output. On the other hand, preload and afterload are themselves **determined by** the cardiac output and by certain vascular characteristics. Preload and afterload may be designated **coupling factors,** because they constitute a functional coupling between the heart and blood vessels.

To understand the regulation of cardiac output, therefore, it is important to appreciate the nature of the coupling between the heart and the vascular system. Guyton and colleagues developed graphic techniques that we have modified to analyze the interactions between the cardiac and vascular components of the circulatory system. The graphic analysis involves two simultaneous functional relationships between **cardiac output** and **central venous pressure** (i.e., the

pressure in the right atrium and thoracic venae cavae).

The curve that defines one of these relationships will be called the **cardiac function curve.** It is an expression of the well-known Frank-Starling relationship (p 97) and reflects the dependence of cardiac output on preload (i.e., central venous, or right atrial, pressure). *The cardiac function curve is a characteristic of the heart itself* and it has been studied in hearts completely isolated from the rest of the circulatory system (see Chapters 3 and 4).

The second curve, which we shall call the **vascular function curve,** defines the dependence of central venous pressure on cardiac output. This relationship depends only on certain vascular system characteristics, namely, peripheral resistance, arterial and venous compliances, and blood volume. *The vascular function curve is entirely independent of the characteristics of the heart* and it could be studied even if the heart were replaced by a mechanical pump.

■ VASCULAR FUNCTION CURVE

The vascular function curve defines the changes in central venous pressure evoked by changes in cardiac output; that is, central ve-

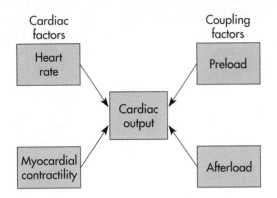

Figure 9-1 ■ The four factors that determine cardiac output.

nous pressure is the **dependent variable** (or **response**), and cardiac output is the **independent variable** (or **stimulus**). This contrasts with the cardiac function curve, for which central venous pressure (or preload) is the independent variable and cardiac output is the dependent variable.

The simplified model of the circulation illustrated in Figure 9-2 helps explain how cardiac output determines the level of central venous pressure. The essential components of the cardiovascular system have been lumped into four elements. The right and left sides of the heart, as well as the pulmonary vascular bed, are considered simply as a **pump,** much as that employed during open heart surgery. The high-resistance microcirculation is designated the **peripheral resistance.** Finally, the compliance of the system is subdivided into two components, **arterial compliance,** C_a, and **venous compliance,** C_v. As defined in Chapter 6, compliance (C) is the increment of volume (ΔV) accommodated per unit change of pressure (ΔP); that is,

$$C = \Delta V/\Delta P \qquad (1)$$

The venous compliance is about 20 times as great as the arterial compliance. In the example to follow, the ratio of C_v to C_a will be set at 19:1

to simplify certain calculations. Thus, if it were necessary to add x ml of blood to the arterial system to produce a 1 mm Hg increment in arterial pressure, it would be necessary to add 19x ml of blood to the venous system to raise venous pressure by the same amount.

To illustrate why central venous pressure varies inversely with cardiac output, let us first give our model the characteristics that resemble those of an average adult person (Figure 9-2, *A*). Let the flow (Q_h) generated by the heart (i.e., cardiac output) be 5 L/min; let mean arterial pressure, P_a, be 102 mm Hg; and let central venous pressure, P_v, be 2 mm Hg. The peripheral resistance, R, is the ratio of pressure difference ($P_a - P_v$) to flow (Q_r) through the resistance vessels; this ratio equals 20 mm Hg/L/min. An arteriovenous pressure difference of 100 mm Hg is sufficient to force a flow (Q_r) of 5 L/min through a peripheral resistance of 20 mm Hg/L/min; this flow *(peripheral runoff)* is precisely equal to the flow (Q_h) generated by the heart. From heartbeat to heartbeat, the volume (V_a) of blood in the arteries and the volume (V_v) of blood in the veins remain constant because the volume of blood transferred from the veins to the arteries by the heart equals the volume of blood that flows from the arteries through the resistance vessels and into the veins.

Figure 9-2, *B* illustrates the status of the circulation at the very beginning of an episode of cardiac arrest; i.e., $Q_h = 0$. Initially, the volumes of blood in the arteries (V_a) and veins (V_v) have not had time to change. The arterial and venous pressures depend on V_a and V_v, respectively. Therefore, these pressures are identical to the respective pressures in panel *A* (i.e., $P_a = 102$ and $P_v = 2$). The arteriovenous pressure gradient of 100 mm Hg will force a flow (the peripheral runoff) of 5 L/min through the peripheral resistance of 20 mm Hg/L/min. Thus, although cardiac output now equals 0 L/min, the flow through the microcirculation equals 5 L/min. In other words, the

A Control state

$Q_h = 5$ L/min

Veins · Pump · Arteries

C_v · Peripheral resistance · C_a

$P_v = 2$ · $P_a = 102$

$Q_r = 5$ L/min

$R = (102 - 2) \div 5 = 20$ mm Hg/L/min

Control state. The flow (Q_r) across the peripheral resistance is equal to the flow (Q_h) generated by the heart. The mean arterial pressure (P_a) is 102 mm Hg, the central venous pressure (P_v) is 2 mm Hg, and the peripheral resistance is 20 mm Hg/L/min.

B Beginning of cardiac arrest

$Q_h = 0$ L/min

$P_v = 2$ · $P_a = 102$

$Q_r = 5$ L/min

At the very beginning of cardiac arrest (i.e., $Q_h = 0$ L/min), P_a and P_v have not yet changed. Hence Q_r is still 5 L/min through a resistance of 20 mm Hg/L/min. Because of the disparity between Q_h and Q_r, P_a will begin to decrease rapidly and P_v will begin to rise rapidly.

C Cardiac arrest: steady state

$Q_h = 0$ L/min

$P_v = 7$ · $P_a = 7$

$Q_r = 0$ L/min

When the effects of cardiac arrest have attained the steady state, P_a will have fallen to 7 mm Hg and P_v will have risen to the same value. Because $P_a - P_v = 0$, flow across the resistance will cease (i.e., $Q_r = 0$).

D Beginning of cardiac resuscitation

$Q_h = 1$ L/min

$P_v = 7$ · $P_a = 7$

$Q_r = 0$ L/min

The heart is resuscitated and it begins to pump at a constant value of $Q_h = 1$ L/min. At the very beginning of resuscitation, P_a and P_v have not had time to change, and therefore Q_r is still 0 L/min. Because Q_h exceeds Q_r by 1 L/min, P_a will rise rapidly and P_v will fall rapidly. A new equilibrium will be attained when P_a increases to 26 mm Hg and P_v falls to 6 mm Hg. When $P_a - P_v = 20$ mm Hg, the flow (Q_r) through the resistance will be 1 L/min, which equals the cardiac output (Q_h).

Figure 9-2 ■ **Simplified model of the cardiovascular system, consisting of a pump, arterial compliance *(C_a)*, peripheral resistance, and venous compliance *(C_v)*.**

potential energy stored in the arteries by the previous pumping action of the heart causes blood to be transferred from arteries to veins, initially at the control rate, even though the heart can no longer transfer blood from the veins into the arteries.

As time passes, the blood volume in the arteries progressively decreases and the blood volume in the veins progressively increases. Because the vessels are elastic structures, arterial pressure falls gradually and venous pressure rises gradually. This process will continue until the arterial and venous pressures become equal (Figure 9-2, *C*). Once this condition is reached, the flow (Q_r) from the arteries to the veins through the resistance vessels will be zero, as is the cardiac output (Q_h).

At zero flow equilibrium (Figure 9-2, *C*), the pressure attained in the arteries and veins depends on the relative compliances of these vessels. Had the arterial (C_a) and venous (C_v) compliances been equal, the decline in P_a would have been equal to the rise in P_v because the decrement in arterial volume equals the increment in venous volume (principle of conservation of mass). P_a and P_v would have both attained the average of P_a and P_v in panels *A* and *B*; i.e., $P_a = P_v$ = (102 + 2)/2 = 52 mm Hg.

However, the veins are much more compliant than the arteries; the compliance ratio is approximately equal to the ratio (C_v:C_a = 19) that we have assumed for the model. Hence, the transfer of blood from arteries to veins at equilibrium would induce a fall in arterial pressure 19 times as great as the concomitant rise in venous pressure. As Figure 9-2, *C* shows, P_v would increase by 5 mm Hg (from 2 to 7 mm Hg), whereas P_a would fall by 19 × 5 = 95 mm Hg (from 102 to 7 mm Hg). This equilibrium pressure that prevails in the circulatory system in the absence of flow is often referred to as the **mean circulatory pressure,** or **static pressure.** The pressure in the static system reflects the total volume

of blood in the system and the overall compliance of the entire system.

The example of cardiac arrest in Figure 9-2 provides the basis for understanding the vascular function curves. Two important points on the curve have already been derived, as shown in Figure 9-3. One point *(A)* represents the normal status (depicted in Figure 9-2, *A*). At that point, when cardiac output was 5 L/min, P_v was 2 mm Hg. Then, when flow stopped (cardiac output = 0), P_v became 7 mm Hg at equilibrium; this pressure is the mean circulatory pressure, P_{mc}.

The inverse relation between P_v and cardiac output in Figure 9-3 simply denotes that when cardiac output is suddenly decreased, the peripheral runoff from arteries to veins is temporarily greater than the rate at which the heart pumps it from the veins back into the arteries.

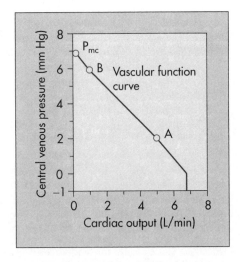

Figure 9-3 ■ Changes in central venous pressure produced by changes in cardiac output. The mean circulatory pressure (or static pressure), *P_{mc},* **is the equilibrium pressure throughout the cardiovascular system when cardiac output is 0. Points *B* and *A* represent the values of venous pressure at cardiac outputs of 1 and 5 L/min, respectively.**

During that transient period, a net volume of blood is translocated from arteries to veins; hence, P_a falls and P_v rises.

An example of a sudden increase in cardiac output, but with peripheral resistance remaining constant, will illustrate how a third point *(B)* on the vascular function curve is derived. Consider that the arrested heart is suddenly restarted and immediately begins pumping blood from the veins into the arteries at a rate of 1 L/min (Figure 9-2, *D*). When the heart first begins to beat, the arteriovenous pressure gradient is zero, and hence no blood flows from the arteries into the veins. Thus, when beating has just resumed, blood is being depleted from the veins at the rate of 1 L/min, and the arterial volume is being repleted at the same rate. Hence, P_v begins to fall and P_a begins to rise. Because of the difference in compliances, P_a will rise 19 times more rapidly than P_v will fall.

The resultant pressure gradient will cause blood to flow through the resistance. If the heart maintains a constant output of 1 L/min, P_a will continue to rise and P_v will continue to fall until the pressure gradient becomes 20 mm Hg. This gradient will force a flow of 1 L/min through a resistance of 20 mm Hg/L/min. This gradient will be achieved by a 19 mm Hg rise (to 26 mm Hg) in P_a and a 1 mm Hg fall (to 6 mm Hg) in P_v. This equilibrium value of $P_v = 6$ mm Hg for a cardiac output of 1 L/min also appears *(B)* on the vascular function curve of Figure 9-3. It reflects a net transfer of blood from the venous to the arterial side of the circuit after the heart has been restarted, and a consequent reduction of P_v.

The reduction of P_v that can be achieved by an increase in cardiac output is limited. At some critical maximal value of cardiac output, sufficient fluid will be translocated from the venous to the arterial side of the circuit to reduce P_v below the ambient pressure. In a system of very distensible vessels, such as the venous system, the vessels will be collapsed when the intravas-cular pressure falls below the extravascular pressure. This venous collapse constitutes an impediment to venous return to the heart. Hence, it will limit the maximal value of cardiac output to 7 L/min in this example (Figure 9-3), regardless of the capabilities of the pump. For readers interested in the mathematical derivation of these results, the basic equations are presented in the box.

Mathematical Analysis of the Vascular Function Curve

From the definition of **peripheral resistance** (p 123):

$$R = (P_a - P_v)/Q_r \qquad (2)$$

where R is resistance, P_a is arterial pressure, P_v is venous pressure, and Q_r is blood flow through the resistance vessels.

At equilibrium, Q_r equals cardiac output, Q_h. Assume that R = 20 and that Q_h had been 0, but that it had then been increased to a constant value of 1 L/min (Figure 9-4, arrow *1*). If we solve equation 2 for P_a when the system is in equilibrium (i.e., $Q_r = Q_h$):

$$P_a = P_v + Q_r R = P_v + (1 \times 20) \qquad (3)$$

Thus, P_a will increase to a value 20 mm Hg greater than P_v. It will continue to be 20 mm Hg above P_v, as long as the pump output is maintained at 1 L/min and the peripheral resistance remains at 20 mm Hg/L/min.

We can calculate what the actual changes in P_a and P_v will be when Q_r attains a constant value of 1 L/min. The arterial volume increment needed to achieve the required level of P_a depends entirely on the arterial compliance, C_a. For a rigid arterial system (low compliance), this volume will be small; for a distensible system, the volume will be large. Whatever the magnitude, however, the change in volume represents the translocation of some quantity of blood from the venous to the arterial side of the circuit.

For a given total blood volume, any increment in arterial volume (ΔV_a) must equal the decrement in venous volume (ΔV_v); that is,

$$\Delta V_a = -\Delta V_v \qquad (4)$$

From the definition of compliance,

$$C_a = \Delta V_a / \Delta P_a \qquad (5)$$

and

$$C_v = \Delta V_v / \Delta P_v \qquad (6)$$

By substitution into equation 4,

$$\frac{\Delta P_v}{\Delta P_a} = -\frac{C_a}{C_v} \qquad (7)$$

Given that C_v is 19 times as great as C_a, the increment in P_a will be 19 times as great as the decrement in P_v; that is,

$$\Delta P_a = -19\Delta P_v \qquad (8)$$

To calculate the absolute values of P_a and P_v, let ΔP_a represent the difference between the prevailing P_a and the mean circulatory pressure (P_{mc}); that is, let

$$\Delta P_a = P_a - P_{mc} \qquad (9)$$

and let ΔP_v represent the difference between the prevailing P_v and the mean circulatory pressure.

$$\Delta P_v = P_v - P_{mc} \qquad (10)$$

Substituting these values for ΔP_a and ΔP_v into equation 8:

$$P_a - P_{mc} = -19 (P_v - P_{mc}) \qquad (11)$$

By solving equations 3 and 11 simultaneously:

$$P_a = P_{mc} + 19 \qquad (12)$$

and

$$P_v = P_{mc} - 1 \qquad (13)$$

Hence, for a mean circulatory pressure of 7 mm Hg, P_a increases to 26 mm Hg and P_v decreases to 6 mm Hg when Q_h increases from 0 to 1 L/min (Figure 9-4). These pressure changes pro-vide the required arteriovenous pressure gradient of 20 mm Hg.

If the pump output is abruptly increased to a constant level of 5 L/min (Figure 9-4, arrow *2*) and peripheral resistance remains constant at 20 mm Hg/L/min, an additional volume of blood again will be translocated from the venous to the arterial side of the circuit. It will progressively accumulate in the arteries until P_a reaches a level of 100 mm Hg above P_v, as shown by substitution into equation 3:

$$P_a = P_v + Q_r R = P_v + (5 \times 20) \qquad (14)$$

By solving equations 11 and 14 simultaneously, we find that P_a rises to a value of 95 mm Hg above P_{mc}, and P_v falls to a value 5 mm Hg below P_{mc}. In Figure 9-4, therefore, P_v declines to 2 mm Hg and P_a rises to 102 mm Hg. The resultant pressure gradient of 100 mm Hg will force a cardiac output of 5 L/min through a constant peripheral resistance of 20 mm Hg/L/min.

The following equation for P_v as a function of Q_r in the model is derived from equations 2, 7, 9, and 10 above:

$$P_v = -\frac{RC_a}{C_a + C_v} Q_r + P_{mc} \qquad (15)$$

Note that the slope depends only on R, C_a and C_v. Note also that when $Q_r = 0$, $P_v = P_{mc}$; that is, at zero flow, P_v equals the mean circulatory pressure.

Venous Pressure Dependence on Cardiac Output

Experimental and clinical observations have shown that changes in cardiac output do indeed evoke the alterations in P_a and P_v that have been predicted above for our simplified model. In an experiment on an anesthesized dog, a mechanical pump was substituted for the right ventricle (Figure 9-5). As the cardiac output, Q, was diminished in a series of small steps, P_a fell and P_v rose.

Figure 9-5 ■ **Changes in arterial** (P_a) **and central venous** (P_v) **pressures produced by changes in systemic blood flow** (Q_r) **in a canine right-heart bypass preparation. Stepwise changes in** Q_r **were produced by altering the rate of a mechanical pump.** (From Levy MN: *Circ Res* 44:739, 1979. By permission of the American Heart Association, Inc.)

Figure 9-4 ■ **Changes in arterial** (P_a) **and venous** (P_v) **pressures in the circulatory model shown in Figure 9-3. The total peripheral resistance is 20 mm Hg/L/min, and the ratio of** C_v **to** C_a **is 19:1. The cardiac output** *(CO)* **is 0 to the left of arrow *1*. It is increased to 1 L/min at arrow *1*, and to 5 L/min at arrow *2*.**

Similarly, a major coronary artery may suddenly become occluded in a human patient. The resultant acute **myocardial infarction (death of myocardial tissue)** often diminishes cardiac output, which is attended by a fall in arterial pressure and a rise in central venous pressure.

Blood Volume

The vascular function curve is affected by variations in total blood volume. During circulatory standstill (zero cardiac output), the mean circulatory pressure depends only on total vascular compliance and blood volume, as stated previously. Thus, for a given vascular compliance the mean circulatory pressure will be increased when the blood volume is expanded **(hypervolemia)** and decreased when the blood vol-

ume is diminished **(hypovolemia).** This is illustrated by the Y-axis intercepts in Figure 9-6, where the mean circulatory pressure is 5 mm Hg after hemorrhage and 9 mm Hg after transfusion, as compared with the value of 7 mm Hg at the normal blood volume **(normovolemia).**

From Figure 9-6 it is also apparent that the cardiac output at which $P_v = 0$ varies directly with the blood volume. Therefore, the maximal value of cardiac output becomes progressively more limited as the total blood volume is reduced. However, the pressure ($P_v = 0$) at which the veins collapse (sharp change in slope of the vascular function curve) is not altered appreciably by changes in blood volume. This pressure depends only on the pressure surrounding the central veins.

Furthermore, the differences in P_v during hypervolemia, normovolemia, and hypovolemia in the static system are preserved at each level of cardiac output such that the vascular function curves parallel each other (Figure 9-6). To illustrate, consider the example of hypervolemia, in which the mean circulatory pressure is 9 mm Hg. In Figure 9-6, both P_a and P_v would be 9 mm Hg, instead of 7 mm Hg, when the cardiac output is zero. With a sudden increase in cardiac output to 1 L/min (at arrow *1*, Figure 9-4), if the peripheral resistance were still 20 mm Hg/L/min, an arteriovenous pressure gradient of 20 mm Hg would still be necessary for 1 L/min to flow through the resistance vessels. This does not differ from the example for normovolemia. Assuming the same ratio of C_v to C_a of 19:1, the pressure gradient would be achieved by a 1 mm Hg decline in P_v and a 19 mm Hg rise in P_a. Hence, a change in cardiac output from 0 to 1 L/min would evoke the same 1 mm Hg reduction in P_v irrespective of the blood volume, as long as C_a, C_v, and the peripheral resistance were independent of blood volume. Equation 15 also discloses that the slope of the vascular function curve remains constant as long as R, C_v, and C_a do not change.

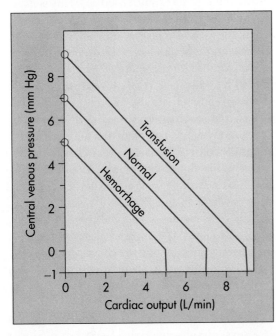

Figure 9-6 ■ **Effects of increased blood volume *(transfusion curve)* and of decreased blood volume *(hemorrhage curve)* on the vascular function curve. Similar shifts in the vascular function curve are produced by increases and decreases, respectively, in venomotor tone.**

Venomotor Tone

The effects of changes in venomotor tone on the vascular function curve closely resemble those for changes in blood volume. In Figure 9-6, for example, the transfusion curve could just as well represent increased venomotor tone, whereas the hemorrhage curve could represent decreased tone. During circulatory standstill, for a given blood volume, the pressure within the vascular system will rise as the tension exerted by the smooth muscle within the vascular walls increases. It is principally the arteriolar and venous smooth muscle that is under any notable nervous or humoral control. The fraction of the blood volume located within the arterioles is very small, whereas the blood volume in the veins is large (see Table 1-1). Therefore, only changes in venous tone can alter the mean circulatory pressure appreciably. Hence, mean circulatory pressure rises with increased venomotor tone and falls with diminished tone.

Experimentally, the pressure attained shortly after abrupt circulatory standstill is usually above 7 mm Hg, even when blood volume is normal. This is attributable to the generalized venoconstriction elicited by cerebral ischemia, activation of the chemoreceptors, and reduced excitation of the baroreceptors. If resuscitation is not successful, this reflex response subsides as central nervous activity ceases. At normal blood volume the mean circulatory pressure usually approaches a value close to 7 mm Hg.

Blood Reservoirs

Venoconstriction is considerably greater in certain regions of the body than in others. In effect, large vascular beds that undergo appreciable venoconstriction constitute blood reservoirs. The vascular bed of the skin is one of the major blood reservoirs in humans. Blood loss evokes profound subcutaneous venoconstriction, which produces the characteristic pale appearance of the skin. The resulting diversion of blood away from the skin liberates several hundred milliliters of blood to be perfused through more vital regions. The vascular beds of the liver, lungs, and spleen are also important blood reservoirs. In the dog the spleen is packed with red blood cells and can constrict to a small fraction of its normal size. During hemorrhage, this mechanism autotransfuses blood of high erythrocyte content into the general circulation. However, in humans the volume changes of the spleen are considerably smaller.

Peripheral Resistance

The changes in the vascular function curve induced by changes in arteriolar tone are shown in Figure 9-7. The arterioles contain only about 3% of the total blood volume (see Table 1-1). Hence, changes in the contractile state of these vessels do not significantly alter the mean circulatory pressure, as stated previously. Thus, the family of vascular function curves representing different peripheral resistances converges at a common point on the ordinate.

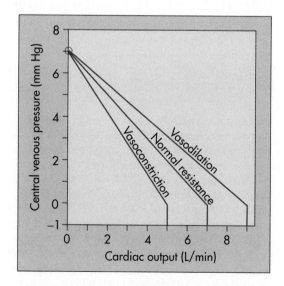

Figure 9-7 ■ **Effects of arteriolar vasodilation and vasoconstriction on the vascular function curve.**

At any given cardiac output, P_v varies inversely with the arteriolar tone, all other factors remaining constant. Arteriolar constriction sufficient to double the peripheral resistance will cause a twofold rise in P_a (see Chapter 6). In the example shown in Figure 9-4, a change in the cardiac output from 0 to 1 L/min (arrow *1*) caused P_a to rise from 7 to 26 mm Hg, an increment of 19 mm Hg. If peripheral resistance had been twice as great, the same change in cardiac output would have evoked twice as great an increment in P_a.

To achieve this greater rise in P_a, twice as great an increment in blood volume would be required on the arterial side of the circulation, if the arterial compliance remained constant. Given a constant total blood volume, this larger arterial volume signifies a corresponding reduction in venous volume. Hence, the decrement in venous volume would be twice as great when the peripheral resistance was doubled. If venous compliance remained constant, a twofold reduction in venous volume would be reflected by a twofold decline in P_v. Therefore, in Figure 9-4, an increase in cardiac output from 0 L/min to 1 L/min (arrow *1*) would have caused a 2 mm Hg decrement in P_v, to a level of 5 mm Hg, instead of the 1 mm Hg decrement that occurred with normal peripheral resistance. Similarly, greater increases in cardiac output would have evoked proportionately greater decrements in P_v under conditions of increased peripheral resistance than with normal levels of resistance.

This relationship between the peripheral resistance and the decrement in P_v, together with the failure of peripheral resistance to affect the mean circulatory pressure, accounts for the clockwise rotation of the vascular function curves with increased peripheral resistance (Figure 9-7). Conversely, arteriolar vasodilation produces a counterclockwise rotation from the same vertical axis intercept. A higher maximal level of cardiac output is attainable when the resistance vessels are dilated than when they are constricted.

■ INTERRELATIONSHIPS BETWEEN CARDIAC OUTPUT AND VENOUS RETURN

Cardiac output and venous return are inextricably interdependent. Clearly, except for small, transient disparities, the heart is unable to pump any more blood than is delivered to it through the venous system. Similarly, because the circulatory system is a closed circuit, the venous return must equal the cardiac output over any appreciable time interval. The flow around the entire closed circuit depends on the capability of the pump, the characteristics of the circuit, and the total volume of fluid in the system. Cardiac output and venous return are simply two terms for the flow around the closed circuit. Cardiac output is the volume of blood being pumped by the heart per unit time. Venous return is the volume of blood returning to the heart per unit time. At equilibrium, these two flows are equal.

The techniques of circuit analysis will be applied in an effort to gain some insight into the control of flow around the circuit. Acute changes in cardiac contractility, peripheral resistance, or blood volume may transiently affect cardiac output and venous return disparately. Except for such brief disparities, however, such factors simply alter flow around the entire circuit. Whether one thinks of that flow as "cardiac output" or "venous return" is irrelevant. Commonly, authors have ascribed the reduction in cardiac output during some intervention, such as hemorrhage, to a decrease in venous return. It will become clear that such an explanation is a blatant example of circular reasoning. Hemorrhage reduces flow around the entire circuit, for reasons to be elucidated. To attribute the reduction in cardiac output to a curtailment of venous return is equivalent to ascribing the decrease in total flow to a decrease in total flow!

■ COUPLING BETWEEN HEART AND VASCULATURE

In accordance with Starling's law of the heart, cardiac output is intimately dependent on the right atrial (or central venous) pressure. Furthermore, right atrial pressure is approximately equal to right ventricular end-diastolic pressure, because the normal tricuspid valve constitutes a low resistance junction between the right atrium and ventricle. In the discussion to follow, graphs of cardiac output as a function of central venous pressure (P_v) will be called **cardiac function curves.** Extrinsic regulatory influences may be expressed as shifts in such curves, as indicated previously (see Figure 4-19).

A typical cardiac function curve is plotted on the same coordinates as a normal vascular function curve in Figure 9-8. *The cardiac function*

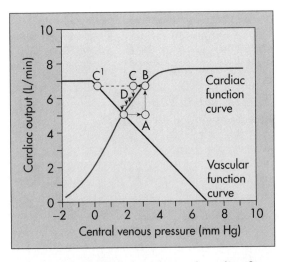

Figure 9-8 ■ Typical vascular and cardiac function curves plotted on the same coordinate axes. Note that to plot both curves on the same graph, it is necessary to reverse the X and Y axes for the vascular function curves shown in Figures 9-3, 9-6, and 9-7. The coordinates of the equilibrium point, at the intersection of the cardiac and vascular function curves, represent the stable values of cardiac output and central venous pressure at which the system tends to operate. Any perturbation (e.g., when venous pressure is suddenly increased to point *A*) institutes a sequence of changes in cardiac output and venous pressure that restore these variables to their equilibrium values.

curve is plotted according to the usual convention; that is, the variable (P_v) plotted along the abscissa is the **independent variable** (stimulus), and the variable (cardiac output) plotted along the ordinate is the **dependent variable** (response). In accordance with the Frank-Starling mechanism, the cardiac function curve reveals that a rise in P_v causes an increase in cardiac output.

Conversely, the vascular function curve describes an inverse relationship between cardiac output and P_v; that is, a rise in cardiac output causes a reduction in P_v. P_v is the dependent variable (or response) and cardiac output is the independent variable (or stimulus) for the vascular function curve. By convention, P_v should be scaled along the Y axis and cardiac output should be scaled along the X axis. Note that this convention is observed for the vascular function curves displayed in Figures 9-3, 9-6, and 9-7.

However, to include the vascular function curve on the same set of coordinate axes with the cardiac function curve (Figure 9-8), it is necessary to violate the plotting convention for one of these curves. *We have arbitrarily violated the convention for the vascular function curve.* Note that the vascular function curve in Figure 9-8 reflects how P_v (scaled along the X axis) varies in response to a change of cardiac output (scaled along the Y axis).

The **equilibrium point** of a system represented by a given pair of cardiac and vascular function curves is defined by the intersection of these two curves. The coordinates of this equilibrium point represent the values of cardiac output and P_v at which such a system tends to operate. Only transient deviations from such values for cardiac output and P_v are possible, as long as the given cardiac and vascular function curves accurately describe the system.

The tendency for the cardiovascular system to operate about such an equilibrium point may best be illustrated by examining its response to a sudden perturbation. Consider the changes elicited by a sudden rise in P_v from the equilib-

rium point to point A in Figure 9-8. Such a change might be induced by rapid injection, during ventricular diastole, of a given volume of blood on the venous side of the circuit, accompanied by withdrawal of an equal volume from the arterial side so that total blood volume would remain constant.

As defined by the cardiac function curve, this elevated P_v would increase cardiac output (A to B) during the very next ventricular systole. The increased cardiac output, in turn, would result in the net transfer of blood from the venous to the arterial side of the circuit, with a consequent reduction in P_v.

In one heartbeat, the reduction in P_v would be small (B to C) because the heart would transfer only a tiny fraction of the total venous blood volume over to the arterial side. Because of this reduction in P_v, the cardiac output during the very next beat diminishes (C to D) by an amount dictated by the cardiac function curve. Because D is still above the intersection point, the heart will pump blood from the veins to the arteries at a rate greater than that at which the blood will flow across the peripheral resistance from arteries to veins. Hence, P_v will continue to fall. This process will continue in diminishing steps until the point of intersection is reached. Only one specific combination of cardiac output and venous pressure (denoted by the coordinates of the point of intersection) will satisfy simultaneously the requirements of the cardiac and vascular function curves.

Myocardial Contractility

Combinations of cardiac and vascular function curves help explain the effects of alterations in ventricular contractility. In Figure 9-9 the lower cardiac function curve represents the control state, whereas the upper curve reflects an improved contractility. This pair of curves is analogous to the family of ventricular function curves shown in Figure 4-19. The enhancement of ventricular contractility might be achieved by electrical stimulation of the cardiac sympathetic nerves. If the effects of such stimulation were restricted to the heart, the vascular function curve would be unaffected. Therefore, one vascular function curve would suffice, as shown in Figure 9-9.

During the control state the equilibrium values for cardiac output and P_v are designated by point *A*. Cardiac sympathetic nerve stimulation would abruptly raise cardiac output to point *B*, because of the enhanced contractility, before P_v would change appreciably. However, this high cardiac output would increase the net transfer of blood from the venous to the arterial side of the circuit, and consequently P_v would then begin to fall (point *C*). Cardiac output would continue to fall until a new equilibrium point *(D)* was reached; this point is located at the intersection of the vascular function curve with the new cardiac function curve. The new equilibrium point

(D) lies above and to the left of the control equilibrium point *(A)*. This shift reveals that sympathetic stimulation evokes a greater cardiac output at a lower level of P_v.

Such a change accurately describes the true response. In the experiment depicted in Figure 9-10 the left stellate ganglion was stimulated between the two arrows. During stimulation, aortic flow (cardiac output) rose quickly to a peak value and then fell gradually to a steady-state value significantly greater than the control level. The increased aortic flow was accompanied by reductions in right and left atrial pressures (P_{RA} and P_{LA}). The initial abrupt rise in cardiac output in this experiment represents the shift from *A* to *B* in Figure 9-9, whereas the subsequent, more

Figure 9-10 ■ **During electrical stimulation of the left stellate ganglion (containing cardiac sympathetic nerve fibers), aortic blood flow increased while pressures in the left atrium *(P_{LA})* and right atrium *(P_{RA})* diminished. These data conform with the conclusions derived from Figure 9-9, in which the equilibrium values of cardiac output and venous pressure are observed to shift from point *A* to point *D* during cardiac sympathetic nerve stimulation.** (Redrawn from Sarnoff SJ, Brockman SK, Gilmore JP, Linden RJ, Mitchell JH: *Circ Res* 8:1108, 1960.)

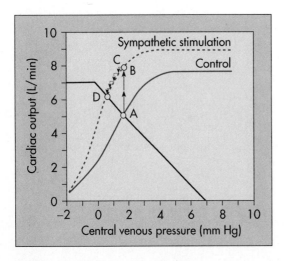

Figure 9-9 ■ **Enhancement of myocardial contractility, as by cardiac sympathetic nerve stimulation, causes the equilibrium values of cardiac output and P_v to shift from the intersection (point *A*) of the control vascular and cardiac function curves *(continuous lines)* to the intersection (point *D*) of the same vascular function curve with the cardiac function curve *(dashed line)* that represents enhanced myocardial contractility.**

gradual reductions in cardiac output and atrial pressure in the experiment represent the progressive shift from *B* to *D*.

Blood Volume

Changes in blood volume affect the vascular function curve in the manner shown in Figure 9-6. To understand the circulatory alterations evoked by a given change in blood volume, the appropriate cardiac function curve should be plotted along with the vascular function curves that represent the control and experimental states.

Figure 9-11 illustrates the response to a blood transfusion. Equilibrium point *B*, which denotes the values for cardiac output and P_v after transfusion, lies above and to the right of the control equilibrium point *A*. Thus, transfusion increases both cardiac output and P_v. Hemorrhage has the opposite effect. Mechanistically, the change in ventricular filling pressure (central venous pressure) evoked by a given change in blood volume alters cardiac output by changing the sensitivity of the

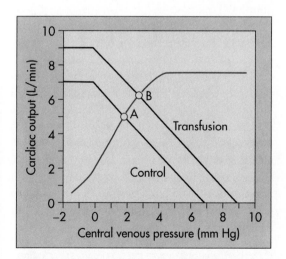

Figure 9-11 ■ **After a blood transfusion, the vascular function curve is shifted to the right. Therefore, cardiac output and venous pressure are both increased, as denoted by the translocation of the equilibrium point from *A* to *B*.**

contractile proteins to the prevailing level of intracellular Ca^{++}, as explained in Chapters 3 and 4. Pure increases or decreases in venomotor tone elicit responses analogous to those evoked by augmentations or reductions, respectively, of the total blood volume, for reasons discussed on page 202.

Heart Failure

Heart failure is the general term that refers to a number of conditions in which the heart is not able to provide adequate blood flow to the tissues of the body. Heart failure may be acute or chronic. Acute heart failure may be caused by toxic quantities of drugs and anesthetics or by certain pathologic conditions, such as a sudden coronary artery occlusion. Chronic heart failure may occur in such conditions as essential hypertension or ischemic heart disease. In these various forms of heart failure, myocardial contractility is impaired. Consequently, the cardiac function curve is shifted downward and to the right, as depicted in Figure 9-12.

In **acute heart failure,** blood volume does not change immediately. Therefore, the equilibrium point of the cardiac and vascular function curves will shift from the intersection of the normal curves (Figure 9-12, point *A*) to the intersection of the normal vascular function curve with a cardiac function curve that denotes impaired contractility (point *B* or *C*).

In **chronic heart failure,** both the cardiac function and vascular function curves shift. The vascular function curve shifts because of an increase in blood volume caused in part by fluid retention by the kidneys. The fluid retention is related to the concomitant reduction in glomerular filtration rate and to the increased secretion of aldosterone by the adrenal cortex. The resultant hypervolemia is reflected by a rightward shift of the vascular function curve, as shown in Figure 9-12. Hence, with moderate degrees of heart failure, P_v will be elevated, but cardiac output will be approximately normal (point *D*). With more severe degrees of heart failure, P_v will be still higher, but cardiac output will be subnormal (point *E*).

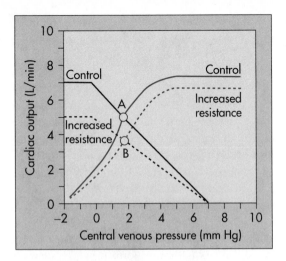

Figure 9-12 ■ With moderate or severe heart failure, the cardiac function curves are shifted to the right. Before any change in blood volume, cardiac output decreases and central venous pressure rises (from control equilibrium point *A* to point *B* or point *C*). After the increase in blood volume that usually occurs in heart failure, the vascular function curve is shifted to the right. Hence, central venous pressure may be elevated with no reduction in cardiac output (point *D*) or (in severe heart failure) with some diminution in cardiac output (point *E*).

Figure 9-13 ■ An increase in peripheral resistance shifts the cardiac and vascular function curves downward. At equilibrium the cardiac output is less *(B)* when the peripheral resistance is high than when it is normal *(A)*.

Peripheral Resistance

Predictions concerning the effects of changes in peripheral vascular resistance are also complex because both the cardiac and vascular function curves shift. With increased peripheral resistance (Figure 9-13), the vascular function curve is rotated counterclockwise, but it converges to the same P_v-axis intercept as the control curve (Figure 9-7); the direction of rotation differs in Figures 9-7 and 9-13 because the axes were switched for the vascular function curves in the two figures. The cardiac function curve is also shifted downward because (1) as peripheral resistance increases, arterial pressure (afterload) tends to rise; and (2) at any given P_v the heart is able to pump less blood against a greater after-

load. Because the cardiac and vascular function curves are both displaced downward, the new equilibrium point, *B*, will fall below the control point, *A*.

Whether point *B* will fall directly below point *A* or will lie to the right or left of point *A* depends on the magnitude of the shift in each curve. For example, if a given increase in peripheral resistance shifts the vascular function curve more than the cardiac function curve, equilibrium point *B* will fall below and to the left of *A*; that is, both cardiac output and P_v will diminish. Conversely, if the cardiac function curve is displaced more than the vascular function curve, point *B* will fall below and to the right of point *A*; that is, cardiac output will decrease but P_v will rise somewhat.

■ FUNCTION OF THE RIGHT VENTRICLE

Although the interrelations between cardiac output and central venous pressure are complicated and perplexing even in the simplified circulation

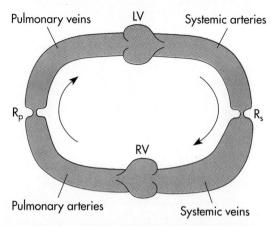

Figure 9-14 ■ **Simplified cardiovascular system model that consists of left** *(LV)* **and right** *(RV)* **ventricles, systemic** *(R_s)* **and pulmonary** *(R_p)* **vascular resistances, systemic arterial and venous compliances, and pulmonary arterial and venous compliances.**

model that includes just one pump and only the systemic circulation, the interrelations are much more complex when the systemic and pulmonary circulations and the left and right ventricles are included in the analysis. However, the systemic and pulmonary vascular systems are important components of the cardiovascular systems in mammals, and therefore the more complete model does merit some analysis.

Figure 9-14 shows a more complete, but still oversimplified, cardiovascular system model that contains two pumps in series (the left and right ventricles) and two vascular beds in series (the systemic and pulmonary vasculature). The series arrangement requires that the flows pumped by the two ventricles be virtually equal to each other over any substantial period; otherwise, the blood would ultimately accumulate in one or the other of the vascular systems. Because the cardiac function curves for the two ventricles differ substantially, the filling (atrial) pressures for the two ventricles must differ appropriately to ensure equal stroke volumes (see Figure 4-20).

Two basic tenets about ventricular function are that the left ventricle is the pump that forces blood through the systemic vasculature, and the right ventricle is the pump that forces blood through the pulmonary vasculature. Although these assertions are essentially correct, it is still instructive to examine right ventricular function in more detail.

Any change in contractility that affects the two ventricles disparately will alter the distribution of blood volume in the two vascular systems. For example, if a coronary artery to the left ventricle becomes occluded suddenly, left ventricular contractility will be impaired and **left ventricular failure** will ensue. Instantaneously, left atrial pressure will not change and the left ventricle will begin to pump a diminished flow. If the right ventricle is not affected by the acute coronary artery occlusion, the right ventricle will initially continue to pump the normal flow. The disparate right and left ventricular outputs will result in a progressive increase in left atrial pressure and a progressive decrease in right atrial pressure. Therefore, left ventricular output will increase toward the normal value and the right ventricular output will fall below the normal value. This process will continue until the outputs of the two ventricles become equal to each other again. At this new equilibrium, the outputs of the two ventricles will be subnormal. The elevated left atrial pressure will be accompanied by an equally elevated pulmonary venous pressure, which can have serious clinical consequences. The high pulmonary venous pressure can increase lung stiffness and lead to respiratory distress by increasing the mechanical work of pulmonary ventilation. Furthermore, the high pulmonary venous pressure will elevate the hydrostatic pressure in the pulmonary capillaries, and hence may lead to transudation of fluid from the pulmonary capillaries to the pulmonary interstitium or into the alveoli themselves **(pulmonary edema).** The last of these consequences may be lethal.

Consider the effect on the circulatory system model in Figure 9-14 if the right ventricle suddenly ceases to function as a pump, but instead serves as a passive, low-resistance conduit between the systemic veins and the pulmonary arteries. In such a circulatory system, the only pump would then be the left ventricle. The left ventricle would now be required to pump blood through two vascular resistances in series, namely, the systemic and pulmonary resistances (we shall consider the resistance of the right ventricle itself to be negligible).

Normally, pulmonary resistance is about 10% as great as systemic resistance. Because the two resistances are in series with one another, the total resistance would be 10% greater than the systemic resistance alone (see Chapter 5). In a normal cardiovascular system, a 10% increase in systemic vascular resistance would increase mean arterial pressure (and hence left ventricular afterload) by approximately 10%, which would not affect left ventricular function drastically. *However, when the 10% increase in total resistance is achieved by adding a small resistance (namely, the pulmonary resistance) downstream of the systemic resistance, and that resistance is separated from the systemic resistance by a large compliance (the combined systemic venous and pulmonary arterial compliance), the 10% increase in total resistance will then dramatically affect the cardiovascular system.*

The simulated effects of inactivating the pumping action of the right ventricle in a hydraulic analog of the circulatory system are shown in Figure 9-15. In the model, the right and left ventricles generate cardiac outputs that vary directly with their respective filling pressures. Under control conditions, the output of the right ventricle (5 L/min) is equal to that of the left ventricle. The right ventricular pumping action causes the pressure in the pulmonary artery to exceed the pressure in the pulmonary veins by

Figure 9-15 ■ **The changes in cardiac output, systemic arterial pressure *(Pₐₛ)*, systemic venous pressure *(Pᵥₛ)*, and pulmonary venous pressure *(Pᵥₚ)* evoked by simulated right ventricular failure and by simulated fluid infusion in the circulatory model shown in Figure 9-14. At arrow *1*, the pumping action of the right ventricle was discontinued (simulated right ventricular failure) and the right ventricle served only as a low-resistance conduit. At arrow *2*, fluid volume was expanded and the right ventricle continued to serve only as a conduit.** (Modified from Furey SA, Zieske HA, Levy MN: *Am Heart J* 107:404, 1984.)

an amount that will force fluid through the pulmonary vascular resistance at a rate of 5 L/min. When the right ventricle ceases pumping (arrow *1*), the systemic venous and pulmonary arterial systems become a common passive conduit with a large compliance; pulmonary arterial pressure decreases *(not shown)* and systemic venous pressure rises to a common value (5 mm Hg in Figure 9-15). At this low pressure, however, fluid flows from the pulmonary arteries to the pulmonary veins at a greatly reduced rate. At the same time, the left ventricle initially pumps fluid from the pulmonary veins to the systemic arteries at the control rate of 5 L/min. Hence, pulmonary venous pressure drops precipitously. Because pulmonary venous pressure is the preload for the left ventricle, left ventricular (cardiac) output also drops abruptly. This effect in turn results in a rapid reduction in systemic arterial pressure. In summary, cessation of right ventricular pumping causes marked reductions in cardiac output, systemic arterial pressure, and pulmonary venous pressure and a modest rise in systemic venous pressure (Figure 9-15).

Most of the hemodynamic problems induced by inactivating the right ventricle can be reversed by increasing the fluid (blood) volume of the system (arrow *2*, Figure 9-15). If fluid is added until pulmonary venous pressure (left ventricular preload) is raised to its control value, cardiac output and systemic arterial pressure are restored to normal, but systemic venous pressure is abnormally elevated. In a human subject, such a rise in systemic venous pressure may lead to the accumulation of fluid **(edema)** in the dependent regions of the body; such edema is characteristic of **right heart failure.**

In summary, severe contractile failure of the right ventricle is the equivalent of overstressing the left ventricle by adding in series a relatively small (10%) hydraulic resistance (pulmonary vascular resistance) to the normal systemic vascular resistance. Ordinarily, increasing the systemic vascular resistance itself by 10% does not seriously stress the cardiovascular system. However, when the 10% additional resistance is downstream of the systemic venous bed (which has a very large compliance), it may diminish cardiac output drastically. The main compensatory response of the body is to increase blood volume, in part by renal retention of fluid and electrolytes. However, this compensatory response may lead to severe peripheral edema.

With these findings in mind, we might reassess the principal function of the right ventricle as follows. From the viewpoint of providing sufficient flow of blood to all the tissues in the body, the left ventricle alone is adequate to carry out this function; the operation of two ventricles in series is not essential to provide adequate blood flow to the tissues. *The crucial function of the right ventricle is therefore to prevent the rise in systemic venous (and pulmonary arterial) pressure that would be required to force the normal cardiac output through the pulmonary vascular resistance.* By preventing the abnormal rise in systemic venous pressure, extensive dependent edema is averted.

■ ROLE OF HEART RATE

Cardiac output is the product of stroke volume and heart rate. The above analysis of the control of cardiac output was, in reality, restricted to the

---

In humans, **right heart failure** may be caused by occlusive disease predominantly of the coronary vessels to the right ventricle; these vessels are affected much less commonly than are the vessels to the left ventricle. The major hemodynamic effects of acute right heart failure are pronounced reductions in cardiac output and in arterial blood pressure, and the principal treatment consists of infusion of blood or plasma. Bypass of the right ventricle is not infrequently implemented surgically for patients with certain **congenital cardiac defects,** such as severe narrowing of the tricuspid valve or maldevelopment of the right ventricle. The effects of acute right heart failure or of right ventricular bypass are directionally similar to those predicted by the model study (Figure 9-15).

control of stroke volume, and the role of heart rate was neglected.

The effect of changes in heart rate on cardiac output will now be considered. The analysis is complex, because a change in heart rate alters the other three factors (preload, afterload, and contractility) that determine stroke volume (Figure 9-1). An increase in heart rate, for example, would decrease the duration of diastole. Hence, ventricular filling would be diminished; that is, preload would be reduced. If the proposed increase in heart rate did alter cardiac output, the arterial pressure would change; that is, afterload would be altered. Finally, the rise in heart rate would increase the net influx of Ca^{++} per minute into the myocardial cells, and this would enhance myocardial contractility (see Chapter 4).

Heart rate has been varied by artificial pacing in many types of experimental preparations and in humans. The effects on cardiac output have usually resembled the experimental results shown in Figure 9-16. In that experiment, as the atrial pacing frequency was gradually increased in an anesthetized dog, the stroke volume progressively diminished (Figure 9-16, *A*). Presumably, the curtailment of stroke volume was induced by the abridged time for ventricular filling. However, the change in cardiac output induced by a change in heart rate was influenced markedly by the actual level of the heart rate. In this experiment, for example, as the pacing frequency was increased within the range of 50 to 100 beats/min, an increase in heart rate augmented the cardiac output (Q_h). Presumably, over this lower frequency range, the reduction in stroke volume (SV) evoked by a given increase in heart rate (HR) was proportionately less than the increase in heart rate itself; that is, because $Q_h = SV \times HR$, if a given increment in HR exceeds the induced decrement in SV, the induced Q_h will be greater than the initial Q_h.

Over the frequency range from about 100 to 200 beats/min, however, cardiac output was not

Figure 9-16 ■ The changes in stroke volume (A) and cardiac output (B) induced by changing the rate of atrial pacing in an anesthetized dog. (Redrawn from Kumada M, Azuma T, Matsuda K: *Jpn J Physiol* 17:538, 1967.)

affected appreciably by changes in pacing frequency (Figure 9-16, *B*). Hence, as the pacing frequency was increased, the stroke volume needed to decrease proportionately to the increase in heart rate. Finally, at excessively high pacing frequencies (above 200 beats/min), increments in heart rate decreased the cardiac output. Therefore, the induced decrement in SV must have exceeded the increment in HR over this high range of pacing frequencies. Although the relationship of Q_h to HR is characteristically that of an inverted U, the relationship varies quantitatively among subjects and among physiologic states in any given subject.

Attribution of causation to observed correlations between cardiac output and heart rate should be made very cautiously. During physical exercise, for example, cardiac output and

The characteristic relationship between cardiac output and heart rate explains the urgent need for treatment of patients who have excessively slow or excessively fast heart rates. Profound **bradycardias** (slow rates) may occur as the result of a very slow sinus rhythm in patients with **sick sinus syndrome** or as the result of a slow idioventricular rhythm in patients with **complete atrioventricular block.** In either rhythm disturbance, the capacity of the ventricles to fill during a prolonged diastole is limited (often by the noncompliant pericardium). Hence, cardiac output usually decreases substantially, because the very slow heart rate cannot be overcome by a sufficiently great stroke volume. Consequently, these rhythm disturbances often require installation of an artificial pacemaker.

At the other end of the heart rate spectrum, excessively high heart rates in patients with **supraventricular** or **ventricular tachycardias** often require emergency treatment because their cardiac outputs may be critically low. In such patients, the filling time is so restricted at very high heart rates that small additional reductions in filling time elicit disproportionately severe reductions in filling volume. Reversion of the tachycardia to a more normal rhythm can usually be accomplished pharmacologically, but **cardioversion,** delivering a strong electrical current across the thorax or directly to the heart through an implanted device, may be required in emergencies.

heart rate often rise proportionately, and stroke volume may change very little (see Chapter 12). The temptation is great to conclude that the increase in cardiac output must be caused by the observed increase in heart rate, because of the striking correlation between cardiac output and heart rate. However, Figure 9-16 emphasizes that, over a wide range of heart rates, a change in heart rate has little influence on cardiac output. Several studies on exercising subjects have confirmed that, even during exercise, changes in pacing frequency over a substantial frequency range do not alter cardiac output very much.

The principal increase in cardiac output during exercise must therefore be ascribed to (1) the pronounced reduction in peripheral vascular resistance, (2) the positive inotropic effect of the increased sympathetic neural activity on the ventricular myocardium, and (3) the auxiliary pumping action of the contracting skeletal muscles, combined with the directional effects on blood flow effected by the venous valves (as explained toward the end of this chapter). The attendant changes in heart rate are not inconsequential, however. If the heart rate cannot increase normally during exercise, the augmentation of cardiac output and the capacity for exercise may be severely limited. The increase in heart rate does play a *permissive role* in augmenting cardiac output, even if it is not proper to assign it a primary, causative role. The mechanisms responsible for raising heart rate in precise proportion to the increase in cardiac output are undoubtedly neural in origin, but the specific components of the reflex arcs have not yet been elucidated.

■ ANCILLARY FACTORS THAT AFFECT THE VENOUS SYSTEM AND CARDIAC OUTPUT

We have explained the interrelationships between central venous pressure and cardiac output in an oversimplified fashion, and we have described the effects evoked by changes in isolated variables. However, because many feedback control loops regulate the cardiovascular system, an isolated change in a single response rarely occurs. A change in blood volume, for example, reflexly alters cardiac function, peripheral resistance, and venomotor tone. Several auxiliary factors also regulate cardiac output. Such ancillary factors may be considered to modulate the more basic factors that we have considered above.

Gravity

Gravitational forces may affect cardiac output profoundly. It is not unusual for some soldiers standing at attention to faint because of reduced cardiac output. Gravitational effects are exaggerated in airplane pilots during pullouts from dives. The centrifugal force in the footward direction may be several times greater than the force of gravity. Such individuals characteristically black out momentarily during the maneuver, as blood is drained from the cephalic regions and pooled in the lower parts of the body.

The explanation for the reduction in cardiac output under such conditions is often specious. It is argued that when an individual is standing, the forces of gravity impede venous return from the dependent regions of the body. This statement is incomplete, however, because it ignores the facilitative counterforce on the arterial side of the same circuit.

In this sense the vascular system resembles a U tube. To comprehend the action of gravity on flow through such a system, the models depicted in Figures 9-17 and 9-18 will be analyzed. In Figure 9-17, all the U tubes represent rigid cylinders of constant diameter. With both limbs of the U tube oriented horizontally *(A)*, the flow depends only on the pressures at the inflow and outflow ends of the tube (P_i and P_o, respectively), the viscosity of the fluid, and the length and radius of the tube, in accordance with Poiseuille's equation (see Chapter 5). With a constant cross section, the pressure gradient will be uniform; hence, the pressure midway down the tube (P_m) will equal the average of the inflow and outflow pressures.

When the U tube is oriented vertically *(B* to *D)*, hydrostatic forces must be taken into consideration. In tube *B*, both limbs are open to atmospheric pressure and both ends are located at the same hydrostatic level; hence, there is no flow. The pressure at the midpoint of the tube will simply be ρhg. The pressure will depend on the

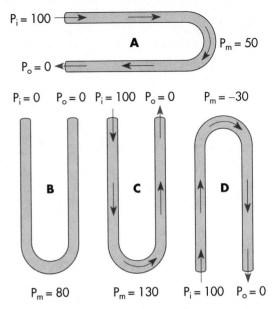

Figure 9-17 ■ **Pressure distributions in rigid U tubes with constant internal diameters, all with the same dimensions. For a given inflow pressure (P_i = 100) and outflow pressure (P_o = 0), the pressure at the midpoint (P_m) depends on the orientation of the U tube, but the flow through the tube is independent of the orientation.**

density of the fluid, ρ; the height of the U tube, h; and the acceleration of gravity, g. In the example, the length of the U tube is such that the midpoint pressure is 80 mm Hg.

Now consider tube *C*, where the tube is oriented the same as tube *B*, but where a 100 mm Hg pressure difference is applied across the two ends. The flow will precisely equal that in *A*, because the pressure gradient, tube dimensions, and fluid viscosity are all the same. Gravitational forces are precisely equal in magnitude but opposite in direction in the two limbs of the U tube. Because the flow will be the same as that in *A*, there will be a pressure drop of 50 mm Hg at the midpoint because of the viscous losses resulting from flow. Furthermore, gravity will tend to increase pressure by 80 mm Hg at the mid-

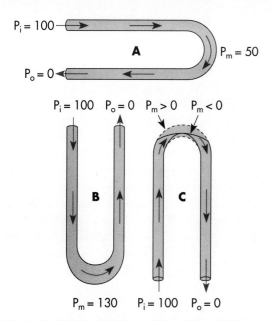

$P_i = 100$ **A** $P_m = 50$

$P_o = 0$

$P_i = 100$ $P_o = 0$ $P_m > 0$ $P_m < 0$

B   **C**

$P_m = 130$ $P_i = 100$ $P_o = 0$

Figure 9-18 ■ **In U tubes with a distensible section at the bend, even when inflow (P_i) and outflow (P_o) pressures are the same, the resistance to flow, and the fluid volume contained within each tube, vary with the orientation of the tube. P_m, Pressure at the midpoint of the tube.**

point, just as in tube B. The actual pressure at the midpoint of tube C will be the result of the viscous loss and hydrostatic gain, or 130 mm Hg in this example.

In D a pressure gradient of 100 mm Hg is applied to the same U tube, but the tube is oriented in the opposite direction. Gravitational forces will be so directed that the pressure at the midpoint will tend to be 80 mm Hg less than that at the end of the U tube. Viscous losses will still produce a 50 mm Hg pressure drop at the midpoint relative to P_i. Hence, with this orientation, pressure at the midpoint of the U tube will be 30 mm Hg below ambient pressure. Flow will, of course, be the same as in tubes A and C, for the reasons stated in relation to C.

In a system of rigid U tubes, gravitational effects will not alter the rate of fluid flow. However, experience shows that gravity does affect the cardiovascular system. The reason is that the vessels are distensible rather than rigid. To explain the gravitational effects, the pressures in a set of U tubes with distensible components (at the bends in the tubes of Figure 9-18) will be examined. In tubes A and B the pressure distributions will resemble those in tubes A and C, respectively, in Figure 9-17. Because the pressure is higher at the bend of tube B than at the bend of tube A in Figure 9-18 and because the segments are distensible in this region, the distension at the bend in tube B will exceed that at the bend in tube A. The extent of the distension will depend on the compliance of these tube segments. Because flow varies directly with the tube diameter, the flow through B will exceed the flow through A for a given pressure difference applied at the ends.

Orienting a U tube with its bend downward actually increases rather than diminishes flow; how then is the observed impairment of cardiovascular function explained when the body is similarly oriented? The explanation is that the cardiovascular system is a closed circuit of constant fluid (blood) volume, whereas the U tube is an open conduit supplied by a fluid source of unlimited volume. In the dependent regions of the cardiovascular system, the distension will occur more on the venous than on the arterial side of the circuit, because the venous compliance is so much greater than the arterial compliance. Such venous distension is readily observed on the back of the hands when the arms are allowed to hang down. The hemodynamic effects of such venous distension (**venous pooling**) resemble those caused by the hemorrhage of an equivalent volume of blood from the body. When an adult person shifts from a supine position to a relaxed standing position, 300 to 800 ml of blood are pooled in the legs. This may reduce cardiac output by about 2 L/min.

The compensatory adjustments to the erect position are similar to the adjustments to blood loss. For example, the diminished baroreceptor excitation reflexly speeds the heart, strengthens the cardiac contraction, and constricts the arterioles and veins. The baroreceptor reflex has a greater effect on the resistance than on the capacitance vessels. Warm ambient temperatures interfere with the compensatory vasomotor reactions, and the absence of muscular activity exaggerates the effects.

When the U tube is rotated so that the bend is directed upward (Figure 9-18, tube *C*), the effects are opposite to those that take place in tube *B*. The pressure at the bend of tube *C* would tend to be −30 mm Hg, just as in tube *D* of Figure 9-17. Because the ambient pressure exceeds the internal pressure, however, the distensible segment of tube *C* will collapse. Flow will then cease, and therefore the pressure decrease associated with viscous flow will not occur. In U tube *C,* when flow stops, the pressure at the top of each limb will be 80 mm Hg less than at the bottom (the hydrostatic pressure difference). Hence, in the left, or inflow, limb the pressure will begin to rise rapidly from a negative value. If the tube remained collapsed at the bend, the pressure to the left of the collapsed segment would rapidly approach 20 mm Hg. However, as soon as this pressure exceeds ambient pressure (0 mm Hg), the collapsed tubing will be forced open and flow will begin. With the onset of flow, however, pressure at the bend will again drop below the ambient pressure. *Thus, the tubing at the bend will flutter; that is, it will fluctuate between the open and closed states.*

When an arm is raised, the cutaneous veins in the hand and forearm collapse, for the reasons described previously. Fluttering does not occur here because the deeper veins are protected from collapse by being tethered to surrounding structures. This protection allows these deeper veins to accommodate the flow ordinarily carried by the collapsed superficial veins. The analogy would be to add a rigid tube (representing the deeper veins) in parallel with the collapsible tube (representing the superficial veins) at the bend of tube *C* in Figure 9-18. The collapsible tube would no longer flutter but would remain closed. All flow would occur through the rigid tube, just as in tube *D* in Figure 9-17.

Muscular Activity and Venous Valves

When a recumbent person stands but remains at rest, the pressure rises in the veins in the dependent regions of the body. The venous pressure in the legs increases gradually and does not reach an equilibrium value until almost 1 minute after standing. The slowness of this rise in P_v is attributable to the venous valves, which permit flow only toward the heart. When the person stands, the valves prevent blood in the veins from actually falling toward the feet. Hence, the column of venous blood is supported at numerous

---

Many of the drugs used to treat **hypertension** also interfere with the reflex adaptation to standing. Similarly, astronauts exposed to weightlessness lose their adaptations after a few days in space, and experience difficulties when they first return to earth. When individuals with impaired reflex adaptations stand, their blood pressure may drop substantially. This response is called **orthostatic hypotension,** which may cause lightheadedness or fainting.

The superficial veins in the neck are ordinarily partially collapsed when a normal individual is upright. Blood returns to the heart from the head mainly through the deeper cervical veins. However, when central venous pressure is abnormally elevated, the superficial neck veins are distended and do not collapse even when the subject sits or stands. Such cervical venous distension is an important clinical sign of **congestive heart failure.**

levels by these valves; temporarily, the venous column consists of many discontinuous segments. However, blood continues to enter the column from many venules and small tributary veins, and the pressure continues to rise. As soon as the pressure in one segment exceeds that in the segment just above it, the intervening valve is forced open. Ultimately, all the valves are open and the column is continuous, similar to the state in the outflow limbs of the U tubes shown in Figures 9-17 and 9-18.

Precise measurement reveals that the final level of P_v in the feet during quiet standing is only slightly greater than that in a static column of blood extending from the right atrium to the feet. This indicates that the pressure drop caused by blood flow from the foot veins to the right atrium is very small. This very low resistance justifies lumping all the veins as a common venous compliance in the circulatory system model illustrated in Figure 9-2.

When an individual who has been standing quietly begins to walk, the venous pressure in the legs decreases appreciably (see Figure 9-19).

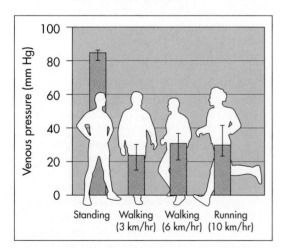

Figure 9-19 ■ Mean pressures (± 95% confidence intervals) in the foot veins of 18 people during quiet standing, walking, and running. (From Stick C, Jaeger H, Witzleb E: *J Appl Physiol* 72:2063, 1992.)

Because of the intermittent venous compression exerted by the contracting leg muscles and because of the presence of the venous valves, blood is forced from the veins toward the heart (see Figure 11-2). Hence, *muscular contraction lowers the mean venous pressure in the legs and serves as an auxiliary pump.* Furthermore, it prevents venous pooling and lowers capillary hydrostatic pressure. Thereby, it reduces the tendency for edema fluid to collect in the feet during standing.

Respiratory Activity

The normal, periodic activity of the respiratory muscles causes rhythmic variations in vena caval flow. Thus, respiration constitutes an auxiliary pump to promote venous return. Coughing, straining at stool, and other activities that require respiratory muscle exertion may affect cardiac output substantially.

The changes in blood flow in the superior vena cava during the normal respiratory cycle are shown in Figure 9-20. During respiration the reduction in intrathoracic pressure is transmitted to the lumina of the intrathoracic blood vessels. The reduction in central venous pressure during inspiration increases the pressure gradient between extrathoracic and intrathoracic veins. The consequent acceleration of venous return to the right

---

This auxiliary pumping mechanism is not very effective in people with **varicose veins** in their legs. The valves in such veins do not operate properly, and therefore when the leg muscles contract, the blood in the leg veins is forced in the retrograde as well as in the antegrade direction. Thus, when an individual with varicose veins stands or walks, the venous pressure in the ankles and feet is excessively high. The consequent high capillary pressure leads to the accumulation of edema fluid in the ankles and feet.

atrium is displayed in Figure 9-20 as an increase in superior vena caval blood flow from 5.2 ml/s during expiration to 11 ml/s during inspiration.

An exaggerated reduction in intrathoracic pressure achieved by a strong inspiratory effort against a closed glottis (called **Müller's maneuver**) does not increase venous return proportionately. The extrathoracic veins collapse near their entry into the chest when their internal pressures fall below the ambient level. As the veins collapse, flow into the chest momentarily stops. The cessation of flow raises pressure upstream, forcing the collapsed segment to open again. The process is repetitive; the venous segments adjacent to the chest alternately open and close.

During normal expiration, flow into the central veins decelerates. However, the mean rate of venous return during normal respiration exceeds the flow during a brief period of **apnea** (cessation of respiration). Hence, normal inspiration apparently facilitates venous return more than

normal expiration impedes it. In part, this must be attributable to the valves in the veins of the extremities and neck. These valves prevent any reversal of flow during expiration. Thus, the respiratory muscles and venous valves constitute an **auxiliary pump** for venous return.

Sustained expiratory efforts increase intrathoracic pressure and thereby impede venous return. Straining against a closed glottis (termed **Valsalva's maneuver**) regularly occurs during coughing, defecation, and heavy lifting. Intrathoracic pressures in excess of 100 mm Hg have been recorded in trumpet players, and pressures over 400 mm Hg have been observed during paroxysms of coughing. Such pressure increases are transmitted directly to the lumina of the intrathoracic arteries. After cessation of coughing the arterial blood pressure may fall precipitously because of the preceding impediment to venous return.

Figure 9-20 ▪ During a normal inspiration, intrathoracic *(ITP)*, right atrial *(RAP)*, and jugular venous *(JVP)* pressures decrease, and flow in the superior vena cava *(SVCF)* increases (from 5.2 to 11 ml/s). All pressures are in millimeters of water, except for femoral arterial pressure *(FAP)*, which is in millimeters of mercury. (Modified from Brecher GA: *Venous return,* New York, 1956, Grune & Stratton.)

The intense, brief increases in intrathoracic pressure induced by coughing constitute an **auxiliary pumping mechanism** for the blood, despite its concurrent tendency to impede venous return momentarily. During certain diagnostic procedures, such as coronary angiography or electrophysiologic testing, patients are at increased risk for **ventricular fibrillation.** Such patients have been trained to cough rhythmically on command. If ventricular fibrillation does occur, substantial arterial blood pressure increments are generated by each cough, and enough cerebral blood flow may be promoted to sustain consciousness and to preserve the viability of the cerebral tissues. The cough raises the intravascular pressure equally in intrathoracic arteries and veins. Blood is propelled through the extrathoracic tissues, however, because the increased pressure is transmitted to the extrathoracic arteries but not to the extrathoracic veins. The venous valves prevent transmission of the intrathoracic pressure to the extrathoracic veins.

Artificial Respiration

In most forms of artificial respiration (mouth-to-mouth resuscitation, mechanical respiration), lung inflation is achieved by applying endotracheal pressures above atmospheric pressure, and expiration occurs by passive recoil of the thoracic cage. Thus, lung inflation is attended by an appreciable rise in intrathoracic pressure. Vena caval flow decreases sharply during the phase of positive-pressure lung inflation (indicated by the progressive rise in endotracheal pressure in the central portion of Figure 9-21). When negative endotracheal pressure (indicated by the abrupt decrease in endotracheal pressure in the right half of Figure 9-21) is used to facilitate deflation, vena caval flow accelerates more than when the lungs are allowed to deflate passively (near the left border of Figure 9-21).

■ SUMMARY

1. Two important relationships between cardiac output (CO) and central venous pressure (P_v) prevail in the cardiovascular system. One applies to the heart and the other to the vascular system.

  a. With respect to the heart, CO varies directly with P_v (or preload) over a very wide range of P_v. This relationship is represented by the cardiac function curve, and it expresses the Frank-Starling mechanism.

  b. With respect to the vascular system, P_v varies inversely with CO. This relationship is represented by the vascular function curve, and it reflects the fact that as CO increases, for example, a greater fraction of the total blood volume resides in the arteries and a smaller volume resides in the veins.

2. The principal mechanism that governs the cardiac function curve is the change in the affinity of the contractile proteins for calcium. This effect is evoked by changes in the cardiac filling pressure (preload).

3. The principal factors that govern the vascular function curve are the arterial and venous

Figure 9-21 ■ During intermittent positive-pressure respiration, the flow in the superior vena cava is approximately 30% greater when the lungs are deflated actively by applying negative endotracheal pressure *(right side)* than when they are allowed to deflate passively against atmospheric pressure *(left side).* (Modified from Brecher GA: *Venous return,* New York, 1956, Grune & Stratton.)

compliances, the peripheral vascular resistance, and the total blood volume.

4. The equilibrium values of CO and P_v that prevail under a given set of conditions are determined by the intersection of the cardiac and vascular function curves.

5. At very low and very high heart rates, the heart is unable to pump an adequate CO. At the very low rates, the increment in filling during diastole cannot compensate for the small number of cardiac contractions per minute. At the very high rates, the large number of contractions per minute cannot compensate for the inadequate filling time.

6. Gravity influences CO because the veins are so compliant, and substantial quantities of blood tend to pool in the veins of the dependent portions of the body.

7. Respiration changes the pressure gradient between the intrathoracic and extrathoracic veins. Hence, respiration serves as an auxiliary pump, which may alter the mean level of CO and may induce rhythmic changes in stroke volume during the various phases of the respiratory cycle.

■ KEY WORDS AND CONCEPTS

- Determinants of cardiac output
- Central venous pressure
- Cardiac function curve
- Vascular function curve
- Arterial compliance
- Venous compliance
- Peripheral runoff
- Mean circulatory pressure
- Static circulatory pressure
- Venous pressure dependence on cardiac output
- Vascular hypervolemia
- Vascular hypovolemia
- Venomotor tone

- Blood reservoirs
- Total peripheral vascular resistance
- Coupling between heart and vessels
- Heart failure
- Aldosterone
- Effect of heart rate on cardiac output
- Function of the right ventricle
- Right ventricular failure
- Left ventricular failure
- Pulmonary edema
- Effect of gravity on cardiac output
- Venous pooling
- Orthostatic hypotension
- Role of venous valves
- Skeletal muscles as auxiliary blood pumps
- Effect of respiration on cardiac output
- Müller's maneuver
- Valsalva's maneuver

■ SELF-STUDY PROBLEMS

1. Is the ventricular preload a determinant of cardiac performance, or does cardiac performance determine the preload?

2. What effect does the arterial blood pressure have on cardiac performance?

3. If isoproterenol was infused into the left coronary artery at such a rate that it would influence myocardial contractility exclusively, what effects would that infusion have on cardiac output and central venous pressure?

4. If 2 L of blood were infused into a normal human subject, what influence would that transfusion have on cardiac output and central venous pressure?

5. If a person with a healthy myocardium suddenly develops complete atrioventricular block and the ventricular rate becomes 35 beats/min, what will happen to cardiac output and central venous pressure?

6. If a person is strapped to a tilt table in such a manner that he or she will not have to use the skeletal muscles when tilted to the upright position, what will happen to the cardiac out-

put, mean arterial pressure, central venous pressure, and pressure in a foot vein when the person is tilted to that position?

■ BIBLIOGRAPHY

Journal articles

Aukland K: Why don't our feet swell in the upright position? *News Physiol Soc* 9:214, 1994.

Ferlinz J: Right ventricular function in adult cardiovascular disease, *Prog Cardiovasc Dis* 25:225, 1982.

Freeman GL, Little WC, O'Rourke RA: Influence of heart rate on left ventricular performance in conscious dogs, *Circ Res* 61:455, 1987.

Furey SA, Zieske HA, Levy MN: The essential function of the right ventricle, *Am Heart J* 107:404, 1984.

Geddes LA, Wessale JL: Cardiac output, stroke volume, and pacing rate, *J Cardiovasc Electrophysiol* 2:408, 1991.

Lacolley PJ, Pannier BM, Cuche J-L et al: Microgravity and orthostatic intolerance: carotid hemodynamics and peripheral responses, *Am J Physiol* 264:H588, 1993.

Levy MN: The cardiac and vascular factors that determine systemic blood flow, *Circ Res* 44:739, 1979.

Monos E, Berczi V, Nadasy G: Local control of veins: biomechanical, metabolic, and humoral aspects, *Physiol Rev* 75:611, 1995.

Risöe C, Tan W, Smiseth OA: Effect of carotid sinus baroreceptor reflex on hepatic and splenic vascular capacitance in vagotomized dogs, *Am J Physiol* 266:H1528, 1994.

Rothe CF: Mean circulatory filling pressure: its meaning and measurement, *J Appl Physiol* 74:499, 1993.

Seymour RS, Hargens AR, Pedley TJ: The heart works against gravity, *Am J Physiol* 265:R715, 1993.

Sheriff DD, Zhou XP, Scher AM, Rowell LB: Dependence of cardiac filling pressure on cardiac output during rest and dynamic exercise in dogs, *Am J Physiol* 265:H316, 1993.

Shoukas AA: Overall systems analysis of the carotid sinus baroreceptor reflex control of the circulation, *Anesthesiology* 79:1402, 1993.

Shoukas AA, Bohlen HG: Rat venular pressure-diameter relationships are regulated by sympathetic activity, *Am J Physiol* 259:H674, 1990.

Stick C, Jaeger H, Witzleb E: Measurement of volume changes and venous pressure in the human lower leg during walking and running, *J Appl Physiol* 72:2063, 1992.

Tyberg JV: Venous modulation of ventricular preload, *Am Heart J* 123:1098, 1992.

Ursino M, Antonucci M, Belardinelli E: Role of active changes in venous capacity by the carotid baroreflex: analysis with a mathematical model, *Am J Physiol* 267:H2531, 1994.

Books and monographs

Guyton AC, Jones CE, Coleman TG: *Circulatory physiology: cardiac output and its regulation,* ed 2, Philadelphia, 1973, WB Saunders.

Rothe CF: *Venous system: physiology of the capacitance vessels.* In *Handbook of physiology,* Section 2: *The cardiovascular system—peripheral circulation and organ blood flow,* vol III, Bethesda, Md., 1983, American Physiological Society.

Smith JJ, editor: *Circulatory response to the upright posture,* Boca Raton, Fla., 1990, CRC Press.

Yin FCP, editor: *Ventricular/vascular coupling,* New York, 1987, Springer-Verlag.

Coronary Circulation

■ FUNCTIONAL ANATOMY OF CORONARY VESSELS

The right and left coronary arteries, which arise at the root of the aorta behind the right and left cusps of the aortic valve, respectively, provide the entire blood supply to the myocardium. The right coronary artery supplies principally the right ventricle and atrium; the left coronary artery, which divides near its origin into the anterior descending and the circumflex branches, supplies principally the left ventricle and atrium, but there is some overlap. In humans the right coronary artery is dominant in 50% of individuals, the left coronary artery is dominant in another 20%, and the flow delivered by each main artery is about equal in the remaining 30%. The epicardial distribution of the coronary arteries and veins is illustrated in Figure 10-1.

Coronary blood flow is most commonly measured in humans by thermodilution. Thermodilution is the same procedure used for the measurement of cardiac output (p 78), except that the indicator (cold saline) is ejected at the tip of a catheter inserted into the coronary sinus via a peripheral vein. The thermal sensor (thermistor) is located on the catheter a few centimeters from the catheter tip. The greater the coronary sinus outflow, the less is the temperature decrease produced by the cold saline injection. This method does not measure total coronary blood flow because only about two thirds of coronary arterial inflow returns to the venous circulation through the coronary sinus. However, almost all the blood flow that does empty into the coronary sinus comes from the left ventricle. Hence, the thermodilution method provides a good estimate of left ventricular coronary blood flow. Right and left coronary artery inflow, as well as inflow of the major branches of the left coronary artery, can be measured with reasonable accuracy by injection of a radioactive tracer (e.g., ^{133}Xe) through a catheter threaded into the coronary artery via a peripheral artery. Myocardial clearance of the isotope is monitored with a detector appropriately placed over the precordium.

In the major coronary arteries, blood flow can also be measured by the pulsed Doppler technique. An ultrasound signal is emitted from a crystal at the tip of a cardiac catheter that is inserted, via a peripheral artery (e.g., femoral), into the origin of the coronary artery to be studied. The sound is reflected by the flowing blood, and the frequency shift of the reflected sound is proportional to the velocity of the blood flow. From

223

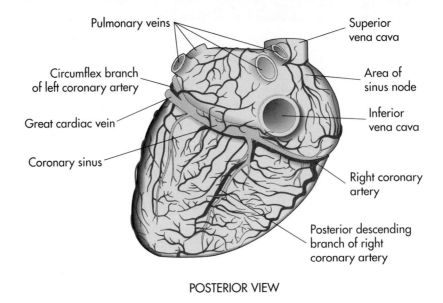

Figure 10-1 ■ Anterior and posterior surfaces of the heart, illustrating the location and distribution of the principal coronary vessels.

an estimate of the cross-sectional area of the coronary artery and the measured flow velocity, the blood flow can be calculated. Coronary blood flow can also be estimated by videodensitometry in which the movement of a bolus of a radiopaque substance injected into the coronary artery can be monitored by rapid sequential radiographs. Similarly, intracoronary injection of microbubbles and tracking of their movement by echocardiography is used to measure coronary blood flow. Also, cine computed tomography and magnetic resonance imaging are used for determination of total and regional myocardial blood flow.

After passage through the capillary beds, most of the venous blood returns to the right atrium through the coronary sinus, but some reaches the right atrium by way of the anterior coronary veins. There are also vascular communications directly between the vessels of the myocardium and the cardiac chambers; these make up the **arteriosinusoidal, arterioluminal,** and **thebesian vessels.** The arteriosinusoidal channels consist of small arteries or arterioles that lose their arterial structure as they penetrate the chamber walls and divide into irregular, endothelium-lined sinuses (50 to 250 μm). These sinuses anastomose with other sinuses and with capillaries, and communicate with the cardiac chambers. The arterioluminal vessels are small arteries or arterioles that open directly into the atria and ventricles. The thebesian vessels are small veins that connect capillary beds directly with the cardiac chambers and also communicate with cardiac veins and other thebesian veins. On the basis of anatomic studies, intercommunication appears to exist among all the minute vessels of the myocardium in the form of an extensive plexus of subendocardial vessels. However, the myocardium does not receive significant nutritional blood flow directly from the cardiac chambers.

■ FACTORS THAT INFLUENCE CORONARY BLOOD FLOW
Physical Factors
The primary factor responsible for perfusion of the myocardium is the aortic pressure, which is, of course, generated by the heart itself. Changes in aortic pressure generally evoke parallel directional changes in coronary blood flow. However, alterations of cardiac work, produced by an increase or decrease in aortic pressure, have a considerable effect on coronary resistance. Increased metabolic activity of the heart results in a decrease in coronary resistance, and a reduction in cardiac metabolism produces an increase in coronary resistance. If a cannulated coronary artery is perfused by blood from a pressure-controlled reservoir, perfusion pressure can be altered without changing aortic pressure and cardiac work. Under these conditions, abrupt variations in perfusion pressure produce equally abrupt changes in coronary blood flow in the same direction. However, maintenance of the perfusion pressure at the new level is associated with a return of blood flow toward the level observed before the induced change in perfusion pressure (Figure 10-2). This phenomenon is an example of autoregulation of blood flow and is discussed in Chapter 8. Under normal conditions, blood pressure is kept within relatively narrow limits by the baroreceptor reflex mechanisms, so that changes in coronary blood flow are primarily caused by caliber changes of the coronary resistance vessels in response to metabolic demands of the heart.

In addition to providing the head of pressure to drive blood through the coronary vessels, the heart also influences its blood supply by the squeezing effect of the contracting myocardium on the blood vessels that course through it (**extravascular compression** or **extracoronary resistance**). This force is so great during early ventricular systole that blood flow, as measured in a large coronary artery that supplies the left ventricle, is briefly reversed. Maximal left coronary inflow occurs in early diastole, when the ventricles have relaxed and extravascular compression of the coronary vessels is virtually absent. This flow pattern is seen in the phasic coronary flow curve for the left coronary artery (Figure 10-3). After an initial reversal in early systole, left coronary blood flow follows the aortic pressure until early diastole, when it rises abruptly and then declines slowly as aortic pressure falls during the remainder of diastole.

Figure 10-2 ■ **Pressure-flow relationships in the coronary vascular bed. At constant aortic pressure, cardiac output, and heart rate, coronary artery perfusion pressure was abruptly increased or decreased from the control level indicated by the point where the two lines cross. The closed circles represent the flows that were obtained immediately after the change in perfusion pressure; the open circles represent the steady-state flows at the new pressures. There is a tendency for flow to return toward the control level (autoregulation of blood flow), and this is most prominent over the intermediate pressure range (about 60 to 180 mm Hg).** (From Berne RM, Rubio R: *Coronary circulation.* In *Handbook of physiology,* Section 2: *The cardiovascular system—the heart,* vol 1, Bethesda, Md., 1979, American Physiological Society.)

Figure 10-3 ■ **Comparison of phasic coronary blood flow in the left and right coronary arteries.**

The minimal extravascular resistance and absence of left ventricular work during diastole can be used to improve myocardial perfusion in patients with damaged myocardium and low blood pressure. The method is called **counterpulsation** and consists of the insertion of an inflatable balloon into the thoracic aorta through a femoral artery. The balloon is inflated during ventricular diastole and deflated during systole. This procedure enhances coronary blood flow during diastole by raising diastolic pressure at a time when coronary extravascular resistance is lowest. Furthermore, it reduces cardiac energy requirements by lowering aortic pressure during ventricular ejection.

Left ventricular myocardial pressure (pressure within the wall of the left ventricle) is greatest near the endocardium and lowest near the epicardium. However, under normal conditions, this pressure gradient does not impair endocardial blood flow, because a greater blood flow to the endocardium during diastole compensates for the greater blood flow to the epicardium during systole. In fact, when 10-μm diameter radioactive spheres are injected into the coronary arteries, their distribution indicates that the blood flow to the epicardial and endocardial halves of the left ventricle is approximately equal (slightly higher in the endocardium) under normal conditions. Because extravascular compression is greatest at the endocardial surface of the ventricle, equality of epicardial and endocardial blood flow must mean that the tone of the endocardial resistance vessels is less than the tone of the epicardial vessels.

Flow in the right coronary artery shows a similar pattern (Figure 10-3), but because of the lower pressure developed during systole by the thin right ventricle, reversal of blood flow does not occur in early systole, and systolic blood flow constitutes a much greater proportion of total coronary inflow than it does in the left coronary artery. The extent to which extravascular compression restricts coronary inflow can be readily seen when the heart is suddenly arrested in diastole or with the induction of ventricular fibrillation. Figure 10-4 depicts mean left coronary flow when the vessel was perfused with blood at a constant pressure from a reservoir. At the arrow in record *A,* ventricular fibrillation was electrically induced and an immediate and substantial increase in blood flow occurred. Subsequent increase in coronary resistance over a period of many minutes reduced myocardial blood flow to below the level existing before induction of ventricular fibrillation (record *B,* before stellate ganglion stimulation).

Under abnormal conditions, when diastolic pressure in the coronary arteries is low (such as in severe hypotension, partial coronary artery occlusion, or severe aortic stenosis), the ratio of endocardial to epicardial blood flow falls below a value of 1. This indicates that the blood flow to the endocardial regions is more severely impaired than that to the epicardial regions of the ventricle. The redistribution of coronary blood flow is also reflected in an increase in the gradient of myocardial lactic acid and adenosine concentrations from epicardium to endocardium. For this reason, the myocardial damage observed in arteriosclerotic heart disease (e.g., after coronary occlusion) is greatest in the inner wall of the left ventricle.

Tachycardia and bradycardia have dual effects on coronary blood flow. A change in heart rate is accomplished chiefly by shortening or lengthening of diastole. With tachycardia the proportion of time spent in systole, and consequently the period of restricted inflow, increases. However, this mechanical reduction in mean coronary flow is overridden by the coronary dilation associated with the increased metabolic activity of the more rapidly beating heart. With bradycardia the opposite is true; restriction of coronary inflow is less (more time in diastole), but so are the metabolic (O_2) requirements of the myocardium.

Neural and Neurohumoral Factors

Stimulation of the sympathetic nerves to the heart elicits a marked increase in coronary blood flow. However, the increase in flow is associated with cardiac acceleration and a more forceful systole. The stronger myocardial contractions and the tachycardia (with the consequence that a greater proportion of time is spent in systole) tend to restrict coronary flow, whereas the increase in myocardial metabolic activity, as evidenced by the rate and contractility changes, tends to evoke dilation of the coronary resistance vessels. The increase in coronary blood flow observed with cardiac sympathetic nerve stimulation is the algebraic sum of these factors. In perfused hearts in which the mechanical effect of extravascular compression is eliminated by cardiac arrest or ventricular fibrillation, an initial coronary vasoconstriction is often observed with cardiac sympathetic nerve stimulation before the vasodilation attributable to the metabolic effect comes into play (Figure 10-4, *B*).

Furthermore, after the beta receptors are blocked to eliminate the chronotropic and inotropic effects, direct reflex activation of the sympathetic nerves to the heart increases coronary resistance. These observations indicate that *the primary action of the sympathetic nerve*

Figure 10-4 ■ **A, Unmasking of the restricting effect of ventricular systole on mean coronary blood flow by induction of ventricular fibrillation during constant pressure perfusion of the left coronary artery. B, Effect of cardiac sympathetic nerve stimulation on coronary blood flow and coronary sinus blood O_2 tension in the fibrillating heart during constant pressure perfusion of the left coronary artery.** (Berne RM: Unpublished observations.)

fibers on the coronary resistance vessels is vaso-constriction.

Alpha- and beta-adrenergic drugs and their respective blocking agents reveal the presence of alpha receptors (constrictors) and beta receptors (dilators) on the coronary vessels. Furthermore, the coronary resistance vessels participate in the baroreceptor and chemoreceptor reflexes, and there is sympathetic constrictor tone of the coronary arterioles that can be reflexly modulated. Nevertheless, coronary resistance is predominantly under local nonneural control.

Vagus nerve stimulation slightly dilates the coronary resistance vessels, and activation of the carotid and aortic chemoreceptors can elicit a small decrease in coronary resistance via the vagus nerves to the heart. The failure of strong vagal stimulation to evoke a large increase in coronary blood flow is not because of insensitivity of

the coronary resistance vessels to acetylcholine; intracoronary administration of this agent elicits marked vasodilation.

Reflexes originating in the myocardium and altering vascular resistance in peripheral systemic vessels, including the coronary vessels, have been conclusively demonstrated. However, the existence of extracardiac reflexes, with the coronary resistance vessels as the effector sites, has not been established.

Metabolic Factors

One of the most striking characteristics of the coronary circulation is the close parallelism between the level of myocardial metabolic activity and the magnitude of the coronary blood flow (Figure 10-5). This relationship is also found in the denervated heart or the completely isolated heart, whether in the beating or the fibrillating

Figure 10-5 ■ Relationship between myocardial oxygen consumption and coronary blood flow during a variety of interventions that increased or decreased myocardial metabolic rate. (Redrawn from Berne RM, Rubio R: *Coronary circulation.* In *Handbook of physiology,* Section 2: *The cardiovascular system—the heart,* vol I, Bethesda, Md., 1979, American Physiological Society.)

state. The ventricles will continue to fibrillate for many hours when the coronary arteries are perfused with arterial blood from some external source. With the onset of ventricular fibrillation, an abrupt increase in coronary blood flow occurs because of the removal of extravascular compression (Figure 10-4). Flow then gradually returns toward, and often falls below, the prefibrillation level. The increase in coronary resistance that occurs despite the elimination of extravascular compression is a manifestation of the heart's ability to adjust its blood flow to meet its energy requirements. The fibrillating heart utilizes less O_2 than the pumping heart, and blood flow to the myocardium is reduced accordingly.

The link between cardiac metabolic rate and coronary blood flow remains unsettled. However, it appears that *a decrease in the ratio of oxygen supply to oxygen demand (whether produced by a reduction in oxygen supply or by an increment in oxygen demand) releases a vasodilator substance from the myocardium into the interstitial fluid, where it can relax the coronary resistance vessels.* As diagrammed in Figure 10-6, a decrease in arterial blood oxygen content, coronary blood flow, or both, or an increase in metabolic rate, decreases the oxygen supply/demand ratio. This causes the release of a vasodilator substance such as adenosine, which dilates the arterioles, thereby adjusting oxygen supply to demand. A decrease in oxygen demand would reduce the vasodilator release and permit greater expression of basal tone. Numerous agents, generally referred to as metabolites, have been suggested as mediators of the vasodilation observed with increased cardiac work. Accumulation of vasoactive metabolites may also be responsible for reactive hyperemia, because the duration of coronary flow after release of the briefly occluded vessel is, within certain limits, proportional to the duration of the period of occlusion. Among the substances implicated are CO_2, O_2 (reduced O_2 tension), hydrogen ions (lactic acid), potassium ions, and adenosine. Of these agents, adenosine comes closest to satisfying criteria for the physiologic mediator. According to the adenosine hypothesis, a reduction in myocardial O_2 tension produced by low coronary blood flow, hypoxemia, or increased metabolic activity of the heart leads to the myocardial formation of adenosine. This nucleoside crosses the interstitial fluid space to reach the coronary resistance vessels, and induces vasodilation by activating an adenosine receptor.

Although potassium release from the myocardium can account for about half of the initial decrease in coronary resistance, it cannot be responsible for the increased coronary flow observed with prolonged enhancement of cardiac metabolic activity, because its release from the cardiac muscle is transitory. There is little evidence that CO_2, hydrogen ions, or O_2 play a significant *direct* role in the regulation of coronary

Myocardial oxygen balance

Figure 10-6 ■ Imbalance in the oxygen supply/oxygen demand ratio alters coronary blood flow by the rate of release of a vasodilator metabolite from the cardiomyocytes. A decrease in the ratio elicits an increase in vasodilator release, whereas an increase in the ratio has the opposite effect.

blood flow. Factors that alter coronary vascular resistance are schematized in Figure 10-7.

■ EFFECTS OF DIMINISHED CORONARY BLOOD FLOW

Most of the oxygen in the coronary arterial blood is extracted during one passage through the myocardial capillaries. Thus, the supply of oxgen to the myocardial cells is **flow limited;** that is, any substantial reduction in coronary blood flow will curtail the delivery of oxygen to the myocardium, because the extraction of oxygen from each unit volume of blood is nearly maximal even when blood flow is normal.

Substantial but temporary mechanical dysfunction of the heart may occur if the reduction of coronary flow is neither too prolonged nor too severe to cause myocardial necrosis. A relatively brief period of severe ischemia, followed by reperfusion, may be associated with pronounced mechanical dysfunction (called **myocardial stunning**) of the heart, which eventually will fully recover.

The pathophysiologic basis for myocardial stunning appears to be a combination of calcium overload, initiated during the period of ischemia, combined with the generation of hydroxyl and

Reductions in coronary blood flow (**myocardial ischemia**) may critically impair the mechanical and electrical behavior of the heart. Diminished coronary blood flow as a consequence of coronary artery disease (usually **coronary atherosclerosis**) is one of the most common causes of serious cardiac disease. The ischemia may be global (i.e., it affects an entire ventricle) or regional (i.e., it affects some fraction of the ventricle). The impairment of the mechanical contraction of the affected myocardium is produced not only by the diminished delivery of oxygen and metabolic substrates, but also by the accumulation of potentially deleterious substances (e.g., K^+, lactic acid, H^+) in the cardiac tissues. If the reduction of coronary flow to any region of the heart is sufficiently severe and prolonged, **necrosis** (death) of the affected cardiac cells will result.

superoxide free radicals early in the period of reperfusion. These changes, in turn, are believed to impair the responsiveness of the myofilaments to calcium.

The relationships among coronary perfusion pressure, cardiac behavior, and myocardial metabolic activity in an experimental model of my-

Figure 10-7 ■ Schematic representation of factors that increase (+) or decrease (−) coronary vascular resistance. The intravascular pressure (arterial blood pressure) stretches the vessel wall.

Myocardial stunning may be evident in patients who have had an **acute coronary artery occlusion** (a so-called heart attack). If the patient is treated sufficiently early by **coronary bypass surgery** or **balloon angioplasty** and if adequate blood flow is restored to the ischemic region, the myocardial cells in this region may eventually recover fully. However, for many days or even weeks, the contractility of the myocardium in the affected region may be grossly subnormal.

Myocardial hibernation also occurs mainly in patients with coronary artery disease. Their coronary blood flow is diminished persistently and significantly, and the mechanical function of the heart is impaired concomitantly. However, the metabolic activity of the heart does not reflect the extent of the ischemia; the process is called hibernation, because the down-regulation of metabolism tends to preserve the viability of the cardiac tissues. If coronary blood flow is restored to normal by bypass surgery or angioplasty, mechanical function returns to normal.

ocardial hibernation are shown in Figure 10-8. When the perfusion pressure in isolated hearts was diminished over the range from 160 to about 70 mm Hg, the intraventricular pressure developed by those hearts progressively diminished. However, the intracellular pH and inorganic phosphate concentrations and the efflux of lactic acid remained essentially unaffected. Only when the perfusion pressure was reduced below 60 mm Hg did these metabolic variables change substantially. The changes in developed force and in cardiac metabolism were readily reversible when perfusion pressure was restored. The changes in developed pressure correlated directly with the intracellular Ca^{++} transients measured during each ventricular contraction. However, the reasons why

the Ca^{++} transient diminishes when perfusion pressure is reduced remain to be established.

■ CORONARY COLLATERAL CIRCULATION AND VASODILATORS

In the normal human heart there are virtually no functional intercoronary channels, whereas in the dog there are a few small vessels that link branches of the major coronary arteries. Abrupt occlusion of a coronary artery or one of its branches in a human or dog leads to ischemic necrosis and eventual fibrosis of the areas of myocardium supplied by the occluded vessel. However, if narrowing of a coronary artery occurs

Figure 10-8 ■ The effects of changes in coronary perfusion pressure on myocardial lactate production (panel A), on inorganic phosphate levels *(P$_i$)* and intracellular pH (panel B), and on the pressure developed during left ventricular contraction (panel C) in a group of five ferret hearts. (Modified from Kitikaze M, Marban E: *J Physiol [Lond]* 414:455, 1989.)

slowly and progressively over a period of days, weeks, or longer, collateral vessels develop and may furnish sufficient blood to the ischemic myocardium to prevent or reduce the extent of necrosis. The development of collateral coronary vessels has been extensively studied in dogs, and the clinical picture of coronary atherosclerosis, as it occurs in humans, can be simulated by gradual narrowing of the normal dog's coronary arteries. Collateral vessels develop between branches of occluded and nonoccluded arteries. They originate from preexisting small vessels that undergo proliferative changes of the endothelium and smooth muscle, possibly in response to wall stress and chemical agents released by the ischemic tissue.

Numerous surgical attempts have been made to enhance the development of coronary collateral vessels. However, the techniques used do not increase the collateral circulation over and above that produced by coronary artery narrowing alone. When discrete occlusions or severe narrowing occur in coronary arteries, as in coronary atherosclerosis, the lesions can be bypassed with an artery (internal mammary) or a vein graft. In many cases the narrow segment can be dilated by inserting a balloon-tipped catheter into the diseased vessel via a peripheral artery and inflating the balloon. Distension of the vessel by balloon inflation (**angioplasty**) can produce a lasting dilation of a narrowed coronary artery (Figure 10-9).

A number of drugs that induce coronary vasodilation are available and are used in patients with coronary artery disease to relieve **angina pectoris,** the chest pain associated with myocardial ischemia. Many of these compounds are organic nitrates and nitrites. They are not selective dilators of the coronary vessels, and the mechanism whereby they accomplish their beneficial effects has not been established. The arterioles that would dilate in response to the drugs are undoubtedly already maximally dilated by the ischemia responsible for the symptoms.

In fact, in a patient with marked narrowing of a coronary artery, administration of a vasodilator can fully dilate normal vessel branches parallel to the narrowed segment and reduce the head of pressure to the partially occluded vessel. This will further compromise blood flow to the ischemic myocardium and elicit pain and electrocardiographic changes indicative of tissue injury. This phenomenon is known as **coronary steal,** and it can be observed with vasodilator drugs such as dipyridamole, which acts by blocking cellular uptake and metabolism of endogenous adenosine. Nitrites and nitrates alleviate angina pectoris, at least partly, by reducing cardiac work and myocardial oxygen requirements by relaxing the great veins (decreased preload) and decreasing blood pressure (decreased afterload). In short, the reduction in pressure work and O_2 requirement must be greater than the reduction in coronary blood flow and O_2 supply consequent to the lowered coronary perfusion pressure. It has also been demonstrated that nitrites and nitrates dilate large coronary arteries and coronary collateral vessels, thus increasing blood flow to ischemic myocardium and alleviating precordial pain.

■ CARDIAC OXYGEN CONSUMPTION AND WORK

The volume of O_2 consumed by the heart is determined by the amount and type of activity the heart performs. Under basal conditions, myocardial O_2 consumption is about 8 to 10 ml/min/ 100 g of heart. It can increase several-fold with exercise and decrease moderately under conditions such as hypotension and hypothermia. The cardiac venous blood is normally quite low in O_2 (about 5 ml/dl), and the myocardium can receive little additional O_2 by further O_2 extraction from the coronary blood. Therefore, increased O_2 demands of the heart must be met primarily by an increase in coronary blood flow. When the heartbeat is arrested, as with administration of potassium, but coronary perfusion is maintained experimentally, O_2 consumption falls to 2 ml/ min/100 g or less, which is still six to seven times greater than that for resting skeletal muscle.

Left ventricular work per beat (**stroke work,** p 137) is generally considered to be equal to the product of the stroke volume and the mean aortic pressure against which the blood is ejected by the left ventricle. At resting levels of cardiac output the kinetic energy component is negligible (p 115). However, at high cardiac outputs, as in severe exercise, the kinetic component can account for up to 50% of total cardiac work. One can simultaneously halve the aortic pressure and double the cardiac output, or vice versa, and still arrive at the same value for cardiac work. However, *the O_2 requirements are greater for any given amount of cardiac work when a major fraction is pressure work as opposed to volume work.* An increase in cardiac output at a constant aortic pressure (volume work) is accomplished with a small increase in left ventricular O_2 consumption, whereas increased arterial pressure at constant cardiac output (pressure work) is accompanied by a large increment in myocardial O_2 consumption. Thus, myocardial O_2 consumption may not correlate well with overall cardiac work. The magnitude and duration of left ventricular pressure do correlate with left ventricular O_2 consumption.

Work of the right ventricle is one seventh that of the left ventricle because pulmonary vascular resistance is much less than systemic vascular resistance.

Cusps of aortic valve   Cardiac catheter

A   B

Border of left ventricle

Figure 10-9 ■ **A, Angiogram (intracoronary radiopaque dye) of a person with marked narrowing of the circumflex branch of the left coronary artery *(encircled)*. Reflux of dye into the root of the aorta outlines two of the aortic valve cusps. B, The same segment of the coronary artery after angioplasty.** (Courtesy Dr. Eric R. Powers.)

The greater energy demand of pressure work compared with volume work is of great clinical importance, especially in aortic stenosis, in which left ventricular O_2 consumption is increased because of the high intraventricular pressures developed during systole, but coronary perfusion pressure is normal or reduced because of the pressure drop across the narrowed orifice of the diseased aortic valve.

■ CARDIAC EFFICIENCY

As with an engine, the efficiency of the heart is calculated as the ratio of the work accomplished to the total energy utilized. Assuming an average O_2 consumption of 9 ml/min/100 g for the two ventricles, a 300-g heart consumes 27 ml O_2/min, which is equivalent to 130 small calories at a respiratory quotient of 0.82. Together the two ventricles do about 8 kg-m of work per minute, which is equivalent to 18.7 small calories. Therefore, the gross efficiency is 14%.

$$\frac{18.7}{130} \times 100 = 14\%$$

The net efficiency is slightly higher (18%) and is obtained by subtracting the O_2 consumption of the nonbeating (asystolic) heart (about 2 ml/min/100 g) from the total cardiac O_2 consumption in the calculation of efficiency. It is thus evident that the efficiency of the heart as a pump is relatively low and is comparable with the efficiency of many mechanical devices used in everyday life. With exercise, efficiency improves, because mean blood pressure shows little change, whereas cardiac output and work increase considerably without a proportional increase in myocardial O_2 consumption. The energy expended in cardiac metabolism that does not contribute to the propulsion of blood through the body appears in the form of heat. The energy of the flowing blood is also dissipated as heat, chiefly in passage through the arterioles.

■ SUBSTRATE UTILIZATION

The heart is quite versatile in its use of substrates, and within certain limits the uptake of a particular substrate is directly proportional to its arterial concentration. The utilization of one substrate is also influenced by the presence or absence of other substrates. For example, the addition of lactate to the blood perfusing a heart metabolizing glucose leads to a reduction in glucose uptake, and vice versa. At normal blood concentrations, glucose and lactate are consumed at about equal rates, whereas pyruvate uptake is very low, but so is its arterial concentration. For glucose the threshold concentration is about 4 mM, and below this blood level no myocardial glucose uptake occurs. Insulin reduces this threshold and increases the rate of glucose uptake by the heart. A very low threshold exists for cardiac utilization of lactate; insulin does not affect its uptake by the myocardium. With hypoxia, glucose utilization is facilitated by an increase in the rate of transport across the myocardial cell wall, whereas lactate cannot be metabolized by the hypoxic heart and is in fact produced by the heart under anaerobic conditions. Associated with lactate production by the hypoxic heart is the breakdown of cardiac glycogen.

Of the total cardiac O_2 consumption, only 35% to 40% can be accounted for by the oxidation of carbohydrate. Thus, the heart derives the major part of its energy from oxidation of noncarbohydrate sources. The chief noncarbohydrate fuel used by the heart is esterified and nonesterified fatty acid, which accounts for about 60% of myocardial O_2 consumption in the postabsorptive state. The various fatty acids show different thresholds for myocardial uptake but are generally utilized in direct proportion to their arterial concentration. Ketone bodies, especially acetoacetate, are readily oxidized by the heart and contribute a major source of energy in diabetic acidosis. As is true of carbohydrate substrates, utilization of a specific noncarbohydrate substrate is influenced by the presence of other substrates, both noncarbohydrate and carbohydrate. Therefore, within certain limits, the heart uses preferentially that substrate which is available in the largest concentration. Most evidence indicates that the contribution to myocardial energy expenditure provided by the oxidation of amino acids is small.

Normally the heart derives its energy by oxidative phosphorylation, in which each mole of glucose yields 36 moles of adenosine triphosphate (ATP). However, during hypoxia, glycolysis supervenes and 2 moles of ATP are provided by each mole of glucose; beta oxidation of fatty acids is also curtailed. If hypoxia is prolonged, cellular creatine phosphate and eventually ATP are depleted.

In ischemia, lactic acid accumulates (lack of washout) and causes a decrease in intracellular pH. This condition inhibits glycolysis, fatty acid use, and protein synthesis, which results in cel-

lular damage and eventually in necrosis of myocardial cells.

■ SUMMARY

1. The physical factors that influence coronary
   blood flow are the viscosity of the blood, the
   frictional resistance of the vessel walls, the
   aortic pressure, and the extravascular compression of the vessels within the walls of the
   left ventricle. Left coronary blood flow is restricted during ventricular systole as a result
   of extravascular compression, and flow is
   greatest during diastole when the intramy-
   ocardial vessels are not compressed.
2. Neural regulation of coronary blood flow is
   much less important than is metabolic regulation. Activation of the cardiac sympathetic
   nerves directly constricts the coronary resistance vessels. However, the enhanced myocardial metabolism caused by the associated
   increase in heart rate and contractile force
   produces vasodilation, which overrides the direct constrictor effect of sympathetic nerve
   stimulation. Stimulation of the cardiac
   branches of the vagus nerves slightly dilates
   the coronary arterioles.
3. A striking parallelism exists between metabolic
   activity of the heart and coronary blood flow. A
   decrease in oxygen supply or an increase in
   oxygen demand apparently releases a vasodilator that decreases coronary resistance. Of the
   known factors (CO_2, O_2, H^+, K^+, adenosine)
   that can mediate this response, adenosine appears to be the most likely candidate.
4. Prolonged, severe reduction in coronary
   blood flow leads to myocardial cell necrosis
   and thereby impairs cardiac contraction. Moderate, sustained reductions in coronary blood
   flow may evoke myocardial hibernation,
   which is a reversible impairment of mechanical performance associated with a down-regulation of cardiac metabolism. Transient periods of severe ischemia followed by reper-

fusion may induce myocardial stunning,
which is a temporary stage of impaired mechanical performance by the heart.

5. In response to gradual occlusion of a coronary artery, collateral vessels from adjacent
   unoccluded arteries develop and supply
   blood to the compromised myocardium distal
   to the point of occlusion.
6. The myocardium functions only aerobically
   and in general utilizes substrates in proportion to their arterial concentration.

■ KEY WORDS AND CONCEPTS

- Coronary vessels
- Arteriosinusoidal vessels
- Arterioluminal vessels
- Thebesian vessels
- Perfusion pressure
- Autoregulation of blood flow
- Phasic coronary flow
- Extravascular compression
- Counterpulsation
- Tachycardia
- Bradycardia
- Sympathetic stimuli
- Alpha-adrenergic receptors
- Beta-adrenergic receptors
- Myogenic factor
- Metabolic factors
- Oxygen supply/demand ratio
- Coronary collateral circulation
- Myocardial ischemia
- Myocardial stunning
- Myocardial hibernation
- Bypass surgery
- Angioplasty
- Adenosine
- Nitrites and nitrates
- Cardiac work
- Pressure work
- Volume work

- Stroke work
- Oxygen consumption
- Cardiac efficiency
- Substrate utilization

■ SELF-STUDY PROBLEMS

1. What is the effect of cardiac sympathetic nerve stimulation on coronary blood flow?
2. What is meant by metabolic regulation of coronary blood flow?
3. How do tachycardia and bradycardia affect coronary blood flow?
4. With regard to the various disturbances in cardiac function induced by diminished coronary blood flow, distinguish among myocardial infarction, stunning, and hibernation.

■ BIBLIOGRAPHY

Journal articles

Baron JF, Vicaut E, Hou X, Duvelleroy M: Independent role of arterial O_2 tension in local control of coronary blood flow, *Am J Physiol* 258:H1388, 1990.

Belardinelli L, Linden J, Berne RM: The cardiac effects of adenosine, *Prog Cardiovasc Dis* 32:73, 1989.

Berne RM: Role of adenosine in the regulation of coronary artery blood flow, *Circ Res* 47:807, 1980.

Bolli R: Myocardial "stunning" in man, *Circulation* 86:1671, 1992.

Feigl EO: Coronary physiology, *Physiol Rev* 63:1, 1983.

Hoffman JIE, Spaan JAE: Pressure-flow relations in coronary circulation, *Physiol Rev* 70:331, 1990.

Klocke FJ, Ellis AK: Control of coronary blood flow, *Annu Rev Med* 31:489, 1980.

Klocke FJ, Mates RE, Canty JM Jr, Ellis AK: Coronary pressure-flow relationships—controversial issues and probable implications, *Circ Res* 56:310, 1985.

Kusuoka H, Marban E: Cellular mechanisms of myocardial stunning, *Annu Rev Physiol* 54:243, 1992.

Manor D, Williams S, Ator R, Bryant K, Scheel KW: Modulation of coronary flow by left ventricular volume in the presence and absence of vasomotor tone, *Am J Physiol* 269:H2010, 1995.

Marban E: Myocardial stunning and hibernation: the physiology behind the colloquialisms, *Circulation* 83:681, 1991.

Mohabir R, Lee HC, Kurz RW, Clusin WT: Effects of ischemia and hypercarbic acidosis on myocyte calcium transient, contraction, and pH_i in perfused rabbit hearts, *Circ Res* 69:1525, 1991.

Mohri M, Tomoike H, Noma M, Inoue T, Hisano K, Nakamura M: Duration of ischemia is vital for collateral development: repeated brief coronary artery occlusions in conscious dogs, *Circ Res* 64:287, 1989.

Morgan JP: Abnormal intracellular modulation of calcium as a major cause of cardiac contractile dysfunction, *N Engl J Med* 325:625, 1991.

Olsson RA, Bunger R: Metabolic control of coronary blood flow, *Prog Cardiovasc Dis* 29:369, 1987.

Olsson RA, Pearson JD: Cardiovascular purinoceptors, *Physiol Rev* 70:761, 1990.

Symons JD, Firoozmand E, Longhurst JC: Repeated dipyridamole administration enhances collateral-dependent flow and regional function during exercise: a role for adenosine, *Circ Res* 73:503, 1993.

Wearn JT, Mettier SR, Klumpp TG, Zschiesche LJ: The nature of the vascular communications between the coronary arteries and the chambers of the heart, *Am Heart J* 9:143, 1933.

White CW, Wilson RF, Marcus ML: Methods of measuring myocardial blood flow in humans, *Prog Cardiovasc Dis* 31:79, 1988.

Books and monographs

Berne RM, Rubio R: *Coronary circulation.* In *Handbook of physiology,* Section 2: *The cardiovascular system—the heart,* vol I, Bethesda, Md., 1979, American Physiological Society.

Gregg DE: *Coronary circulation in health and disease,* Philadelphia, 1950, Lea & Febiger.

Marcus ML: *The coronary circulation in health and disease,* New York, 1983, McGraw-Hill.

Olsson RA, Bunger R, Spaan JAE: *The coronary circulation.* In Fozzard HA et al, editors: *The heart and cardiovascular system,* ed 2, New York, 1991, Raven Press.

Schaper W, Bernotat-Danielowski S, Niennaber C, Schaper J: *Collateral circulation.* In Fozzard HA et al, editors: *The heart and cardiovascular system,* ed 2, New York, 1991, Raven Press.

Sparks HV Jr, Wangler RD, Gorman MW: *Control of the coronary circulation.* In Sperelakis N, editor: *Physiology and pathophysiology of the heart,* ed 2, Boston, 1989, Wolters-Kluwer.

Special Circulations

■ CUTANEOUS CIRCULATION

The oxygen and nutrient requirements of the skin are relatively small and, in contrast to most other body tissues, the supply of these essential materials is not the chief governing factor in the regulation of cutaneous blood flow. The primary function of the cutaneous circulation is maintenance of a constant body temperature. Consequently, the skin shows wide fluctuations in blood flow, depending on the need for loss or conservation of body heat. Mechanisms responsible for alterations in skin blood flow are primarily activated by changes in ambient and internal body temperatures.

Regulation of Skin Blood Flow

There are essentially two types of resistance vessels in skin: arterioles and **arteriovenous (AV) anastomoses.** The arterioles are similar to those found elsewhere in the body. AV anastomoses shunt blood from the arterioles to venules and venous plexuses; hence, they bypass the capillary bed. They are found primarily in the fingertips, palms of the hands, toes, soles of the feet, ears, nose, and lips. AV anastomoses differ morphologically from the arterioles in that they are either short, straight, or long, coiled vessels about

20 to 40 μm in lumen diameter, with thick muscular walls richly supplied with nerve fibers (Figure 11-1). These vessels are almost exclusively under sympathetic neural control and become maximally dilated when their nerve supply is interrupted. Conversely, reflex stimulation of the sympathetic fibers to these vessels may produce constriction to the point of complete obliteration of the vascular lumen. Although AV anastomoses do not exhibit **basal tone** (tonic activity of the vascular smooth muscle independent of innervation), they are highly sensitive to vasoconstrictor agents such as epinephrine and norepinephrine. Furthermore, AV anastomoses do not appear to be under metabolic control, and they fail to show reactive hyperemia or autoregulation of blood flow. *Thus, the regulation of blood flow through these anastomotic channels is governed principally by the nervous system in response to reflex activation by temperature receptors or from higher centers of the central nervous system.*

Most of the skin resistance vessels exhibit some basal tone and are under dual control of the sympathetic nervous system and local regulatory factors, in much the same manner as are resistance vessels in other vascular beds. How-

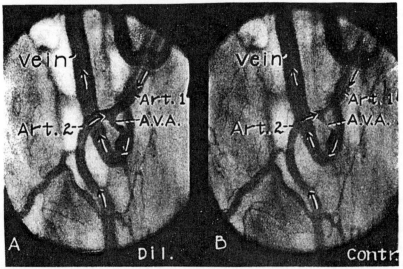

Figure 11-1 ■ *Top,* Arteriovenous *(AV)* anastomosis in the human ear injected with Berlin blue. *A,* Artery; *V,* vein; arrow points to AV anastomosis. The walls of the AV anastomosis in the fingertips are thicker and more cellular. (From Pritchard MML, Daniel PM: *J Anat* 90:309, 1956.) *Bottom,* Two frames from a motion picture record of the same relatively large arteriovenous anastomosis *(A.V.A.)* in a stable rabbit ear chamber installed 3½ months previously. *Frame A,* A.V.A. dilated; *Frame B,* contracted. On this day the lumen of the A.V.A. measured 51 μm dilated and 5 μm contracted at its narrowest point. (From Clark ER, Clark EL: *Am J Anat* 54:229, 1934.)

ever, in the case of skin, neural control plays a more important role than local factors. Stimulation of sympathetic nerve fibers to skin blood vessels (arteries and veins, as well as arterioles) induces vasoconstriction, and severance of the sympathetic nerves induces vasodilation. With chronic denervation of the cutaneous blood vessels, the degree of tone that existed before denervation is gradually regained over a period of several weeks. This is accomplished by an enhancement of basal tone that compensates for the degree of tone previously contributed by sympathetic nerve fiber activity. Epinephrine and norepinephrine elicit only vasoconstriction in cutaneous vessels. Denervation of the skin vessels results in enhanced sensitivity to circulating catecholamines **(denervation hypersensitivity).**

Parasympathetic vasodilator nerve fibers do not supply the cutaneous blood vessels. However, stimulation of the sweat glands, which are innervated by cholinergic fibers of the sympathetic nervous system, results in dilation of the skin resistance vessels. Sweat contains an enzyme that acts on a protein moiety in the tissue fluid to produce **bradykinin,** a polypeptide with potent vasodilator properties. Bradykinin formed in the tissue can act locally to dilate the arterioles and increase blood flow to the skin.

The skin vessels of certain regions, particularly the head, neck, shoulders, and upper chest, are

under the influence of the higher centers of the central nervous system. Blushing, as with embarrassment or anger, and blanching, as with fear or anxiety, are examples of cerebral inhibition and stimulation, respectively, of the sympathetic nerve fibers to the affected regions.

In contrast to AV anastomoses in the skin, the cutaneous resistance vessels show autoregulation of blood flow and reactive hyperemia. If the arterial inflow to a limb is stopped with an inflated blood pressure cuff for a brief period, the skin shows a marked reddening below the point of vascular occlusion when the cuff is deflated. This increased cutaneous blood flow (reactive hyperemia) is also manifested by distension of the superficial veins in the erythematous extremity. Autoregulation of blood flow in the skin is best explained by a myogenic mechanism (see p 175).

Ambient and Body Temperature in Regulation of Skin Blood Flow *Because the primary function of the skin is to preserve the internal milieu and protect it from adverse changes in the environment, and because ambient temperature is one of the most important external variables the body must contend with, it is not surprising that the vasculature of the skin is chiefly influenced by environmental temperature.* Exposure to cold elicits a generalized cutaneous vasoconstriction that is most pronounced in the hands and feet. This response is chiefly mediated by the nervous system, because arrest of the circulation to a hand with a pressure cuff and immersion of that hand in cold water results in vasoconstriction in the skin of the other extremities that are exposed to room temperature. With the circulation to the chilled hand unoccluded, the reflex vasoconstriction is caused in part by the cooled blood returning to the general circulation and stimulating the temperature-regulating center in the anterior hypothalamus. Direct application of cold to this region of the brain produces cutaneous vasoconstriction.

The fingers (and sometimes the toes) of some individuals are very sensitive to cold. Upon exposure to cold the arteries and arterioles to the hands constrict, producing ischemia of the fingers characterized by blanching of the skin associated with tingling, numbness, and pain. The blanching is followed by cyanosis and later by redness as the arterial spasm subsides. This condition, called **Raynaud's disease,** is of unknown cause and occurs most frequently in young women.

The skin vessels of the cooled hand also show a direct response to cold. Moderate cooling or exposure for brief periods to severe cold (0° to 15° C) results in constriction of the resistance and capacitance vessels, including AV anastomoses. However, prolonged exposure of the hand to severe cold has a secondary vasodilator effect. Prompt vasoconstriction and severe pain are elicited by immersion of the hand in water near 0° C, but are soon followed by dilation of the skin vessels with reddening of the immersed part and alleviation of the pain. With continued immersion of the hand, alternating periods of constriction and dilation occur, but the skin temperature rarely drops to as low a degree as it did with the initial vasoconstriction. Prolonged severe cold, of course, results in tissue damage. The rosy faces of people working or playing in a cold environment are examples of cold vasodilation. However, the blood flow through the skin of the face may be greatly reduced despite the flushed appearance. The red color of the slowly flowing blood is in large measure the result of reduced oxygen uptake by the cold skin and the cold-induced shift to the left of the oxyhemoglobin dissociation curve.

Direct application of heat to the skin produces not only local vasodilation of resistance and capacitance vessels and AV anastomoses but also reflex dilation in other parts of the body. The local effect is independent of the vascular nerve supply, whereas the reflex vasodilation is a combination of anterior hypothalamic stimulation by the returning warmed blood and of stimulation of receptors in the heated part. However, evidence for a reflex from peripheral temperature receptors is not as definitive for warm stimulation as it is for cold stimulation.

The close proximity of the major arteries and veins to each other permits considerable heat exchange (***countercurrent***) *between artery and vein.* Cold blood that flows in veins from a cooled hand toward the heart takes up heat from adjacent arteries, resulting in warming of the venous blood and cooling of the arterial blood. Heat exchange is of course in the opposite direction with exposure of the extremity to heat. Thus, heat conservation is enhanced and heat gain is minimized during exposure of extremities to cold and warm environments, respectively.

Skin Color: Relationship to Skin Blood Volume, Oxyhemoglobin, and Blood Flow

The color of the skin is caused in large part by pigment, but in all but very dark skin, the degree of pallor or ruddiness is mainly a function of the amount of blood in the skin. With little blood in the venous plexus the skin appears pale, whereas with moderate to large quantities of blood in the venous plexus the skin shows color. Whether this color is bright red, blue, or some shade between is determined by the degree of oxygenation of the blood in the subcutaneous vessels. For example, a combination of vasoconstriction and reduced hemoglobin can produce an ashen gray color of the skin, whereas a combination of venous engorgement and reduced hemoglobin can result in a dark purple hue. Skin color provides little information about the rate of cutaneous blood flow. There may coexist rapid blood flow and pale skin when the AV anastomoses are open, and slow blood flow and red skin when the extremity is exposed to cold.

■ SKELETAL MUSCLE CIRCULATION

The rate of blood flow in skeletal muscle varies directly with the contractile activity of the tissue and the type of muscle. Blood flow and capillary density in red (slow-twitch, high-oxidative) muscle are greater than in white (fast-twitch, low-oxidative) muscle. In resting muscle the precapillary arterioles exhibit asynchronous intermittent contractions and relaxations, so that at any given moment a very large percentage of the capillary bed is not perfused. Consequently, total blood flow through quiescent skeletal muscle is low (1.4 to 4.5 ml/min/100 g). With exercise the resistance vessels relax and the muscle blood flow may increase manyfold (up to 15 to 20 times the resting level), the magnitude of the increase depending largely on the severity of the exercise.

Regulation of Skeletal Muscle Blood Flow

Control of muscle circulation is achieved by neural and local factors. As with all tissues, physical factors such as arterial pressure, tissue pressure, and blood viscosity influence muscle blood flow. However, another physical factor comes into play during exercise—the squeezing effect of the active muscle on the vessels. With intermittent contractions, inflow is restricted and venous outflow is enhanced during each brief contraction (Figure 11-2). The presence of the venous valves prevents backflow of blood in the veins between contractions, thereby aiding in the forward propulsion of the blood (see also p 216). With strong sustained contractions the vascular bed can be compressed to the point where blood flow actually ceases temporarily.

Neural Factors Although the resistance vessels of muscle possess a high degree of basal tone, they also display tone attributable to continuous low-frequency activity in the sympathetic vasoconstrictor nerve fibers. The basal frequency of firing in the sympathetic vasoconstrictor fibers is quite low (about 1 to 2 per second), and maximal vasoconstriction is observed at frequencies as low as 8 to 10 per second. Stim-

When the valves of the superficial leg veins are incompetent, as may occur with pregnancy, thrombophlebitis, or obesity, the veins become dilated and tortuous. Such **varicose veins** can be treated by surgical removal, by injection of sclerosing solutions, or merely by the use of elastic stockings.

Figure 11-2 ■ **Action of the muscle pump in venous return from the legs. A, Standing at rest the venous valves are open and blood flows upward toward the heart by virtue of the pressure generated by the heart and transmitted through the capillaries to the veins from the arterial side of the vascular system (vis a tergo). B, Contraction of the muscle compresses the vein so that the increased pressure in the vein drives blood toward the thorax through the upper valve and closes the lower valve in the uncompressed segment of the vein just below the point of muscular compression. C, Immediately after muscle relaxation, the pressure in the previously compressed venous segment falls, and the reversed pressure gradient causes the upper valve to close. The valve below the previously compressed segment opens because pressure below it exceeds that above it and the segment fills with blood from the foot. As blood flow continues from the foot, the pressure in the previously compressed segment rises. When it exceeds the pressure above the upper valve, this valve opens and continuous flow occurs as in A.**

ulation of the sympathetic nerve fibers to skeletal muscle elicits vasoconstriction caused by the release of norepinephrine at the fiber endings. Intraarterial injection of norepinephrine elicits only vasoconstriction, whereas low doses of epinephrine produce vasodilation in muscle and large doses cause vasoconstriction.

The tonic activity of the sympathetic nerves is greatly influenced by reflexes from the baroreceptors. An increase in carotid sinus pressure results in dilation of the vascular bed of the muscle, and a decrease in carotid sinus pressure elicits vasoconstriction (Figure 11-3). When the existing sympathetic constrictor tone is high, as in the experiment illustrated in Figure 11-3, the decrease in blood flow associated with common carotid artery occlusion is small, but the increase after the release of occlusion is large. The vasodilation produced by baroreceptor stimulation is caused by inhibition of sympathetic vasoconstrictor activity. Because muscle is the major body component on the basis of mass and thereby represents the largest vascular bed, the participation of its resistance vessels in vascular reflexes plays an important role in maintaining a constant arterial blood pressure.

A comparison of the vasoconstrictor and vasodilator effects of the sympathetic nerves to blood vessels of muscle and skin is summarized in Figure 11-4. Note the lower basal tone of the skin vessels, their greater constrictor response, and the absence of active cutaneous vasodilation.

Local Factors Whether neural or local factors predominate in the regulation of skeletal muscle blood flow depends on the activity of the muscle. In resting muscle the neural factors predominate and superimpose neurogenic tone on the nonneural basal tone (Figure 11-4). Section of the sympathetic nerves to muscle abolishes the neural component of vascular tone and unmasks the intrinsic basal tone of the blood vessels. *Neural and local blood flow regulating*

Figure 11-3 ■ **Evidence for participation of the muscle vascular bed in vasoconstriction and vasodilation mediated by the carotid sinus baroreceptors after common carotid artery occlusion and release. In this preparation the sciatic and femoral nerves constituted the only direct connection between the hind leg muscle mass and the rest of the dog. The muscle was perfused by blood at a constant pressure that was completely independent of the animal's arterial pressure.** (Redrawn from Jones RD, Berne RM: *Am J Physiol* 204:461, 1963.)

mechanisms oppose each other, and during muscle contraction the local vasodilator mechanism supervenes. However, during exercise, strong sympathetic nerve stimulation slightly reduces the vasodilation induced by locally released metabolites.

■ CEREBRAL CIRCULATION

Blood reaches the brain through the internal carotid and vertebral arteries. The latter join to form the basilar artery, which, in conjunction with branches of the internal carotid arteries, forms the **circle of Willis.** A unique feature of

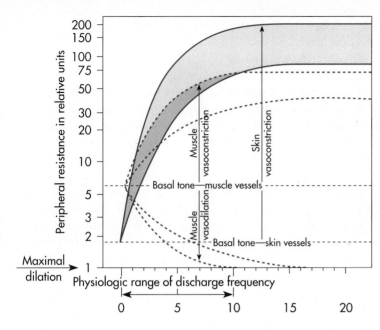

Figure 11-4 ■ Basal tone and the range of response of the resistance vessels in muscle *(dashed lines)* and skin *(shaded area)* to stimulation and section of the sympathetic nerves. Peripheral resistance plotted on a logarithmic scale. (Redrawn from Celander O, Folkow B: *Acta Physiol Scand* 29:241, 1953.)

the cerebral circulation is that it all lies within a rigid structure, the cranium. Because intracranial contents are incompressible, any increase in arterial inflow, as with arteriolar dilation, must be associated with a comparable increase in venous outflow. The volume of blood and of extravascular fluid can vary considerably in most tissues. In brain the volume of blood and extravascular fluid is relatively constant; changes in either of these fluid volumes must be accompanied by a reciprocal change in the other. In contrast to most other organs, the rate of total cerebral blood flow is held within a relatively narrow range; in humans it averages 55 ml/min/100 g of brain.

Estimation of Cerebral Blood Flow

Total cerebral blood flow can be measured in humans by the nitrous oxide (N_2O) method, which is based on the Fick principle (see p 76). The subject breathes a gas mixture of 15% N_2O, 21% O_2, and 64% N_2 for 10 minutes, which is sufficient time to permit equilibration of the N_2O between the brain tissue and the blood leaving the brain. Simultaneous samples of arterial (any

artery) blood and mixed cerebral venous (internal jugular vein) blood are taken at the start of N_2O inhalation and at 1-minute intervals throughout the 10-minute period of N_2O administration. From these data, the cerebral blood flow can be calculated by the Fick equation:

Cerebral blood flow =

$$\frac{\text{Amount of } N_2O \text{ taken up by brain during time } (t_2 - t_1)}{\text{AV difference of } N_2O \text{ across brain during time } (t_2 - t_1)}$$

The development of multiple collimated scintillation detectors built into a helmet that fits over the cranium has made possible the measurement of regional blood flow (cortical blood flow) in animals and humans. An inert radioactive gas (e.g., ^{133}Xe) is injected into an internal carotid artery, and from its rate of washout from the brain, regional cerebral blood flow can be determined. The radioactive gas may also be given by inhalation, but more sophisticated techniques are required to eliminate noncerebral blood flow and to distinguish between blood flow to cortical (gray matter) and deep cerebral (white matter) tissue.

Regulation of Cerebral Blood Flow

Of the various body tissues, the brain is the least tolerant of ischemia. Interruption of cerebral blood flow for as little as 5 seconds results in loss of consciousness, and ischemia lasting just a few minutes results in irreversible tissue damage. Fortunately, regulation of the cerebral circulation is primarily under direction of the brain itself. Local regulatory mechanisms and reflexes originating in the brain tend to maintain cerebral circulation relatively constant in the presence of possible adverse extrinsic effects such as sympathetic vasomotor nerve activity, circulating humoral vasoactive agents, and changes in arterial blood pressure. Under certain conditions the brain also regulates its blood flow by initiating changes in systemic blood pressure.

Neural Factors The cerebral vessels receive innervation from the cervical sympathetic nerve fibers that accompany the internal carotid and vertebral arteries into the cranial cavity. The importance of neural regulation of the cerebral circulation is controversial, but the prevalent belief is that, relative to other vascular beds, sympathetic control of the cerebral vessels is weak and that the contractile state of the cerebrovascular smooth muscle depends primarily on local metabolic factors. There are no known sympathetic vasodilator nerves to the cerebral vessels, but the vessels do receive parasympathetic fibers from the facial nerve, which produce a slight vasodilation on stimulation.

> Elevation of intracranial pressure results in an increase in systemic blood pressure. This response, called **Cushing's phenomenon,** is apparently caused by ischemic stimulation of vasomotor regions in the medulla. It helps maintain cerebral blood flow in such conditions as expanding intracranial tumors.

Local Factors *Generally, total cerebral blood flow is constant. However, regional cortical blood flow is associated with regional neural activity.* For example, movement of one hand results in increased blood flow only in the hand area of the contralateral sensorimotor and premotor cortex. Also, talking, reading, and other stimuli to the cerebral cortex are associated with increased blood flow in the appropriate regions of the contralateral cortex (Figure 11-5). Stimulation of the retina with flashes of light increases blood flow only in the visual cortex. Glucose uptake also corresponds with regional cortical neuronal activity. For example, when the retina is stimulated by light, uptake of ^{14}C-2-deoxyglucose is enhanced in the visual cortex.

It is well known that the cerebral vessels are very sensitive to carbon dioxide tension. Increases in arterial blood CO_2 tension ($Paco_2$) elicit marked cerebral vasodilation; inhalation of 7% CO_2 results in a twofold increment in cerebral blood flow. By the same token, decreases in $Paco_2$, such as elicited by hyperventilation, produce a decrease in cerebral blood flow. CO_2 produces changes in arteriolar resistance by altering perivascular (and probably intracellular vascular smooth muscle) pH. By independently changing Pco_2 and bicarbonate concentration, it has been demonstrated that pial vessel diameter (and presumably blood flow) and pH are inversely related, regardless of the level of the Pco_2.

Carbon dioxide can diffuse to the vascular smooth muscle from the brain tissue or from the lumen of the vessels, whereas hydrogen ions in the blood are prevented from reaching the arteriolar smooth muscle by the **blood-brain barrier.** Hence, the cerebral vessels dilate when the hydrogen ion concentration of the cerebrospinal fluid is increased but show only minimal dilation in response to an increase in the hydrogen ion concentration of the arterial blood.

With respect to K^+, such stimuli as hypoxia, electrical stimulation of the brain, and seizures

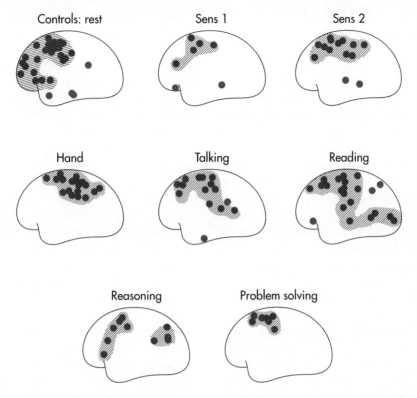

Figure 11-5 ■ **Effects of different stimuli on regional blood flow in the contralateral human cerebral cortex.** *Sens 1,* **low-intensity electrical stimulation of the hand;** *Sens 2,* **high-intensity electrical stimulation of the hand (pain).** (Redrawn from Ingvar DH: *Brain Res* 107:181, 1976.)

elicit rapid increases in cerebral blood flow and are associated with increases in perivascular K^+. The increments in K^+ are similar to those that produce pial arteriolar dilation when K^+ is applied topically to these vessels. However, the increase in K^+ is not sustained throughout the period of stimulation. Hence, only the initial increment in cerebral blood flow can be attributed to the release of K^+.

Adenosine levels of the brain increase with ischemia, hypoxemia, hypotension, hypocapnia, electrical stimulation of the brain, and induced seizures. When applied topically, adenosine is a potent dilator of the pial arterioles. In short, any intervention that either reduces the O_2 supply to the brain or increases the O_2 need of the brain results in rapid (within 5 seconds) formation of adenosine in the cerebral tissue. Unlike pH or K^+, the adenosine concentration of the brain increases with initiation of the stimulus and remains elevated throughout the period of O_2 imbalance. The adenosine released into the cerebrospinal fluid during conditions associated with inadequate brain O_2 supply is available to the brain tissue for reincorporation into cerebral tissue adenine nucleotides.

All three factors, pH, K^+, and adenosine may act in concert to adjust the cerebral blood flow to the metabolic activity of the brain.

The cerebral circulation shows reactive hyperemia and excellent autoregulation between pressures of about 60 and 160 mm Hg. Mean arterial pressures below 60 mm Hg result in reduced cerebral blood flow and syncope, whereas mean pressures above 160 may lead to increased permeability of the blood-brain barrier and cerebral edema. Autoregulation of cerebral blood flow is abolished by hypercapnia or any other potent vasodilator, and none of the candidates for metabolic regulation of cerebral blood flow has been shown to be responsible for this phenomenon. Hence, autoregulation of cerebral blood flow is probably attributable to a myogenic mechanism, although experimental proof is still lacking.

■ PULMONARY CIRCULATION

The pulmonary and systemic vascular beds are in series with each other. Therefore, under steady-state conditions, the total pulmonary and systemic blood flows are virtually identical. Despite this similarity in the rate of blood flow, the anatomic, hemodynamic, and physiologic characteristics of these two sections of the cardiovascular system differ substantially.

Functional Anatomy

Pulmonary Vasculature The pulmonary vascular system is a low-resistance network of highly distensible vessels. The main pulmonary artery is much shorter than the aorta. The walls of the pulmonary artery and its branches are much thinner than the walls of the aorta, and they contain less smooth muscle and elastin. Contrary to systemic arterioles, which have very thick walls composed mainly of circularly arranged smooth muscle, the pulmonary arterioles are thin and contain little smooth muscle. The pulmonary arterioles do not have the same capacity for vasoconstriction as do their counterparts in the systemic circulation. The pulmonary venules and veins are also very thin and possess little smooth muscle.

The pulmonary capillaries differ markedly from the systemic capillaries. Whereas the systemic capillaries constitute an interconnecting network of tubular vessels, the pulmonary capillaries are aligned so that the blood flows in thin sheets between adjacent alveoli (Figure 11-6). Hence, the capillary blood is exposed optimally to the alveolar gases. The total surface area for exchange between alveoli and blood is about 50 to 70 m^2. Only thin layers of vascular and alveolar endothelium separate the blood and alveolar gas. The thickness of the sheets of blood between adjacent alveoli depends on the intravascular pressure and intraalveolar pressure. Ordinarily, the width of an interalveolar sheet of blood is about equal to the diameter of a red blood cell (Figure 11-6). During pulmonary vascular congestion, as when left atrial pressure is elevated, the width of the sheet may increase several-fold. Conversely, when local alveolar pressure exceeds the adjacent capillary pressure, the capillaries may collapse and blood will not flow to those alveoli. Hydrostatic factors participate in this phenomenon, particularly with respect to the regional distribution of blood flow to the lungs, as described below.

Bronchial Vasculature The bronchial arteries are branches of the thoracic aorta. These arteries and their branches, down to the arterioles, have the structural characteristics of most systemic arteries; that is, they have much thicker walls and more smooth muscles than do the pulmonary arterial vessels of equivalent caliber. The bronchial vessels supply blood to the tracheobronchial tree down to the terminal bronchioles.

The bronchial veins drain partly into the pulmonary venous system and partly into the azygos veins, which are a part of the systemic venous system. The bronchial circulation normally constitutes about 1% of the cardiac output. Therefore, the fraction of the bronchial blood flow that returns to the left atrium (via the pulmonary veins) rather than to the right atrium (via the azygos veins) constitutes at most 1% of the

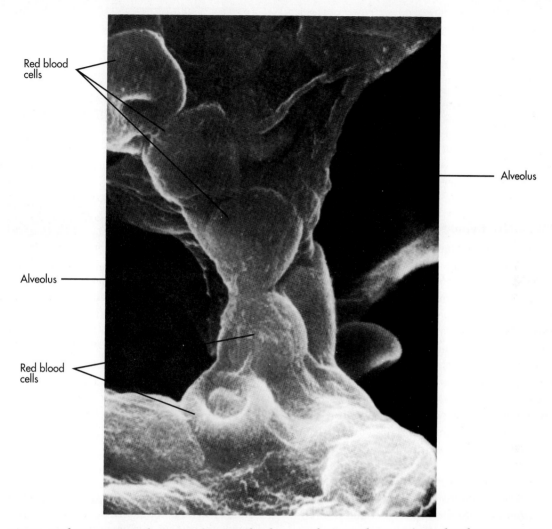

Red blood cells

Alveolus

Alveolus

Red blood cells

Figure 11-6 ■ Scanning electron micrograph of mouse lung to show an interalveolar septum. Note that the membranes that separate an alveolus from a capillary are so thin that the shapes of the erythrocytes in the capillary can easily be discerned. (From Greenwood MF, Holland P: *Lab Invest* 27:296, 1972.)

venous return to the heart. This small quantity of bronchial venous blood, plus a small amount of coronary venous blood that drains directly into the left atrium or left ventricle, "contaminates" the pulmonary venous blood, which is ordinarily fully saturated with O_2. Hence, the aortic blood is very slightly desaturated. This small quantity of venous drainage directly into the left side of the heart also accounts for the fact that, even under true equilibrium conditions, the output of the left ventricle slightly exceeds that of the right ventricle.

Sustained abridgment of the pulmonary arterial blood supply to a lung, after **pulmonary embolism,** for example, usually increases the precapillary (arterial) communications between vessels of the systemic and pulmonary circuits. Certain inflammatory and degenerative pulmonary diseases, such as **emphysema,** are often associated with increased bronchial blood flow, and significant admixtures of blood take place between the two systems.

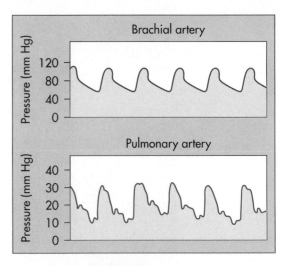

Figure 11-7 ■ Pressures recorded in the brachial and pulmonary arteries of a normal human subject. (Modified from Harris P, Heath D: *Human pulmonary circulation,* Edinburgh, 1962, E and S Livingstone.)

Pulmonary Hemodynamics

Pressures in the Pulmonary Circulation
In normal individuals the average systolic and diastolic pressures in the pulmonary artery are about 25 and 10 mm Hg, respectively, and the mean pressure is about 15 mm Hg (Figure 11-7). These pressures are much lower than those in systemic arteries (Figure 11-7), because the pulmonary vascular resistance is only about one tenth the resistance of the systemic vascular bed. The mean pressure in the left atrium is normally about 5 mm Hg, and so the total pulmonary arteriovenous pressure gradient is only about 10 mm Hg. The mean hydrostatic pressure in the pulmonary capillaries lies between the pulmonary arterial and pulmonary venous values but somewhat closer to the latter.

Pulmonary Blood Flow
At equilibrium the pulmonary and systemic blood flows are equal, except for the small disparity contributed by the bronchial circulation. Because of the low pressures in the pulmonary blood vessels and their great distensibility, gravity affects the regional distribution of blood flow in the lungs.

Three distinct flow patterns may be found at different hydrostatic levels in the lung, as illustrated in Figure 11-8. Consider that the pulmonary artery delivers blood at a steady pressure of 15 mm Hg and that pulmonary venous pressure remains constant at 5 mm Hg. In those pulmonary arterial and venous branches that are 13

The mean left atrial pressure is an index of the left ventricular filling pressure. To determine whether a patient suffers from **left heart failure,** it is desirable but difficult to measure the left atrial pressure directly. However, a flexible, balloon-tipped catheter can easily be guided into the pulmonary artery. If the catheter is advanced until the tip is wedged into a small branch of the pulmonary artery, the **pulmonary artery wedge pressure** serves as a useful estimate of the pressure in the left atrium. The wedged catheter halts flow in the small vessels distal to the catheter. These vessels then serve as an extension of the catheter and thereby allow the catheter to communicate with the pulmonary veins and left atrium.

cm below (zone *C*) the hydrostatic level of the main pulmonary vessels, the respective pressures will be 10 mm Hg (equivalent of 13 cm of blood) greater than those in the main vessels, by virtue of gravitational effects. Conversely, in pulmonary arterial and venous branches that are 13 cm

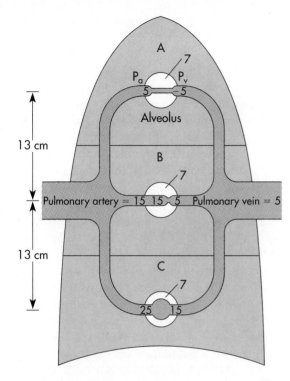

Figure 11-8 ■ Schematic representation of the three types of flow regimens that might exist in the pulmonary circulation. In zone *A*, alveolar pressure exceeds intravascular pressures. Pulmonary capillaries in this zone will not be perfused. In zone *B*, alveolar pressure is intermediate between pulmonary arterial and venous pressures. Pulmonary capillaries will flutter between the open and closed states. In zone *C*, intravascular pressures exceed alveolar pressure. The pulmonary capillaries are always open, but the flow resistances in individual vessels vary with the hydrostatic pressure in the vessel.

Ordinarily, the mean pressure in the alveoli is atmospheric. Therefore, the conditions depicted in zone *A* do not ordinarily prevail in any region of the lungs. In **hypovolemic shock,** however, the mean pulmonary artery pressure is often very low. Therefore, vascular pressures in the lung apices might be subatmospheric. The atmospheric pressure in the alveoli would then compress the apical capillaries, so that virtually no blood would flow to that zone from the pulmonary circulation. However, the bronchial circulation, which operates at much higher pressures, would be unaffected.

above (zone *A*) the main vessels, the respective pressures will be 10 mm Hg less than those in the main vessels. At the same hydrostatic level (zone *B*) as the main vessels, the respective pressures in the branches will be approximately equal to those in the main vessels.

Consider that the alveolar pressure equals 7 mm Hg in all alveoli. Such an alveolar pressure might exist in an individual receiving positive-pressure ventilation. In zone *A* the alveolar pressure would exceed the local arterial and venous pressures (Figure 11-8). The pulmonary capillary pressures lie between those of the arteries and veins, and therefore alveolar pressure would also exceed capillary pressure. Capillaries lying between adjacent alveoli would be collapsed. Those alveoli would not be perfused, and gas would not be exchanged.

In zone *B* the alveolar pressure lies between the local arterial and venous pressures (Figure 11-8). Again, if alveolar pressure equals 7 mm Hg, a capillary in that region will flutter between the open and closed state. When the capillary is open, blood will flow through it, and the capillary pressure will decrease progressively from the arterial to the venous end. The pressure at the venous end will be less than the alveolar pressure, and therefore the capillary will collapse at that end. With the cessation of flow, the arterial and capillary pressures at a given hydrostatic level will equalize. Thus, the capillary pressure will quickly rise to that in the local small arteries, which exceeds the prevailing alveolar pressure. Hence, the capillary will then be forced open. With the restitution of flow, however, the pressure will drop along the length of the capillary. As the pressure at the venous end drops below the ambient alveolar pressure, the capillary will again close. Hence, the capillary will flutter between the open and closed states.

The critical pressure gradient for flow in zone *B* is the arterioalveolar pressure difference, not the arteriovenous pressure difference, as it is for most vessels in the body. As long as venous pressure is less than alveolar pressure, venous pressure does not influence the flow. Such a flow condition is called a **waterfall effect,** because the height of a waterfall has no influence on the flow.

In Zone *C* the arterial and venous pressures both exceed the alveolar pressure. Hence, the pressure everywhere along the capillary exceeds the alveolar pressure, and the capillary remains permanently open. In this zone the flow is determined by the arteriovenous pressure gradient, and the resistance may be calculated by the conventional analog of Ohm's law. The large and small pulmonary vessels, including the capillaries, are very distensible, as noted above. The pressure difference that determines the caliber of a distensible tube is the **transmural pressure,** that is, the difference between the internal and external pressures. In an erect individual the intravascular pressures in the lungs increase from apex to base. The transmural pressures increase accordingly, and the diameter of the pulmonary vessels increases from apex to base. Because resistance to flow varies inversely with vessel caliber, resistance decreases and flow increases in zone *C* in the apex-to-base direction. Such predicted changes in flow have been verified in humans.

Regulation of the Pulmonary Circulation

The total volume of blood pumped by the heart passes through the pulmonary circulation. Therefore, the various cardiac and vascular factors that determine cardiac output in general also determine total pulmonary blood flow. These factors have been discussed in Chapter 9.

The autonomic nervous system innervates the pulmonary blood vessels. Although the small pulmonary vessels contain little smooth muscle, small changes in smooth muscle tone may alter vascular resistance substantially, because the pressures in the pulmonary circulation are so low. Baroreceptor stimulation can dilate the pulmonary resistance vessels reflexly. Conversely, peripheral chemoreceptor stimulation constricts the pulmonary vessels. The importance of such neural regulation remains to be established, however.

Hypoxia has the most important influence on pulmonary vasomotor tone. Acute and chronic hypoxia both increase pulmonary vascular resistance (Figure 11-9). Regional reductions in alveolar O_2 tension constrict the nearby arterioles. This response helps maintain an optimal **ventilation-perfusion ratio.** The O_2 tension in poorly ventilated alveoli will approach the Po_2 in the pulmonary arterial blood. Blood flowing by such alveoli will not be well oxygenated, and therefore the O_2 tension of the blood returning to the left atrium will decrease.

Figure 11-9 ■ **Effect of hypoxia on vascular resistance of an isolated rat lung. The lung was perfused with blood at a constant flow. When the O_2 tension of the inspired air was reduced** *(between the arrows),* **the pulmonary resistance vessels constricted, as indicated by the substantial rise in perfusion pressure.** (Modified from Grover RF, Wagner WW Jr, McMurtry IF, Reeves JT: *Pulmonary circulation.* In *Handbook of physiology,* Section 2: *The cardiovascular system—peripheral circulation and organ blood flow,* vol III, Bethesda, Md., 1983, American Physiological Society.)

Arteriolar vasoconstriction reduces the blood flow to such poorly ventilated alveoli, and thereby reduces the contamination of the pulmonary venous blood with poorly oxygenated blood. Thus, this mechanism shunts pulmonary blood flow from the poorly ventilated regions to the better ventilated regions of the lungs, and thereby improves the O_2 saturation of the systemic arterial blood. The mechanism by which hypoxia raises pulmonary vascular resistance has not yet been established. Electrophysiologic studies on pulmonary vascular smooth muscle cells indicate that hypoxia inhibits an outward potassium current. The resulting depolarization of the cell membrane augments the influx of calcium into the smooth muscle cells and thereby induces contraction. These results therefore suggest that in an intact pulmonary blood vessel, hypoxia would lead to vasoconstriction.

■ RENAL CIRCULATION
Anatomy

The primary branches of the **renal artery** divide into a number of **interlobar arteries.** These interlobar branches (Figure 11-10) proceed radially from the hilus toward the corticomedullary junction, between adjacent medullary pyramids. As an interlobar artery approaches the corticomedullary junction (horizontal dashed line, Figure 11-10), it branches into a number of **arcuate arteries,** which travel in various directions over the bases of the adjacent medullary pyramids, in the zone between the cortex and medulla. The arcuate branches that arise from adjacent interlobar arteries do not interconnect. Hence, occlusion of an interlobar artery destroys a pyramid-shaped region of the kidney.

From the arcuate arteries, a number of **interlobular branches** travel toward the capsular surface of the kidney (Figure 11-10). The **afferent arterioles** to the **glomeruli** are branches of these interlobular arteries. Each human kidney has approximately 1 million glomeruli. The af-

ferent arteriole to each glomerulus divides into several vessels that form discrete capillary loops (Figure 11-11). The proximal and distal limbs of each loop are interconnected by many smaller capillaries. The distal limbs of each capillary loop within a glomerulus rejoin to form the **efferent arteriole,** the diameter of which is usually less than that of the afferent arteriole. The entire glomerular capillary tuft is enveloped by **Bowman's capsule,** which collects the glomerular filtrate.

The efferent arterioles divide into another capillary network, the **peritubular capillaries.** The architecture of the peritubular capillary network varies, depending on whether the efferent arteriole arises from glomeruli close to the medullary border (the **juxtamedullary glomeruli**) or from glomeruli in the more peripheral regions of the renal cortex (Figure 11-10).

Capillaries that originate from the regular cortical glomeruli surround relatively short renal tubules, which are located almost entirely in the renal cortex itself. The capillary networks of neighboring cortical nephrons freely communicate with one another. Most of the capillaries arising from the efferent arterioles of juxtamedullary glomeruli form long hairpin loops **(vasa recta)** that accompany the loops of Henle deep into the renal medulla, sometimes to the tips of the renal papillae. The vasa recta participate in the countercurrent exchange system responsible for concentrating the urine. In general, the renal venous system parallels the arterial distribution to the renal tissues (Figure 11-10).

Renal Hemodynamics

Segmental Resistance The pressure drops only slightly in the interlobar, arcuate, and interlobular arteries: the main preglomerular resistance resides in the afferent arterioles (Figure 11-12). The pressure in the glomerular capillaries is normally about 50 to 60 mm Hg. Thus, the net balance of forces across the capillary wall favors

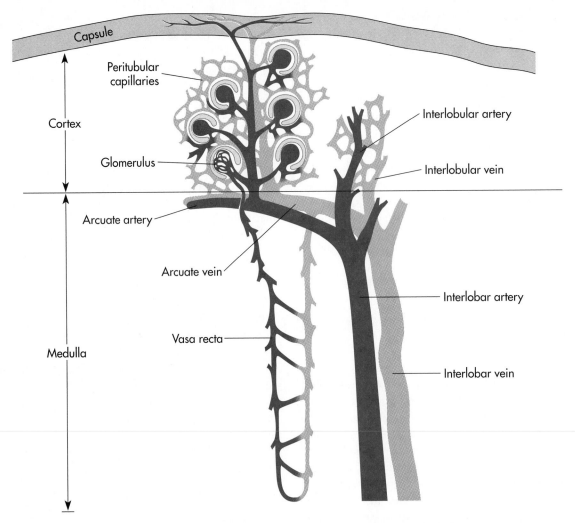

Figure 11-10 ■ Anatomy of the vasculature to one lobe of the kidney.

the outward filtration of plasma water along the entire length of the capillary loop. Furthermore, the filtration coefficient of the glomerular capillaries exceeds that of most other capillaries in the body. Hence, *about 20% of the plasma water that enters the glomerular capillaries is filtered into Bowman's capsule.* The greatest hydraulic resistance in the renal circulation is in the efferent arterioles. Consequently, the pressure in the peritubular capillaries is normally about 10 to 20 mm Hg. Such pressures favor net reabsorption of the large quantities of fluid that pass from the renal tubules to the interstitial spaces of the kidney. The peritubular capillaries also are considerably more permeable than most of the other capillaries in the body.

Renal Blood Flow *The weight of the kidneys constitutes only about 0.5% of total body weight, yet the kidneys receive about 20% of cardiac output.* Most of this rich blood supply

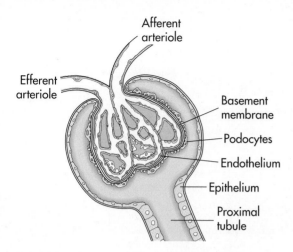

Figure 11-11 ■ **Anatomy of the mammalian glomerulus.**

Figure 11-12 ■ **Intravascular pressures in the renal artery *(RA)*, afferent arterioles *(AA)*, glomerular capillaries *(GI)*, efferent arterioles *(EA)*, peritubular capillaries *(PC)*, venules *(V)*, and renal vein *(RV)*.** (From Frohnert PP: *Renal blood flow.* In Knox FG, editor: *Textbook of renal pathophysiology,* Hagerstown, Md., 1978, Harper & Row. Based on data from Brenner BM: *J Clin Invest* 50:1776, 1971.)

perfuses the renal cortex; blood flow per unit weight to the inner medulla and papillae is only about one tenth of that to the cortex. Nevertheless, even these medullary tissues receive as much blood per unit weight as does the brain.

The kidney has one of the highest metabolic rates in the body. The large renal blood flow is not essential to subserve the great metabolic rate, however. The kidney extracts less than 10% of the O_2 present in the renal arterial blood. Therefore, the renal blood flow is at least ten times greater than that needed to deliver the required O_2 and nutrients. The excessively high renal blood flow is so important because it delivers large volumes of blood to the glomeruli for the process of ultrafiltration.

Regulation of the Renal Circulation

Autoregulation Renal blood flow tends to remain constant, despite fluctuations in arterial perfusion pressure. In the experiment represented in Figure 11-13, for example, arterial pressure was suddenly raised from 140 to 190 mm Hg. This stepwise change in pressure rapidly increased the renal blood flow, from 135 to 165

ml/min. This rise in renal blood flow was transitory, however, and flow returned close to the control level in less than 1 minute. Over a pressure range of about 75 to 170 mm Hg, the steady-state level of renal blood flow is relatively insensitive to changes in arterial pressure (Figure 11-14). Beyond this range, however, renal blood flow varies directly with perfusion pressure.

This ability of the renal blood flow to remain constant, despite fluctuations in perfusion pres-

Figure 11-13 ■ Changes in renal blood flow evoked by a sudden increase in arterial perfusion pressure from 140 to 190 mm Hg in an isolated dog kidney. The kidney was perfused from a peripheral artery of another dog. (Modified from Semple SJG, deWardener HE: *Circ Res* 7:643, 1959. With permission of the American Heart Association.)

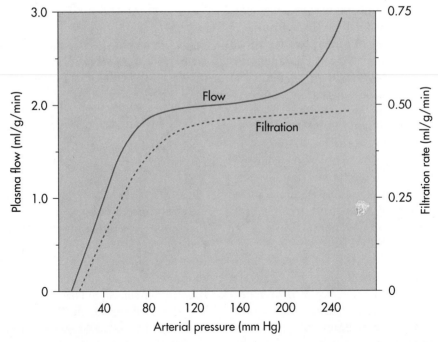

Figure 11-14 ■ Renal plasma flow and glomerular filtration rate as a function of arterial perfusion pressure in an anesthetized dog. (Adapted from Shipley RE, Study RS: *Am J Physiol* 167:676, 1951.)

sure, is a process intrinsic to the kidney itself; it has been demonstrated even in isolated kidney preparations (Figure 11-13). Concomitant measurement of glomerular filtration rate (GFR) reveals that the tendency for GFR to be autoregulated is equally pronounced (Figure 11-14). Therefore, the resistance change induced by an alteration in perfusion pressure must occur mainly in the afferent arteriole. As the perfusion pressure is raised, for example, afferent arteriolar constriction not only limits the increase in renal blood flow but also restricts the rise in glomerular capillary pressure and the concomitant increment in GFR.

Renal autoregulation has been studied extensively, but the mechanism remains controversial. The two principal mediators appear to be the **myogenic mechanism** and **tubuloglomerular feedback.** The myogenic mechanism is the intrinsic property of vascular smooth muscle to contract in response to a stretching force, such as an increase in transmural pressure (see Chapter 8). Tubuloglomerular feedback involves a feedback loop in which a change in the flow of renal tubular fluid is detected by the **macula densa** of the **juxtaglomerular apparatus,** and the juxtaglomerular apparatus then sends a signal to the afferent arterioles to restore basal levels of renal blood flow and GFR. The precise nature of the signal that regulates the caliber of the afferent arterioles is controversial. Many vasoactive substances, such as prostaglandins, catecholamines, adenosine, nitric oxide, and the components of the renin-angiotensin system, may participate in the process of tubuloglomerular feedback.

The juxtaglomerular apparatus is the source of one of the principal humoral mechanisms, the **renin-angiotensin system,** involved in the regulation of blood volume and blood pressure. In response to various types of signals, such as a reduction in GFR, the juxtaglomerular apparatus releases the enzyme **renin.** This enzyme acts on a substrate, **angiotensinogen,** which circulates in the blood, to release the decapeptide peptide **angiotensin I.** This peptide is then split by a **converting enzyme,** mainly in the lungs, to form an octapeptide, **angiotensin II.** This peptide is not only a potent arteriolar vasoconstrictor, but it also affects many other vital functions, such as the regulation of certain renal tubular transport processes and the release of adrenocortical hormones.

Neural Regulation Stimulation of the renal sympathetic nerves decreases renal blood flow substantially but reduces GFR only slightly. The neural activity constricts the afferent and efferent arterioles and the proximal segments of the vasa recta. Presumably, the reduction of renal blood flow exceeds the reduction of GFR because the postglomerular constriction is greater than the preglomerular constriction.

In resting subjects the basal level of renal sympathetic tone is low; abolition of that tone scarcely affects renal blood flow. The arterial baroreceptor reflexes influence the renal vasculature only slightly. Activation of low-pressure vascular receptors elicits much larger reflex effects on the renal circulation. A reduction in left atrial pressure, for example, increases renal nerve activity and renal vascular resistance greatly. Emotional reactions, such as anxiety, fear, and rage, also curtail renal blood flow dramatically.

■ SPLANCHNIC CIRCULATION

The splanchnic circulation consists of the blood supply to the gastrointestinal tract, liver, spleen, and pancreas. Several features distinguish the splanchnic circulation, the most noteworthy being that two large capillary beds are partially in series with one another. The small splanchnic arterial branches supply the capillary beds in the gastrointestinal tract, spleen, and pancreas. From these capillary beds, the venous blood ultimately flows into the portal vein, which normally provides most of the blood supply to the liver. However, the hepatic artery also supplies blood to the liver.

Intestinal Circulation

Anatomy The gastrointestinal tract is supplied by the celiac, superior mesenteric, and inferior mesenteric arteries. The superior mesenteric artery is the largest of all the aortic branches and carries over 10% of the cardiac output. Small mesenteric arteries form an extensive vascular network in the submucosa (Figure 11-15). Their branches penetrate the longitudinal and circular muscle layers and give rise to third-

and fourth-order arterioles. Some third-order arterioles in the submucosa become the main arterioles to the tips of the villi.

The direction of the blood flow in the capillaries and venules in a villus is opposite to that in the main arteriole (Figure 11-16). This arrangement constitutes a **countercurrent exchange system.** An effective countercurrent multiplier in the villus facilitates the absorption of sodium and water. The countercurrent exchange also permits diffusion of O_2 from arterioles to venules. At low flow rates, a substantial fraction of the O_2 may be shunted from arterioles to venules near the base of the villus. Thus, the supply of O_2 to the mucosal cells at the tip of the villus may be curtailed. When intestinal blood flow is reduced, the shunting of O_2 is exaggerated, which may cause extensive necrosis of the intestinal villi.

Neural Regulation The neural control of the mesenteric circulation is almost exclusively sympathetic. Increased sympathetic activity constricts the mesenteric arterioles, precapillary sphincters, and capacitance vessels. These responses are mediated by alpha-adrenergic receptors, which are prepotent in the mesenteric circulation; however, beta-adrenergic receptors are also present. Infusion of a beta-receptor agonist, such as isoproterenol, causes vasodilation.

During fighting or in response to artificial stimulation of the hypothalamic "defense" area, pronounced vasoconstriction occurs in the mesenteric vascular bed. This shifts blood flow from the temporarily less important intestinal circulation to the more crucial skeletal muscles, heart, and brain.

Autoregulation Autoregulation in the intestinal circulation is not as well developed as in certain other vascular beds, such as those in the brain and kidney. The principal mechanism responsible for autoregulation is metabolic, although a myogenic mechanism probably also participates (see Chapter 8). The adenosine con-

Figure 11-15 ■ Distribution of small blood vessels to the rat intestinal wall. *SA,* Small artery; *SV,* small vein: *1A* to *5A,* first- to fifth-order arterioles; *1V* to *4V,* first- to fourth-order venules; *CC* and *LC,* capillaries in circular and longitudinal muscle layers; *MA* and *CV,* main arteriole and collecting venule of a villus; *DA,* distribution arteriole; *2VM,* second-order mucosal venule; *PC,* precapillary sphincter; *MC,* mucosal capillary. (From Gore RW, Bohlen HG: *Am J Physiol* 233:H685, 1977.)

centration in the mesenteric venous blood rises fourfold after brief arterial occlusion. Adenosine is a potent vasodilator in the mesenteric vascular bed and may be the principal metabolic mediator of autoregulation. However, potassium and altered osmolality may also contribute to the overall response.

The O_2 consumption of the small intestine is more rigorously controlled than is the blood flow. In one series of experiments, the O_2 uptake of the small intestine remained constant when arterial perfusion pressure was varied between 30 and 125 mm Hg.

Functional Hyperemia Food ingestion increases intestinal blood flow. The secretion of certain gastrointestinal hormones contributes to this hyperemia. Gastrin and cholecystokinin augment intestinal blood flow, and they are secreted when food is ingested. The absorption of food affects intestinal blood flow. Undigested food has no vasoactive influence, whereas several prod-

ucts of digestion are potent vasodilators. Among the various constituents of chyme, the principal mediators of mesenteric hyperemia are glucose and fatty acids.

Hepatic Circulation

Anatomy The blood flow to the liver is normally about 25% of cardiac output. The flow is derived from two sources, the portal vein and the hepatic artery. Ordinarily, the portal vein provides about three fourths of the blood flow. The portal venous blood has already passed through the gastrointestinal capillary bed, and therefore much of the O_2 has been extracted. The hepatic artery delivers the remaining one fourth of the blood, which is fully saturated with O_2. Hence, about three fourths of the O_2 used by the liver is derived from the hepatic arterial blood.

The small branches of the portal vein and hepatic artery give rise to terminal portal venules and hepatic arterioles (Figure 11-17). These ter-

Figure 11-16 ■ **Scanning electron micrographs of rabbit intestinal villi** *(left panel)* **and corrosion cast of the microcirculation in the villus** *(right panel)***. *A,* Arteriole; *V,* venule.** (From Gannon BJ, Gore RW, Rogers PAW: *Biomed Res* 2(suppl):235, 1981.)

Figure 11-17 ■ Microcirculation to a hepatic acinus. *THA*, Terminal hepatic arteriole; *TPV*, terminal portal venule; *BD*, bile ductule; *THV*, terminal hepatic venule; *LY*, lymphatic. The hepatic arterioles empty either directly *(1)* or through the peribiliary plexus *(2)* into the sinusoids that run from the terminal portal venule to the terminal hepatic venules. (From Rappaport AM: *Microvasc Res* 6:212, 1973.)

minal vessels enter the hepatic acinus (the functional unit of the liver) at its center. Blood flows from these terminal vessels into the sinusoids, which constitute the capillary network of the liver. The sinusoids radiate toward the periphery of the acinus, where they connect with the terminal hepatic venules. Blood from these terminal venules drains into progressively larger branches of the hepatic veins, which are tributaries of the inferior vena cava.

Hemodynamics The mean blood pressure in the portal vein is about 10 mm Hg and that in the hepatic artery about 90 mm Hg. The resis-

tance of the vessels upstream to the hepatic sinusoids is considerably greater than that of the downstream vessels. Consequently, the pressure in the sinusoids is only 2 or 3 mm Hg greater than that in the hepatic veins and inferior vena cava. The ratio of presinusoidal to postsinusoidal resistance in the liver is much greater than is the ratio of precapillary to postcapillary resistance for almost any other vascular bed. Hence, drugs and other interventions that alter the presinusoidal resistance usually affect the pressure in the sinusoids only slightly. Such changes in presinusoidal resistance have little effect on the fluid exchange across the sinusoidal wall. Conversely, changes in hepatic venous (and in central venous) pressure are transmitted almost quantitatively to the hepatic sinusoids and profoundly affect the transsinusoidal exchange of fluids.

Regulation of Flow Blood flows in the portal venous and hepatic arterial systems vary reciprocally. When blood flow is curtailed in one system, the flow increases in the other system. However, the ensuing increase in flow in one system usually does not fully compensate for the initiating reduction in flow in the other system.

The portal venous system does not autoregulate. As portal venous pressure and flow are raised, resistance either remains constant or decreases. The hepatic arterial system does autoregulate, however.

When central venous pressure is elevated, as in **congestive heart failure,** large quantities of plasma water transude from the liver into the peritoneal cavity; such a fluid accumulation in the abdomen is known as **ascites.** Extensive fibrosis of the liver, as in the various types of **hepatic cirrhosis,** leads to a pronounced increase in hepatic vascular resistance, which raises the pressure substantially in the portal venous system. The consequent increase in capillary hydrostatic pressure throughout the splanchnic circulation also leads to extensive fluid transudation into the abdominal cavity (i.e., ascites). Furthermore, the pressure may rise substantially in other veins that anastomose with the portal vein. A noteworthy example is that of the esophageal veins. These veins may enlarge considerably to form **esophageal varices,** which may rupture and thereby lead to severe, and frequently fatal, internal bleeding. To obviate these grave problems associated with elevated portal venous pressure, an anastomosis **(portacaval shunt)** is often created surgically between the portal vein and inferior vena cava to lower portal venous pressure.

The liver tends to maintain a constant O_2 consumption, because the extraction of O_2 from the hepatic blood is very efficient. As the rate of O_2 delivery to the liver is varied, the liver compensates by an appropriate change in the fraction of O_2 extracted from the blood. This extraction is facilitated by the distinct separation of the presinusoidal vessels at the acinar center from the postsinusoidal vessels at the periphery of the acinus (Figure 11-17). The substantial distance between these types of vessels prevents a countercurrent exchange of O_2, contrary to the condition that exists in an intestinal villus (Figure 11-16).

The sympathetic nerves constrict the presinusoidal resistance vessels in the portal venous and hepatic arterial systems. Neural effects on the capacitance vessels are more important, however. The liver contains about 15% of the total blood volume of the body. Under appropriate conditions, such as in response to hemorrhage, about half of the hepatic blood volume can be rapidly expelled by virtue of a constriction of the capacitance vessels. Hence, the liver constitutes an important blood reservoir in humans. In certain other species, such as the dog, the spleen is a more important blood reservoir.

■ FETAL CIRCULATION

The circulation of the fetus shows a number of differences from that of the postnatal infant. The fetal lungs are functionally inactive, and the fetus depends completely on the placenta for O_2 and nutrient supply. Oxygenated fetal blood from the placenta passes through the umbilical vein to the liver. Approximately half passes through the liver, and the remainder bypasses the liver and reaches the inferior vena cava through the **ductus venosus** (Figure 11-18). In the inferior vena cava, blood from the ductus venosus joins blood returning from the lower trunk and extremities, and this combined stream is in turn joined by blood from the liver through the hepatic veins.

The streams of blood tend to maintain their identity in the inferior vena cava and are divided into two streams of unequal size by the edge of the interatrial septum **(crista dividens).** The larger stream, which is mainly blood from the umbilical vein, is shunted to the left atrium through the **foramen ovale,** which lies between the in-

ferior vena cava and the left atrium (inset, Figure 11-18). The other stream passes into the right atrium, where it is joined by superior vena caval blood returning from the upper parts of the body and by blood from the myocardium.

Figure 11-18 ■ **Schematic diagram of the fetal circulation. The numbers represent the percentage of O$_2$ saturation of the blood flowing in the indicated blood vessel. The insert at upper left illustrates the direction of flow of a major portion of the inferior vena cava blood through the foramen ovale to the left atrium.** (Values for O$_2$ saturations are from Dawes GS, Mott JC, Widdicombe JG: *J Physiol* 126:563, 1954.)

In contrast to the adult, in whom the right and left ventricles pump in series, the ventricles in the fetus operate essentially in parallel. Because of the large pulmonary resistance, only one tenth of right ventricular output goes through the lungs. The remainder passes through the **ductus arteriosus** from the pulmonary artery to the aorta at a point distal to the origins of the arteries to the head and upper extremities. Blood flows from pulmonary artery to aorta because the pulmonary resistance is high and the diameter of the ductus arteriosus is as large as that of the descending aorta.

The large volume of blood coming through the foramen ovale into the left atrium is joined by blood returning from the lungs, and it is pumped out by the left ventricle into the aorta. Most of the blood in the ascending aorta goes to the head, upper thorax, and arms; the remainder joins blood from the ductus arteriosus and supplies the rest of the body and the placenta. The amount of blood pumped by the left ventricle is about half of that pumped by the right ventricle. The major fraction of the blood that passes down the descending aorta comes from the ductus arteriosus and right ventricle and flows by way of the two umbilical arteries to the placenta.

Figure 11-18 indicates the O_2 saturations of the blood at various points of the fetal circulation. Fetal blood leaving the placenta is 80% saturated, but the saturation of the blood passing through the foramen ovale is reduced to 67% by mixing with desaturated blood returning from the lower part of the body and the liver. Addition of the desaturated blood from the lungs reduces the O_2 saturation of left ventricular blood to 62%, which is the level of saturation of the blood reaching the head and upper extremities.

The blood in the right ventricle, a mixture of desaturated superior vena caval blood, coronary venous blood, and inferior vena caval blood, is only 52% saturated with O_2. When the major portion of this blood traverses the ductus arteriosus and joins that pumped out by the left ventricle, the resulting O_2 saturation of blood traveling to the lower part of the body and back to the placenta is 58%. Thus, it is apparent that the tissues receiving blood of the highest O_2 saturation are the liver, heart, and upper parts of the body, including the head.

At the placenta the chorionic villi dip into the maternal sinuses, and O_2, CO_2, nutrients, and metabolic waste products exchange across the membranes. The barrier to exchange is quite large, and the equilibrium of Po_2 between the two circulations is not reached at normal rates of blood flow. Therefore, the O_2 tension of the fetal blood leaving the placenta is very low. Were it not for the fact that fetal hemoglobin has a greater affinity for O_2 than does adult hemoglobin, the fetus would not receive an adequate O_2 supply. The fetal oxyhemoglobin dissociation curve is shifted to the left so that at equal pressures of O_2 fetal blood carries significantly more O_2 than does maternal blood.

In early fetal life the high cardiac glycogen levels that prevail may protect the heart from acute periods of hypoxia. The glycogen levels decrease in late fetal life and reach adult levels by term.

Circulatory Changes That Occur at Birth

The umbilical vessels have thick muscular walls that are very reactive to trauma, tension, sympathomimetic amines, bradykinin, angiotensin, and changes in Po_2. In animals in which the umbilical cord is not tied, hemorrhage of the newborn

---

If the mother is subjected to hypoxia, the reduced blood O_2 tension is reflected in the fetus by tachycardia and an increase in blood flow through the umbilical vessels. If the hypoxia persists or if flow through the umbilical vessels is impaired, fetal distress occurs and is first manifested as bradycardia.

is prevented by constriction of these large vessels in response to one or more of these stimuli. Closure of the umbilical vessels produces an increase in total peripheral resistance and of blood pressure. When blood flow through the umbilical vein ceases, the ductus venosus, a thick-walled vessel with a muscular sphincter, closes. The factor that initiates closure of the ductus venosus is still unknown.

The asphyxia that starts with constriction or clamping of the umbilical vessels, together with the cooling of the body, activates the respiratory center of the newborn infant. As the lungs fill with air, pulmonary vascular resistance decreases to about one tenth of the value existing before lung expansion. This resistance change is not caused by the presence of O_2 in the lungs, because the change is just as great if the lungs are filled with nitrogen. However, filling the lungs with liquid does not reduce pulmonary vascular resistance.

The left atrial pressure is raised above that in the inferior vena cava and right atrium by (1) the decrease in pulmonary resistance, with the resulting large flow of blood through the lungs to the left atrium; (2) the reduction of flow to the right atrium caused by occlusion of the umbilical vein; and (3) the increased resistance to left ventricular output produced by occlusion of the umbilical arteries. This reversal of the pressure gradient across the atria abruptly closes the valve over the foramen ovale, and the septal leaflets fuse over several days.

With the decrease in pulmonary vascular resistance, the pressure in the pulmonary artery falls to about one half its previous level (to about 35 mm Hg). This change in pressure, coupled with a slight increase in aortic pressure, reverses the flow of blood through the ductus arteriosus. However, within several minutes the large ductus arteriosus begins to constrict, producing turbulent flow, which is manifested as a murmur in the newborn. Constriction of the ductus arterio-

> The ductus arteriosus occasionally fails to close after birth. This constitutes a congenital cardiovascular abnormality that is amenable to surgical correction.

sus is progressive and is usually complete within 1 to 2 days after birth. Closure of the ductus arteriosus appears to be initiated by the high O_2 tension of the arterial blood passing through it; pulmonary ventilation with O_2 closes the ductus, whereas ventilation with air low in O_2 opens this shunt vessel. Whether O_2 acts directly on the ductus or through the release of a vasoconstrictor substance is not known.

At birth the walls of the two ventricles are approximately of the same thickness, with a possibly slight preponderance of the right ventricle. Also in the newborn, the muscle layer of the pulmonary arterioles is thick, which is partly responsible for the high pulmonary vascular resistance of the fetus. After birth the thickness of the walls of the right ventricle diminishes, as does the muscle layer of the pulmonary arterioles; the left ventricular walls become thicker. These changes are progressive over a period of weeks after birth.

■ SUMMARY
Skin Circulation

1. Most of the resistance vessels in the skin are under dual control of the sympathetic nervous system and local vasodilator metabolites, but the arteriovenous anastomoses found in the hands, feet, and face are solely under neural control.
2. The main function of skin blood vessels is to aid in the regulation of body temperature by constricting to conserve heat and dilating to lose heat.
3. Skin blood vessels dilate directly and reflexly in response to heat, and constrict directly and reflexly in response to cold.

Skeletal Muscle Circulation

1. Skeletal muscle blood flow is regulated centrally by the sympathetic nerves and regulated locally by the release of vasodilator metabolites.
2. At rest, neural regulation of blood flow is paramount, but it yields to metabolic regulation during muscle contractions.

Cerebral Circulation

1. Cerebral blood flow is predominantly regulated by metabolic factors, especially CO_2, K^+, and adenosine.
2. Increased regional cerebral activity produced by stimuli such as touch, pain, hand motion, talking, reading, reasoning, and problem solving are associated with enhanced blood flow in the activated areas of the contralateral cerebral cortex.

Pulmonary Circulation

1. The pulmonary circulation consists of the pulmonary vasculature, whose function is to promote the exchange of O_2 and CO_2 across the pulmonary capillaries, and the bronchial vasculature, whose function is to deliver O_2 and nutrients to the airways.
2. The resistance of the pulmonary vasculature is low. Because of the low pulmonary vascular pressures, the distribution of blood flow to different regions of the lungs is affected by the body's position in space.
3. The smooth muscles in the pulmonary arterioles constrict in response to hypoxia. This response tends to shift blood flow to the well-ventilated alveoli and away from the poorly ventilated alveoli.

Renal Circulation

1. Renal blood flow is very high (about 20% of cardiac output), and the chief resistance to blood flow in the kidneys resides in the afferent and efferent arterioles.
2. Glomerular capillary pressure is high (about 50 to 60 mm Hg), and the glomerular capillaries are very permeable to water; these two factors favor the filtration of large quantities of water from the blood to Bowman's capsule.

Intestinal Circulation

1. The microcirculation in the intestinal villi constitutes a countercurrent exchange system for O_2. This places the villi in jeopardy in states of low blood flow.
2. The splanchnic resistance and capacitance vessels are very responsive to changes in sympathetic neural activity.

Hepatic Circulation

1. The liver receives about 25% of cardiac output; about three fourths of this comes via the portal vein and about one fourth via the hepatic artery. When flow is diminished in either the portal or hepatic system, flow in the other system usually increases, but not proportionately.
2. The liver tends to maintain a constant O_2 consumption, in part because its mechanism for extracting O_2 from the blood is so efficient.
3. The liver normally contains about 15% of total blood volume. It serves as an important blood reservoir for the body.

Fetal Circulation

1. In the fetus a large percentage of right atrial blood passes through the foramen ovale to the left atrium, and a large percentage of pulmonary artery blood passes through the ductus arteriosus to the aorta.
2. At birth the umbilical vessels, ductus venosus, and ductus arteriosus close by contraction of their muscle layers. The reduction in pulmonary vascular resistance caused by lung inflation is the main factor that reverses the pressure gradient between the atria, thereby closing the foramen ovale.

■ **KEY WORDS AND CONCEPTS**

- Arteriovenous (AV) anastomoses
- Reactive hyperemia
- Skin flow, regulation
- Ambient temperature
- Basal tone
- Sympathetic innervation
- Denervation hypersensitivity
- Exposure to cold
- Exposure to heat
- Countercurrent heat exchange
- Skin color and blood flow
- Muscle pump
- Muscle flow, regulation
- Venous valves
- Neural tone
- Metabolic factors
- Local factors
- Cerebral blood flow, regulation
- Cerebral flow, measurement
- Regional cerebral flow
- Carbon dioxide
- Potassium
- Adenosine
- Pulmonary vasculature
- Bronchial vasculature
- Pulmonary embolism
- Pulmonary arterial pressure
- Bronchial arterial pressure
- Gravitational effects on pulmonary blood flow
- Waterfall effect
- Ventilation-perfusion ratio
- Effects of hypoxia on pulmonary blood flow
- Renal vascular anatomy
- Pressure regulation in glomerular capillaries
- Glomerular filtration
- Renal oxygen consumption
- Renal blood flow autoregulation
- Juxtaglomerular apparatus
- Tubuloglomerular feedback

- Renin-angiotensin system
- Anatomy of intestinal circulation
- Neural regulation of intestinal blood flow
- Autoregulation of intestinal blood flow
- Functional splanchnic hyperemia
- Anatomy of hepatic circulation
- Dynamics of hepatic circulation
- Hepatic cirrhosis
- Abdominal ascites
- Esophageal varices
- Portacaval shunt
- Fetal circulation
- Ductus venosus
- Foramen ovale
- Ductus arteriosus
- Fetal hemoglobin
- Cardiac glycogen
- Circulatory changes at birth
- Patent ductus arteriosus

■ **SELF-STUDY PROBLEMS**

1. Compare and contrast the chief factors in the regulation of skin and skeletal muscle blood flow.
2. How is cerebral blood flow regulated?
3. Explain why the spatial distribution of blood flow to the lungs changes when a person shifts from a recumbent to a standing position.
4. Would normal kidneys receive adequate oxygen and nutrients to sustain their viability if renal blood flow was reduced substantially?
5. What changes in renal blood flow, glomerular filtration rate, and renal vascular resistance would you expect to find in a normal kidney if the mean arterial pressure in the renal artery was diminished from 150 to 100 mm Hg?
6. The blood flow to the liver is supplied by the portal vein and hepatic artery. What fraction of blood flow and of oxygen supply is normally derived from these two sources? Explain why the two fractions are not equivalent.

7. What problem in transcapillary fluid exchange in the abdominal viscera occurs as a consequence of chronic inflammatory processes in the liver (hepatic cirrhosis)?

8. What happens to the distribution of right ventricular output when the newborn infant takes his or her first few breaths?

■ BIBLIOGRAPHY

Journal articles

Abboud FM, editor: Regulation of the cerebral circulation (symposium), *Fed Proc* 40:2296, 1981.

Berne RM, Winn HR, Rubio R: The local regulation of cerebral blood flow, *Prog Cardiovasc Dis* 24:243, 1981.

Brunner JJ, Greene AS, Frankle AE, Shoukas AA: Carotid sinus baroreceptor control of splanchnic resistance and capacity, *Am J Physiol* 255:H1305, 1988.

Bshouty Z, Younes M: Distensibility and pressure-flow relationship of the pulmonary circulation, I. Single-vessel model, *J Appl Physiol* 68:1501, 1990.

Clyman RI, Saugstad OD, Mauray F: Reactive oxygen metabolites relax the lamb ductus arteriosus by stimulating prostaglandin production, *Circ Res* 64:1, 1989.

Cowley AW, Mattson DL, Lu S, Roman RJ: Renal medulla and hypertension, *Hypertension* 25 (part 2):663, 1995.

Escourrou P, Raffestin B, Papelier Y et al: Cardiopulmonary and carotid baroreflex control of splanchnic and forearm circulations, *Am J Physiol* 264:H777, 1993.

Farrukh IS, Gurtner GH, Terry PB, Tohidi W, Yang J, Adkinson NF Jr, Michael JR: Effect of pH on pulmonary vascular tone, reactivity, and arachidonate metabolism, *J Appl Physiol* 67:445, 1989.

Greenway CV, Lautt WW: Distensibility of hepatic venous resistance sites and consequences on portal pressure, *Am J Physiol* 254:H452, 1988.

Griendling KK, Murphy TJ, Alexander RW: Molecular biology of the renin-angiotensin system, *Circulation* 87:1816, 1993.

Heymann MA, Iwamoto HS, Rudolf AM: Factors affecting changes in the neonatal systemic circulation, *Annu Rev Physiol* 43:371, 1981.

Holstein-Rathlou NH, Marsh DJ: Renal blood flow regulation and arterial pressure fluctuations: a case study in nonlinear dynamics, *Physiol Rev* 74:367, 1994.

Hyman AL, Kadowitz PJ: Analysis of responses to sympathetic nerve stimulation in the feline pulmonary vascular bed, *J Appl Physiol* 67:371, 1989.

Ito S: Role of nitric oxide in glomerular arterioles and macula densa, *News Physiol Sci* 9:115, 1994.

Iwata F, Joh T, Kawai T, Itoh M: Role of EDRF in splanchnic blood flow of normal and chronic portal hypertensive rats, *Am J Physiol* 263:G149, 1992.

Laughlin MH: Skeletal muscle blood flow capacity: role of muscle pump in exercise hyperemia, *Am J Physiol* 253:H993, 1987.

Leeman M, de Beyl VZ, Delcroix M, Naeije R: Effects of endogenous nitric oxide on pulmonary vascular tone in intact dogs, *Am J Physiol* 266:H2343, 1994.

Maass-Moreno R, Rothe CF: Contribution of large hepatic veins to postsinusoidal vascular resistance, *Am J Physiol* 262:G14, 1992.

Marshall JM: Skeletal muscle vasculature and systemic hypoxia, *News Physiol Sci* 10:274, 1995.

Olsson RA: Local factors regulating cardiac and skeletal muscle blood flow, *Annu Rev Physiol* 43:385, 1981.

Raij L: Nitric oxide and the kidney, *Circulation* 87:V-26, 1993.

Reller MD, Burson MA, Lohr JL, Morton MJ, Thornburg KL: Nitric oxide is an important determinant of coronary flow at rest and during hypoxemic stress in fetal lambs, *Am J Physiol* 269:H2074, 1995.

Schwartz LM, McKenzie JE: Adenosine and active hyperemia in soleus and gracilis muscle of cats, *Am J Physiol* 259:H1295, 1990.

Skarlatos S, Metting PJ, Britton SL: Spontaneous pressure-flow patterns in the kidney of conscious rats, *Am J Physiol* 265:H2151, 1993.

Stamler JS, Loh E, Roddy M-A et al: Nitric oxide regulates basal systemic and pulmonary vascular resistance in healthy humans, *Circulation* 89:2035, 1994.

Tysbenko VA, Yanchuk PI: Central nervous control of hepatic circulation, *J Auton Nerv Syst* 33:255, 1991.

van Tilborg KA, Rabelink TJ, van Rijn HJM et al: Arterial baroreflex control of renal hemodynamics in humans, *Circulation* 90:1883, 1994.

Wanner A: Circulation of the airway mucosa, *J Appl Physiol* 67:917, 1989.

Weir EK, Archer SL: Mechanism of acute hypoxic pulmonary vasoconstriction: the tale of two channels, *FASEB J* 9:183, 1995.

Wong J, Reddy VM, Hendricks-Munoz K, Liddicoat JR, Gerrets R, Fineman JR: Endothelin-1 vasoactive responses in lambs with pulmonary hypertension and increased pulmonary blood flow, *Am J Physiol* 269:H1965, 1995.

Zellers TM, McCormick J, Wu Y: Interaction among ET-1, endothelium-derived nitric oxide, and prostacyclin in pulmonary arteries and veins, *Am J Physiol* 267:H139, 1994.

Books and monographs

Berne RM, Winn HR, Rubio R: *Metabolic regulation of cerebral blood flow.* In *Mechanisms of vasodilation—Second Symposium,* New York, 1981, Raven Press.

Butler J: *Bronchial circulation,* Basel, 1992, Marcel Dekker.

Donald DE: *Splanchnic circulation.* In *Handbook of physiology, Section 2: The cardiovascular system—peripheral circulation and organ blood flow,* vol III, Bethesda, Md., 1983, American Physiological Society.

Faber JJ, Thornburg KK: *Placental physiology,* New York, 1983, Raven Press.

Fishman AP: *The pulmonary circulation,* Philadelphia, 1990, University of Pennsylvania Press.

Granger DN, Kvietys PR, Korthuis RJ, Premen AJ: *Microcirculation of the intestinal mucosa.* In *Handbook of physiology,* Section 6: *The gastrointestinal system—motility and circulation,* vol I, Bethesda, Md., 1989, American Physiological Society.

Greenway CV, Lautt WW: *Hepatic circulation.* In *Handbook of physiology,* Section 6: *The gastrointestinal system—motility and circulation,* vol I, Bethesda, Md., 1989, American Physiological Society.

Grover RF, Wagner WW Jr, McMurtry IF, Reeves JT: *Pulmonary circulation.* In *Handbook of physiology,* Section 2: *The cardiovascular system—peripheral circulation and organ blood flow,* vol III, Bethesda, Md., 1983, American Physiological Society.

Guth PH, Leung FW, Kauffman GL Jr: *Physiology of gastric circulation.* In *Handbook of physiology,* Section 6: *The gastrointestinal system—motility and circulation,* vol I, Bethesda, Md., 1989, American Physiological Society.

Heistad DD, Kontos HA: *Cerebral circulation.* In *Handbook of physiology,* Section 2: *The cardiovascular system—peripheral circulation and organ blood flow,* vol III, Bethesda, Md., 1983, American Physiological Society.

Hellon R: *Thermoreceptors.* In *Handbook of physiology,* Section 2: *The cardiovascular system—peripheral circulation and organ blood flow,* vol III, Bethesda, Md., 1983, American Physiological Society.

Knox FG, Spielman WS: *Renal circulation.* In *Handbook of physiology,* Section 2: *The cardiovascular system—peripheral circulation and organ blood flow,* vol III, Bethesda, Md., 1983, American Physiological Society.

Lewis T: *Blood vessels of the human skin and their responses,* London, 1927, Shaw & Son.

Mott JC, Walker DW: *Neural and endocrine regulation of circulation in the fetus and newborn.* In *Handbook of physiology,* Section 2: *The cardiovascular system—peripheral circulation and organ blood flow,* vol III, Bethesda, Md., 1983, American Physiological Society.

Owman C, Hardebo JE, editors: *Neural regulation of brain circulation,* Amsterdam, 1985, Elsevier.

Phillis JW, editor: *The regulation of cerebral blood flow,* Boca Raton, Fla., 1993, CRC Press.

Roddie EC: *Circulation to skin and adipose tissue.* In *Handbook of physiology,* Section 2: *The cardiovascular system—peripheral circulation and organ blood flow,* vol III, Bethesda, Md., 1983, American Physiological Society.

Shepherd JT: *Circulation to skeletal muscle.* In *Handbook of physiology,* Section 2: *The cardiovascular system—peripheral circulation and organ blood flow,* vol III, Bethesda, Md., 1983, American Physiological Society.

Wagner WW Jr, Weir EK, editors: *Pulmonary circulation and gas exchange,* Armonk, NY, 1994, Futura Publishing.

Interplay of Central and Peripheral Factors in the Control of the Circulation

The primary function of the circulatory system is to deliver the supplies needed for tissue metabolism and growth and to remove the products of metabolism. To explain how the heart and blood vessels serve this function, it has been necessary to analyze the system morphologically and functionally and to discuss the mechanisms of action of the component parts in their contribution to maintaining adequate tissue perfusion under different physiologic conditions. Once the functions of the various components are understood, it is essential that their interrelationships in the overall role of the circulatory system be considered. Tissue perfusion depends on arterial pressure and local vascular resistance, and arterial pressure in turn depends on cardiac output and total peripheral resistance (TPR). Arterial pressure is maintained within a relatively narrow range in the normal individual, a feat accomplished by reciprocal changes in cardiac output and TPR. However, cardiac output and peripheral resistance are each influenced by a number of factors, and it is the interplay among these factors that determines the level of these two variables. The autonomic nervous system and the baroreceptors play the key role in regulating blood pressure. However, from the long-range point of view, the control of fluid balance by the kidney, adrenal cortex, and central nervous system, with maintenance of a constant blood volume, is of the greatest importance.

In a well-regulated system, one way to study the extent and sensitivity of the regulatory mechanism is to disturb the system and observe its response to restore the preexisting steady state. Disturbances in the form of physical exercise and hemorrhage will be used to illustrate the effects of the various factors that go into regulation of the circulatory system.

■ EXERCISE

The cardiovascular adjustments in exercise consist of a combination and integration of neural and local (chemical) factors. The neural factors consist of (1) **central command,** (2) reflexes originating in the contracting muscle, and (3) the baroreceptor reflex. Central command is the cerebrocortical activation of the sympathetic nervous system that produces cardiac acceleration, increased myocardial contractile force, and peripheral vasoconstriction. Reflexes can be activated intramuscularly by stimulation of mechanoreceptors (by stretch, tension) and chemoreceptors (by products of metabolism) in response

269

to muscle contraction. Impulses from these receptors travel centrally via small myelinated (group III) and unmyelinated (group IV) afferent nerve fibers. The group IV unmyelinated fibers may represent the muscle chemoreceptors; no morphologic chemoreceptor has been identified. The central connections of this reflex are unknown, but the efferent limb is the sympathetic nerve fibers to the heart and peripheral blood vessels. The baroreceptor reflex has been described on page 183, and the local factors that influence skeletal muscle blood flow (metabolic vasodilators) are described on pages 177 and 244. Vascular chemoreceptors do not play a significant role in regulation of the cardiovascular system in exercise. The pH, P_{CO_2}, and P_{O_2} of arterial blood are normal during exercise, and the vascular chemoreceptors are located on the arterial side of the circulatory system.

Mild to Moderate Exercise

In humans or in trained animals, anticipation of physical activity inhibits the vagal nerve impulses to the heart and increases sympathetic discharge. The concerted inhibition of parasympathetic areas and activation of sympathetic areas of the medulla on the heart result in an increase in heart rate and myocardial contractility. The tachycardia and the enhanced contractility increase cardiac output.

Peripheral Resistance At the same time that cardiac stimulation occurs, the sympathetic nervous system also elicits vascular resistance changes in the periphery. In skin, kidneys, splanchnic regions, and inactive muscle, sympathetic-mediated vasoconstriction increases vascular resistance, which diverts blood away from these areas (Figure 12-1). This increased resistance in vascular beds of inactive tissues persists throughout the period of exercise.

As cardiac output and blood flow to active muscles increase with progressive increments in the intensity of exercise, visceral blood flow

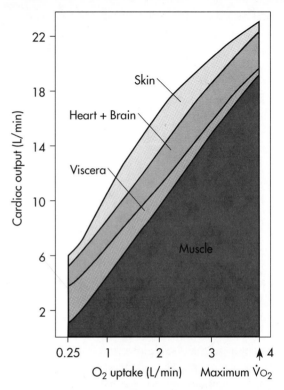

Figure 12-1 ■ Approximate distribution of cardiac output at rest and at different levels of exercise up to the maximal O_2 consumption ($\dot{V}_{O_{2max}}$) in a normal young man. (Redrawn from Ruch HP, Patton TC: *Physiology and biophysics,* ed 12, Philadelphia, 1974, WB Saunders.)

(to the splanchnic and renal vasculatures) decreases. Blood flow to the myocardium increases, whereas that to the brain is unchanged. Skin blood flow initially decreases during exercise and then increases as body temperature rises with increments in duration and intensity of exercise. Skin blood flow finally decreases when the skin vessels constrict as the total body O_2 consumption nears maximum (Figure 12-1).

The major circulatory adjustment to prolonged exercise involves the vasculature of the active muscles. Local formation of vasoactive metabolites induces marked dilation of the resistance vessels, which progresses with increases in the intensity level of exercise. Potassium is one of the vasodilator substances released by contracting muscle, and it may be in part responsible for the initial decrease in vascular resistance in the active muscles. Other contributing factors may be the release of adenosine and a decrease in pH during sustained exercise. The local accumulation of metabolites relaxes the terminal arterioles. Blood flow through the muscle may increase 15 to 20 times above the resting level. This metabolic vasodilation of the precapillary vessels in active muscles occurs very soon after the onset of exercise, and the decrease in TPR enables the heart to pump more blood at a lesser load and more efficiently (less pressure work, p 233) than if TPR were unchanged. Only a small percentage of the capillaries is perfused at rest, whereas in actively contracting muscle all or nearly all of the capillaries contain flowing blood **(capillary recruitment).** The surface available for exchange of gases, water, and solutes is increased manyfold. Furthermore, the hydrostatic pressure in the capillaries is increased because of the relaxation of the resistance vessels. Hence, there is a net movement of water and solutes into the muscle tissue. Tissue pressure rises and remains elevated during exercise as fluid continues to move out of the capillaries and is carried away by the lymphatics. Lymph flow is increased as a result of the increase in capillary hydrostatic pressure and the massaging effect of the contracting muscles on the valve-containing lymphatic vessels (see p 167).

The contracting muscle avidly extracts O_2 from the perfusing blood (increased AV-O_2 difference, Figure 12-2), and the release of O_2 from the blood is facilitated by the nature of oxyhemoglobin dissociation. The reduction in pH caused by the high concentration of CO_2 and the formation of lactic acid and the increase in temperature in the contracting muscle contribute to

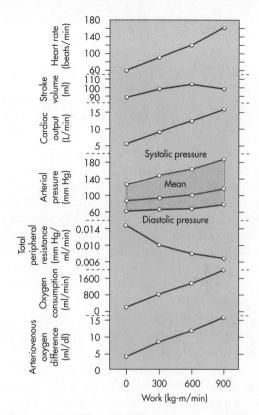

Figure 12-2 ■ Effect of different levels of exercise on several cardiovascular variables. (Data from Carlsten A, Grimby G: *The circulatory response to muscular exercise in man,* Springfield, Ill., 1966, Charles C Thomas.)

shifting the oxyhemoglobin dissociation curve to the right. At any given partial pressure of O_2, less O_2 is held by the hemoglobin in the red cells, and consequently there is more effective O_2 removal from the blood. Oxygen consumption may increase as much as sixtyfold with only a fifteenfold increase in muscle blood flow. Muscle myoglobin may serve as a limited O_2 store in exercise and can release attached O_2 at very low partial pressures. However, it can facilitate O_2 transport from capillaries to mitochondria by serving as an O_2 carrier.

Cardiac Output The enhanced sympathetic drive and the reduced parasympathetic inhibition of the sinoatrial node continue during exercise, and consequently tachycardia persists. If the workload is moderate and constant, the heart rate will reach a certain level and remain there throughout the period of exercise. However, if the workload increases, a concomitant increase in heart rate occurs until a plateau is reached in severe exercise at about 180 beats per minute (Figure 12-2). In contrast to the large increment in heart rate, the increase in stroke volume is only about 10% to 35% (Figure 12-2), the larger values occurring in trained individuals. (In very well trained distance runners, whose cardiac outputs can reach six to seven times the resting level, stroke volume reaches about twice the resting value.)

Thus, it is apparent that the increase in cardiac output observed with exercise is correlated principally with an increase in heart rate. If the baroreceptors are denervated, the cardiac output and heart rate responses to exercise are sluggish compared with the changes in animals with normally innervated baroreceptors. However, in the absence of autonomic innervation of the heart, as produced experimentally in dogs by total cardiac denervation, exercise still elicits an increment in cardiac output comparable with that observed in normal animals, but chiefly by means of an elevated stroke volume. However, if a beta-adrenergic receptor blocking agent is given to dogs with denervated hearts, exercise performance is impaired. The beta-adrenergic receptor blocker apparently prevents the cardiac acceleration and enhanced contractility caused by increased amounts of circulating catecholamines, and hence limits the increase in cardiac output necessary for maximal exercise performance.

Venous Return In addition to the contribution made by sympathetically mediated constriction of the capacitance vessels in both exercising and nonexercising parts of the body, venous return is aided by the working skeletal muscles and the muscles of respiration. The intermittently contracting muscles compress the vessels that course through them and, in the case of veins with their valves oriented toward the heart, pump blood back toward the right atrium. The flow of venous blood to the heart is also aided by the increase in the pressure gradient developed by the more negative intrathoracic pressure produced by deeper and more frequent respirations. In humans, with the exception of the skin, lungs, and liver, there is little evidence that blood reservoirs contribute much to circulating blood volume. In fact, blood volume is usually reduced slightly during exercise, as evidenced by a rise in the hematocrit ratio, because of water loss externally by sweating and enhanced ventilation, and fluid movement into the contracting muscle. The fluid loss from the vascular compartment into contracting muscle reaches a plateau as interstitial fluid pressure rises and opposes the increased hydrostatic pressure in the capillaries of the active muscle. The fluid loss is partially offset by movement of fluid from the splanchnic regions and inactive muscle into the bloodstream. This influx of fluid occurs as a result of a decrease of hydrostatic pressure in the capillaries of these tissues and of an increase in plasma osmolarity because of movement of osmotically active particles into the blood from the contracting muscle. In addition, reduced urine formation by the kidneys helps to conserve body water.

The large volume of blood returning to the heart is so rapidly pumped through the lungs and out into the aorta that central venous pressure remains essentially constant. Thus, the Frank-Starling mechanism of a greater initial fiber length does not account for the greater stroke volume in moderate exercise. Chest x-ray films of individuals at rest and during exercise reveal a decrease in heart size in exercise, which is in harmony with the observations of a constant ventricular filling pressure. However, in maximal or near-maximal exercise, right atrial pressure and end-diastolic ventricular volume do increase. Thus, the Frank-Starling mechanism contributes to the enhanced stroke volume in very vigorous exercise.

Arterial Pressure If the exercise involves a large proportion of the body musculature, such as in running or swimming, the reduction in total vascular resistance can be considerable (Figure 12-2). Nevertheless, arterial pressure starts to rise with the onset of exercise, and the increase in blood pressure roughly parallels the severity of the exercise performed (Figure 12-2). Therefore, the increase in cardiac output is proportionally greater than the decrease in TPR. The vasoconstriction produced in the inactive tissues by the sympathetic nervous system (and to some extent by the release of catecholamines from the adrenal medulla) is important for maintaining normal or increased blood pressure, because sympathectomy or drug-induced block of the adrenergic sympathetic nerve fibers results in a decrease in arterial pressure **(hypotension)** during exercise.

Sympathetic-mediated vasoconstriction also occurs in active muscle when additional muscles are activated after about half of the total skeletal musculature is contracting. In experiments in which one leg is working at maximal levels and then the other leg starts to work, blood flow decreases in the first working leg. Furthermore, blood levels of norepinephrine rise significantly in exercise, and most of it comes from sympathetic nerves in the active muscles.

As body temperature rises during exercise, the skin vessels dilate in response to thermal stimulation of the heat-regulating center in the hypothalamus, and TPR decreases further. This would result in a decline in blood pressure were it not for the increasing cardiac output and constriction of arterioles in the renal, splanchnic, and other tissues.

In general, mean arterial pressure rises during exercise as a result of the increase in cardiac output. However, the effect of enhanced cardiac output is offset by the overall decrease in TPR, so that the mean blood pressure increase is relatively small. Vasoconstriction in the inactive vascular beds contributes to the maintenance of a normal arterial blood pressure for adequate perfusion of the active tissues. The actual pressure attained represents a balance between cardiac output and TPR (p 141). Systolic pressure usually increases more than diastolic pressure, which results in an increase in pulse pressure (Figure 12-2). The larger pulse pressure is primarily attributable to a greater stroke volume, and to a lesser degree to a more rapid ejection of blood by the left ventricle with less peripheral runoff during the brief ventricular ejection period.

Severe Exercise

In severe exercise taken to the point of exhaustion, the compensatory mechanisms begin to fail. Heart rate attains a maximal level of about 180 beats per minute, and stroke volume reaches a plateau and often decreases, resulting in a fall in blood pressure. Dehydration occurs. Sympathetic vasoconstrictor activity supersedes the vasodilator influence on the cutaneous vessels and has the hemodynamic effect of a slight increase in effective blood volume. However, cutaneous vasoconstriction also decreases the rate of heat loss. Body temperature is normally elevated in exercise, and reduction in heat loss through cutaneous vasoconstriction can, under these conditions, lead to very high body temperatures with associated feelings of acute distress. The tissue and blood pH decrease as a result of increased lactic acid and CO_2 production. The reduced pH is probably the key factor that determines the maximal amount of exercise a given individual can tolerate because of muscle pain, subjective feeling of exhaustion, and inability or loss of will to continue. A summary of the neural and local

effects of exercise on the cardiovascular system
is schematized in Figure 12-3.

Postexercise Recovery

When exercise stops, an abrupt decrease in heart
rate and cardiac output occurs—the sympathetic
drive to the heart is essentially removed. In contrast, TPR remains low for some time after the exercise is ended, presumably because of the accumulation of vasodilator metabolites in the
muscles during the exercise period. As a result of
the reduced cardiac output and persistence of
vasodilation in the muscles, arterial pressure falls,
often below preexercise levels, for brief periods.
Blood pressure is then stabilized at normal levels
by the baroreceptor reflexes.

Limits of Exercise Performance

The two main forces that could limit skeletal
muscle performance in the human body are the
rate of O_2 utilization by the muscles and the O_2
supply to the muscles. Muscle O_2 usage is probably not critical, because during exercise maximum O_2 consumption ($\dot{V}o_{2max}$) by a large percentage of the body muscle mass is unchanged
or increases slightly when additional muscles are
activated. In fact, during exercise of a large muscle mass, as in vigorous bicycling, commence-
ment of bilateral arm exercise without change in
the cycling efforts produces only a small increment in cardiac output and $\dot{V}o_{2max}$. However, it
causes a decrease in blood flow to the legs. This
centrally mediated (baroreceptor reflex) vaso-

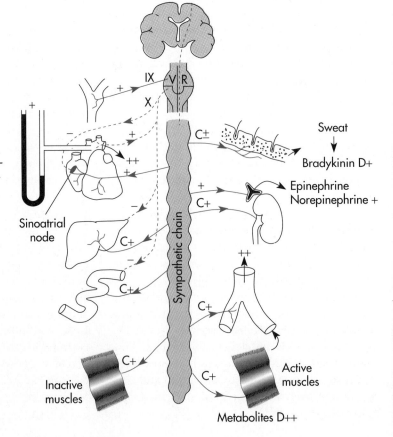

Figure 12-3 ■ Cardiovascular adjustments in exercise. *VR,* Vasomotor region; *C,* vasoconstrictor activity; *D,* vasodilator
activity; *IX,* glossopharyngeal
nerve; *X,* vagus nerve; +, increased activity; −, decreased
activity.

constriction during maximal cardiac output prevents a fall in blood pressure that would otherwise be caused by metabolically induced vasodilation in the active muscles. If muscle O_2 utilization were limiting, recruitment of more contracting muscle would use much more O_2 to meet the enhanced O_2 requirements (about the amount equal to the sum of oxygen consumption of the arms and legs exercised alone).

Limitation of O_2 supply could be caused by inadequate oxygenation of blood in the lungs or limitation of the supply of O_2-laden blood to the muscles. Failure to fully oxygenate blood by the lungs can be excluded, because even with the most strenuous exercise at sea level, arterial blood is fully saturated with O_2. Therefore, O_2 delivery (or blood flow, because arterial blood O_2 content is normal) to the active muscles appears to be the limiting factor in muscle performance. This limitation could be caused by the inability to increase cardiac output beyond a certain level as a result of a limitation of stroke volume, because heart rate reaches maximal levels before $\dot{V}O_{2max}$ is reached. *Hence, the major factor is the pumping capacity of the heart.*

With exercise of a small group of muscles, such as those found in the hand, when the cardiovascular system is not severely taxed, the limiting factor is unknown but lies within the muscle.

Physical Training and Conditioning

The response of the cardiovascular system to regular exercise is to increase its capacity to deliver O_2 to the active muscles and to improve the ability of the muscle to utilize O_2. The $\dot{V}O_{2max}$ is quite reproducible in a given individual and varies with the level of physical conditioning. Training progressively increases the $\dot{V}O_{2max}$, which reaches a plateau at the highest level of conditioning. Highly trained athletes have a lower resting heart rate, greater stroke volume, and lower peripheral resistance than they had

before training or after deconditioning (becoming sedentary). The low resting heart rate is caused by a higher vagal tone and a lower sympathetic tone. With exercise, the maximal heart rate of the trained individual is the same as that in the untrained but is attained at a higher level of exercise.

The trained person also exhibits a low vascular resistance that is inherent in the muscle. For example, if an individual exercises one leg regularly over an extended period and does not exercise the other leg, the vascular resistance is lower and the $\dot{V}O_{2max}$ is higher in the "trained" leg than in the "untrained" leg. Also, the well-trained athlete has a lower resting sympathetic outflow to the viscera than does a sedentary counterpart. Physical conditioning is also associated with greater extraction of O_2 from the blood (greater AV-O_2 difference) by the muscles. With long-term training, capillary density in skeletal muscle increases. Also, an increase in the number of arterioles may account for the decrease in muscle vascular resistance. The numbers of mitochondria increase, as do the oxidative enzymes in the mitochondria. Also, it appears that ATPase activity, myoglobin, and enzymes involved in lipid metabolism increase with physical conditioning.

Endurance training, such as running or swimming, produces an increase in left ventricular volume without producing an increase in left ventricular wall thickness. In contrast, strength exercises, such as weight lifting, appear to produce some increase in left ventricular wall thickness (hypertrophy) with little effect on ventricular volume. However, this increase in wall thickness is small relative to that observed in hypertension, in which there is a persistent elevation of afterload because of the high peripheral resistance.

■ HEMORRHAGE

In an individual who has lost a large quantity of blood, the principal system affected is the cardiovascular system. The arterial systolic, diastolic, and pulse pressures diminish and the arterial pulse is rapid and feeble. The cutaneous veins are collapsed and fill slowly when compressed centrally. The skin is pale, moist, and slightly cyanotic. Respiration is rapid, but the depth of respiration may be shallow or deep.

Course of Arterial Blood Pressure Changes

Cardiac output decreases as a result of blood loss (see Chapter 9). The changes in mean arterial pressure evoked by an acute hemorrhage in experimental animals are illustrated in Figure 12-4. If sufficient blood is withdrawn rapidly to bring mean arterial pressure to 50 mm Hg, the pressure tends to rise spontaneously toward control over the subsequent 20 or 30 minutes. In some ani-

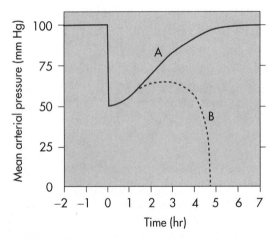

Figure 12-4 ■ Changes in mean arterial pressure after a rapid hemorrhage. At time zero, the animal is bled rapidly to a mean arterial pressure of 50 mm Hg. After a period in which the pressure returns toward the control level, some animals continue to improve until the control pressure is attained (curve *A*). However, in other animals the pressure will begin to decline until death ensues (curve *B*).

mals (curve *A*, Figure 12-4), this trend continues and normal pressures are regained within a few hours. In other animals (curve *B*), after an initial pressure rise, the pressure begins to decline and it continues to fall at an accelerating rate until death ensues. This progressive deterioration of cardiovascular function is termed **hemorrhagic shock.** At some point the deterioration becomes irreversible; a lethal outcome can be retarded only temporarily by any known therapy, including massive transfusions of donor blood.

Compensatory Mechanisms

The changes in arterial pressure immediately after an acute blood loss (Figure 12-4) indicate that certain compensatory mechanisms must be operating. Any mechanism that senses the level of blood pressure and raises the pressure toward normal in response to the reduction in pressure may be designated a **negative feedback mechanism.** It is termed "negative" because the secondary change in pressure is opposite to the initiating change. The following negative feedback responses are evoked: (1) the baroreceptor reflexes, (2) the chemoreceptor reflexes, (3) cerebral ischemia responses, (4) reabsorption of tissue fluids, (5) release of endogenous vasoconstrictor substances, and (6) renal conservation of salt and water.

Baroreceptor Reflexes The reduction in mean arterial pressure and in pulse pressure during hemorrhage decreases the stimulation of the baroreceptors in the carotid sinuses and aortic arch (see Chapter 8). Several cardiovascular responses are thus evoked, all of which tend to restore the normal level of arterial pressure. Reduction of vagal tone and enhancement of sympathetic tone increase heart rate and enhance myocardial contractility.

The increased sympathetic discharge also produces generalized venoconstriction, which has the same hemodynamic consequences as a transfusion of blood (see Chapter 9). Sympathetic activation constricts certain blood reservoirs, which provides an autotransfusion of blood into the circulating bloodstream. In the dog, considerable quantities of blood are mobilized by contraction of the spleen. In humans, the cutaneous, pulmonary, and hepatic vasculatures probably constitute the principal blood reservoirs.

Generalized arteriolar vasoconstriction is a prominent response to the diminished baroreceptor stimulation during hemorrhage. The reflex increase in peripheral resistance minimizes the fall in arterial pressure resulting from the reduction of cardiac output. Figure 12-5 shows the effect of an 8% blood loss on mean aortic pressure in a group of dogs. If both vagi are cut to eliminate the influence of the aortic arch baroreceptors, and only the carotid sinus baroreceptors are operative (left panel), this hemorrhage decreases mean aortic pressure by 14%. This pressure change did not differ significantly from the pressure decline (12%) evoked by the same hemorrhage before vagotomy (not shown). When the

carotid sinuses are denervated and the aortic baroreceptor reflexes are intact, the 8% blood loss decreases mean aortic pressure by 38% (middle panel). Hence, the carotid sinus baroreceptors are more effective than the aortic baroreceptors in attenuating the fall in pressure. The aortic baroreceptors must also be operative, however, because when both sets of afferent baroreceptor pathways are interrupted, an 8% blood loss reduces arterial pressure by 48%.

Although the arteriolar vasoconstriction is widespread during hemorrhage, it is by no means uniform. Vasoconstriction is most severe in the cutaneous, skeletal muscle, and splanchnic vascular beds and is slight or absent in the cerebral and coronary circulations. In many instances the cerebral and coronary vascular resistances are diminished. *Thus, the reduced cardiac output is redistributed to favor flow through the brain and the heart.*

In the early stages of mild to moderate hemorrhage, the changes in renal resistance are usu-

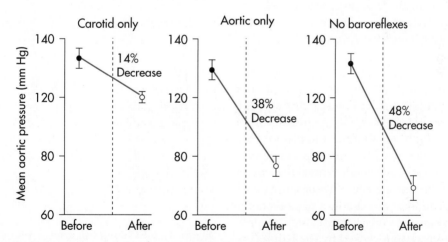

Figure 12-5 ■ Changes in mean aortic pressure in response to an 8% blood loss in a group of eight dogs. *Left panel,* The carotid sinus baroreceptor reflexes were intact and the aortic reflexes were interrupted. *Middle panel,* The aortic reflexes were intact and the carotid sinus reflexes were interrupted. *Right panel,* All sinoaortic reflexes were abrogated. (From Shepherd JT: *Circulation* 50:418, 1974. By permission of the American Heart Association, Inc.; derived from the data of Edis AJ: *Am J Physiol* 221:1352, 1971.)

ally slight. The tendency for increased sympathetic activity to constrict the renal vessels is counteracted by autoregulatory mechanisms (see Chapter 11). With more prolonged and severe hemorrhages, however, renal vasoconstriction becomes intense. The reductions in renal circulation are most severe in the outer layers of the renal cortex. The inner zones of the cortex and outer zones of the medulla are spared.

The severe renal and splanchnic vasoconstriction during hemorrhage favors the heart and brain. However, if such constriction persists too long, it may be detrimental. Frequently, patients survive the acute hypotensive period only to die several days later from kidney failure resulting from renal ischemia. Intestinal ischemia may also have dire effects. In the dog, for example, intestinal bleeding and extensive sloughing of the mucosa occur after only a few hours of hemorrhagic hypotension. Furthermore, the diminished splanchnic flow swells the centrilobular cells in the liver. The resulting obstruction of the hepatic sinusoids raises the portal venous pressure, which intensifies the intestinal blood loss. Fortunately, the pathologic changes in the liver and in the intestine are usually much less severe in humans than in dogs.

Chemoreceptor Reflexes Reductions in arterial pressure below about 60 mm Hg do not evoke any additional responses through the baroreceptor reflexes, because this pressure level constitutes the threshold for stimulation (see Chapter 8). However, low arterial pressure may stimulate peripheral chemoreceptors because of hypoxia in the chemoreceptor tissue consequent to inadequate local blood flow. Chemoreceptor excitation enhances the already existent peripheral vasoconstriction evoked by the baroreceptor reflexes. Also, respiratory stimulation assists venous return by the auxiliary pumping mechanism described in Chapter 9.

Cerebral Ischemia When the arterial pressure is below about 40 mm Hg, the resulting cerebral ischemia activates the sympathoadrenal system. The sympathetic nervous discharge is several times greater than the maximal neural activity that occurs when the baroreceptors cease to be stimulated. Therefore, the vasoconstriction and facilitation of myocardial contractility may be pronounced. With more severe degrees of cerebral ischemia, however, the vagal centers also become activated. The resulting bradycardia may aggravate the hypotension that initiated the cerebral ischemia.

Reabsorption of Tissue Fluids The arterial hypotension, arteriolar constriction, and reduced venous pressure during hemorrhagic hypotension lower the hydrostatic pressure in the capillaries. The balance of these forces promotes the net reabsorption of interstitial fluid into the vascular compartment (see Chapter 7). The rapidity of this response is displayed in Figure 12-6. In a group of cats, 45% of the estimated blood volume was removed over a 30-minute period. The mean arterial blood pressure declined rapidly to about 45 mm Hg. The pressure then re-

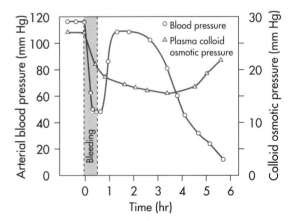

Figure 12-6 ■ Changes in arterial blood pressure and plasma colloid osmotic pressure in response to withdrawal of 45% of the estimated blood volume over a 30-minute period, beginning at time zero. The data are the average values for 23 cats. (Redrawn from Zweifach BW: *Anesthesiology* 41:157, 1974.)

turned rapidly, but only temporarily, to near the control level. The plasma colloid osmotic pressure declined markedly during the bleeding and continued to decrease more gradually for several hours. The reduction in colloid osmotic pressure reflects the dilution of the blood by tissue fluids that contain little protein.

Considerable quantities of fluid may thus be drawn into the circulation during hemorrhage. About 0.25 ml of fluid per minute per kilogram of body weight may be reabsorbed. Approximately 1 L of fluid per hour might be autoinfused into the circulatory system of an average individual from the interstitial spaces after an acute blood loss.

Considerable quantities of fluid may also be slowly shifted from intracellular to extracellular spaces. This fluid exchange is probably mediated by secretion of cortisol from the adrenal cortex in response to hemorrhage. Cortisol appears to be essential for a full restoration of plasma volume after hemorrhage.

Endogenous Vasoconstrictors The **catecholamines** epinephrine and norepinephrine are released from the adrenal medulla in response to the same stimuli that evoke widespread sympathetic nervous discharge. Blood levels of catecholamines are high during and after hemorrhage. When animals are bled to an arterial pressure level of 40 mm Hg, the catecholamines increase as much as 50 times.

Epinephrine comes almost exclusively from the adrenal medulla, whereas norepinephrine is derived from both the adrenal medulla and the peripheral sympathetic nerve endings. These humoral substances reinforce the effects of sympathetic nervous activity listed previously.

Vasopressin, a potent vasoconstrictor, is actively secreted by the posterior pituitary gland in response to hemorrhage. The plasma concentration of vasopressin rises progressively as the arterial blood pressure diminishes (Figure 12-7). The receptors responsible for the augmented

release are the sinoaortic baroreceptors and stretch receptors in the left atrium.

The diminished renal perfusion during hemorrhagic hypotension leads to the secretion of **renin** from the juxtaglomerular apparatus (see Chapter 11). This enzyme acts on a plasma protein, **angiotensinogen,** to form **angiotensin,** a very powerful vasoconstrictor.

Renal Conservation of Salt and Water
Fluid and electrolytes are conserved by the kidneys during hemorrhage in response to various stimuli, including the increased secretion of vasopressin (antidiuretic hormone) noted previously (Figure 12-7). The lower arterial pressure decreases the glomerular filtration rate and thus curtails the excretion of water and electrolytes. Also, the diminished renal blood flow raises the blood levels of angiotensin, as described above. This polypeptide accelerates the release of **aldosterone** from the adrenal cortex. Aldosterone in turn stimulates sodium reabsorption by the renal tubules, and water accompanies the sodium that is actively reabsorbed.

Figure 12-7 ■ **Mean percentage changes in arterial blood pressure and in plasma vasopressin concentration in response to blood loss (0.5 ml/kg/min) in a group of 12 dogs; the maximal volume of blood withdrawn was 30 ml/kg.** (Redrawn from Shen Y-T, Cowley AW Jr, Vatner SF: *Circ Res* 68:1422, 1991. By permission of the American Heart Association, Inc.)

Decompensatory Mechanisms

In contrast to the negative feedback mechanisms just described, latent **positive feedback mechanisms** are also evoked by hemorrhage. Such mechanisms exaggerate any primary change initiated by the blood loss. Specifically, positive feedback mechanisms aggravate the hypotension induced by blood loss and tend to initiate vicious cycles, which may lead to death. The operation of positive feedback mechanisms is manifested in curve *B* of Figure 12-4.

Whether a positive feedback mechanism will lead to a vicious cycle depends on the **gain** of that mechanism. Gain is defined as the ratio of the secondary change evoked by a given mechanism to the initiating change itself. A gain greater than 1 induces a vicious cycle; a gain less than 1 does not. For example, consider a positive feedback mechanism with a gain of 2. If, for any reason, mean arterial pressure were to decrease by 10 mm Hg, the positive feedback mechanism with a gain of 2 would then evoke a secondary pressure reduction of 20 mm Hg, which in turn would cause a further decrement of 40 mm Hg; that is, each change would induce a subsequent change that was twice as great. Hence, mean arterial pressure would decline at an ever-increasing rate until death supervened, much as is depicted by curve *B* in Figure 12-4.

Conversely, a positive feedback mechanism with a gain of 0.5 would indeed exaggerate any change in mean arterial pressure but would not necessarily lead to death. For example, if arterial pressure suddenly decreased by 10 mm Hg, the positive feedback mechanism would initiate a secondary, additional fall of 5 mm Hg. This in turn would provoke a further decrease of 2.5 mm Hg. The process would continue in ever-diminishing steps, with the arterial pressure approaching an equilibrium value asymptotically.

Some of the more important positive feedback mechanisms include (1) cardiac failure, (2) acidosis, (3) central nervous system depres-

sion, (4) aberrations of blood clotting, and (5) depression of the reticuloendothelial system.

Cardiac Failure The role of cardiac failure in the progression of shock during hemorrhage is controversial. All investigators agree that the heart fails terminally, but opinions differ concerning the importance of cardiac failure during earlier stages of hemorrhagic hypotension. Shifts to the right in ventricular function curves (Figure 12-8) constitute experimental evidence of a progressive depression of myocardial contractility during hemorrhage.

The hypotension induced by hemorrhage reduces the coronary blood flow and therefore depresses ventricular function. The consequent reduction in cardiac output leads to a further decline in arterial pressure, a classic example of a positive feedback mechanism. Furthermore, the reduced blood flow to the peripheral tissues leads to an accumulation of vasodilator metabolites, which decreases peripheral resistance and therefore aggravates the fall in arterial pressure.

Acidosis The inadequate blood flow during hemorrhage affects the metabolism of all cells in the body. The resulting stagnant anoxia accelerates the production of lactic acid and other acid metabolites by the tissues. Furthermore, impaired kidney function prevents adequate excretion of the excess H^+, and generalized metabolic acidosis ensues (Figure 12-9). The resulting depressant effect of acidosis on the heart (see Chapter 4) further reduces tissue perfusion and thus aggravates the metabolic acidosis. Acidosis also diminishes the reactivity of the heart and resistance vessels to neurally released and circulating catecholamines, thereby intensifying the hypotension.

Central Nervous System Depression The hypotension in shock reduces cerebral blood flow. Moderate degrees of cerebral ischemia induce a pronounced sympathetic nervous stimulation of the heart, arterioles, and veins, as stated previously. With severe degrees of hypotension, however, the cardiovascular centers in the brain-

Figure 12-8 ■ **Ventricular function curves for the right and left ventricles during the course of hemorrhagic shock. Curves *A* represent the control function curve; curves *B*, 117 min; curves *C*, 247 min; curves *D*, 280 min; curves *E*, 295 min; and curves *F*, 310 min after the initial hemorrhage.** (Redrawn from Crowell JW, Guyton AC: *Am J Physiol* 203:248, 1962.)

Figure 12-9 ■ **Reduction in arterial blood pH (mean ± SD) in a group of 11 dogs whose blood pressure had been held at a level of 35 mm Hg by bleeding into a reservoir, beginning at time zero.** (Modified from Markov AK, Oglethorpe N, Young DB, Hellems HK: *Circ Shock* 8:9, 1981.)

stem eventually become depressed because of inadequate blood flow to the brain. The resulting loss of sympathetic tone then reduces cardiac output and peripheral resistance. The consequent reduction in mean arterial pressure intensifies the inadequate cerebral perfusion.

Various endogenous **opioids,** such as **enkephalins** and **beta-endorphin,** may be released into the brain substance or into the circulation in response to the same stresses that provoke circulatory shock. Opioids exist along with catecholamines in secretory granules in the adrenal medulla and sympathetic nerve terminals, and they are released together in response to stress. Similar stimuli release beta-endorphin and adrenocorticotropic hormone (ACTH) from the anterior pituitary gland. These opioids depress the centers in the brainstem that mediate some of the compensatory autonomic adaptations to blood loss, endotoxemia, and other shock-provoking stresses. Conversely, the opioid antagonist **naloxone** improves cardiovascular function and survival in various forms of shock.

Aberrations of Blood Clotting The alterations of blood clotting after hemorrhage are typically biphasic—an initial phase of hypercoagulability followed by a secondary phase of hypocoagulability and fibrinolysis. In the initial phase, platelets and leukocytes adhere to the vascular endothelium, and intravascular clots, or **thrombi,** develop within a few minutes of the onset of severe hemorrhage. Coagulation may be extensive throughout the minute blood vessels.

Thromboxane A_2 may be released from various ischemic tissues. It aggregates platelets, and more thromboxane A_2 is released from the trapped platelets, which serves to trap additional platelets. This form of positive feedback intensifies and prolongs the clotting tendency. The mortality from certain standard shock-provoking procedures has been reduced considerably by anticoagulants such as heparin.

In the later stages of hemorrhagic hypotension, the clotting time is prolonged and fibrinolysis is prominent. As stated previously, hemorrhage into the intestinal lumen is common after several hours of hemorrhagic hypotension in dogs. Blood loss into the intestinal lumen would of course aggravate the hemodynamic effects of the original hemorrhage.

Reticuloendothelial System During the course of hemorrhagic hypotension, reticuloendothelial system (RES) function becomes depressed. The phagocytic activity of the RES is modulated by an opsonic protein. The opsonic activity in plasma diminishes during shock, which may account in part for the depression of RES function. As a consequence, the antibacterial and antitoxic defense mechanisms are impaired. Endotoxins from the normal bacterial flora of the intestine constantly enter the circulation. Ordinarily they are inactivated by the RES, principally in the liver. When the RES is de-

pressed, these endotoxins invade the general circulation. Endotoxins produce profound, generalized vasodilation, mainly by inducing the abundant synthesis of an isoform of nitric oxide synthase in the smooth muscle of blood vessels throughout the body. The profound vasodilation aggravates the hemodynamic changes caused by blood loss.

In addition to their role in inactivating endotoxin, the macrophages release many of the mediators that are associated with shock. These mediators include acid hydrolases, neutral proteases, oxygen free radicals, certain coagulation factors, and arachidonic acid derivatives: prostaglandins, thromboxanes, and leukotrienes. Macrophages also release certain **monokines** that modulate temperature regulation, intermediary metabolism, hormone secretion, and the immune system.

Interactions of Positive and Negative Feedback Mechanisms

Hemorrhage provokes a multitude of circulatory and metabolic derangements. Some of these changes are compensatory; others are decompensatory. Some of these feedback mechanisms possess a high gain, others a low gain. Furthermore, the gain of any specific mechanism varies with the severity of the hemorrhage. For example, with only a slight loss of blood, mean arterial pressure is within the range of normal and the gain of the baroreceptor reflexes is high. With greater losses of blood, when mean arterial pressure is below about 60 mm Hg (i.e., below the threshold for the baroreceptors), further reductions of pressure have no additional influence through the baroreceptor reflexes. Hence, below this critical pressure, the baroreceptor reflex gain is zero or near zero.

As a general rule, with minor degrees of blood loss, the gains of the negative feedback mechanisms are high, whereas those of the positive feedback mechanisms are low. The converse is true with more severe hemorrhages. The gains of the various mechanisms are additive algebraically. Therefore, whether a vicious cycle develops depends on whether the sum of the various gains exceeds 1. Total gains in excess of 1 are of course more likely with severe losses of blood. Therefore, to avert a vicious cycle, serious hemorrhages must be treated quickly and intensively, preferably by whole blood transfusions, before the process becomes irreversible.

■ SUMMARY

Exercise

1. In anticipation of exercise, the vagus nerve impulses to the heart are inhibited and the sympathetic nervous system is activated by central command. The result is an increase in heart rate, myocardial contractile force, and regional vascular resistance.

2. With exercise, vascular resistance increases in skin, kidneys, splanchnic regions, and inactive muscles and decreases markedly in the active muscles. The overall effect is a pronounced reduction in TPR. This change in resistance, along with the auxiliary pumping action of the contracting skeletal muscles, leads to a large increase in venous return. The increase in heart rate and the enhanced myocardial contractility, both induced by activation of the cardiac sympathetic nerves, enable the heart to transfer the blood to the pulmonary and systemic circulations, thereby increasing cardiac output. Stroke volume increases only slightly. Oxygen consumption and blood oxygen extraction increase, and systolic and mean blood pressure increase slightly.

3. As body temperature rises during exercise, the skin blood vessels dilate. However, when heart rate becomes maximal during severe exercise, the skin vessels constrict. This increases the effective blood volume but causes greater increases in body temperature and a feeling of exhaustion.

4. The limiting factor in exercise performance is the delivery of blood to the active muscles.

Hemorrhage

1. Acute blood loss induces the following hemodynamic changes: tachycardia, hypotension, generalized arteriolar vasoconstriction, and generalized venoconstriction.

2. Acute blood loss invokes a number of negative feedback (compensatory) mechanisms, such as baroreceptor and chemoreceptor reflexes, responses to moderate cerebral ischemia, reabsorption of tissue fluids, release of endogenous vasoconstrictors, and renal conservation of water and electrolytes.

3. Acute blood loss also induces a number of positive feedback (decompensatory) mechanisms, such as cardiac failure, acidosis, central nervous system depression, aberrations of blood coagulation, and depression of the reticuloendothelial system.

4. The outcome of acute blood loss depends on the gains of the various feedback mechanisms and on the interactions between the positive and negative feedback mechanisms.

■ KEY WORDS AND CONCEPTS

- Exercise
- Central command
- Peripheral resistance
- Cardiac output
- Active hyperemia
- Capillary recruitment
- Arterial pressure
- Stroke volume
- Heart rate
- Arteriovenous O_2 difference
- Venous return
- Muscle pump
- Body temperature
- Skin vasodilation

- Baroreceptor
- Exercise limits
- Physical conditioning
- Sedentary state effects
- Training effects
- Maximal O_2 consumption
- Cardiac pumping capacity
- Hemorrhage
- Hemorrhagic hypotension
- Hemorrhagic shock
- Negative feedback mechanisms
- Baroreceptor reflexes
- Chemoreceptor reflexes
- Cerebral ischemia
- Tissue fluids
- Endogenous vasoconstrictors
- Renal conservation of water
- Decompensatory mechanisms
- Cardiac failure
- Acidosis
- Cerebral depression
- Blood clotting disturbances
- Reticuloendothelial function
- Oxygen free radicals

■ SELF-STUDY PROBLEMS

1. What are the major cardiovascular changes that occur with exercise?
2. What is the limiting factor in the performance of strenuous exercise such as distance running or swimming? Why?
3. What are the major compensatory responses to blood loss?
4. What factors tend to aggravate the hemodynamic effects of blood loss?

■ BIBLIOGRAPHY

Journal articles

Abboud FM, Floras JS, Aylward PE et al: Role of vasopressin in cardiovascular and blood pressure regulation, *Blood Vessels* 27:106, 1990.

Astiz ME, Rackow EC, Weil MH: Pathophysiology and treatment of circulatory shock, *Crit Care Clin* 9:183, 1993.

Baker CH, Sutton ET: Arteriolar endothelium-dependent vasodilation occurs during endotoxin shock, *Am J Physiol* 264:H1118, 1993.

Blomqvist CG, Saltin B: Cardiovascular adaptations to physical training, *Annu Rev Physiol* 45:169, 1983.

Booth FW, Thomason DB: Molecular and cellular adaptation of muscle in response to exercise: perspectives of various models, *Physiol Rev* 71:541, 1991.

Brengelmann GL: Circulatory adjustments to exercise and heat stress, *Annu Rev Physiol* 45:191, 1983.

Cameron JD, Dart AM: Exercise training increases total systemic arterial compliance in humans, *Am J Physiol* 266:H693, 1994.

Cheng K-P, Igarashi Y, Little WC: Mechanism of augmented rate of left ventricular filling during exercise, *Circ Res* 70:9, 1992.

Christensen NJ, Galbo H: Sympathetic nervous activity during exercise, *Annu Rev Physiol* 45:139, 1983.

Clausen JP: Effect of physical training on cardiovascular adjustments to exercise in man, *Physiol Rev* 57:779, 1977.

Courneya C-A, Korner PI, Oliver JR, Woods RL: Afferent vascular resistance control during hemorrhage in normal and autonomically blocked rabbits, *Am J Physiol* 261:H380, 1991.

Eldridge FL, Millhorn DE, Kiley JP, Waldrop TG: Stimulation by central command of locomotion, respiration, and circulation during exercise, *Respir Physiol* 59:313, 1985.

Fitts RH: Cellular mechanisms of muscle fatigue, *Physiol Rev* 74:49, 1994.

Geerdes BP, Frederick KL, Brunner MJ: Carotid baroreflex control during hemorrhage in conscious and anesthetized dogs, *Am J Physiol* 265:R195, 1993.

Herd JA: Cardiovascular response to stress, *Physiol Rev* 71:305, 1991.

Kovach AGB, Lefer AM: Endothelial dysfunction in shock states, *News Physiol Sci* 8:145, 1993.

Laughlin MH, Armstrong RB: Muscle and blood flow during locomotory exercise, *Exerc Sport Sci Rev* 13:95, 1985.

Lefer AM, Lefer DJ: Pharmacology of the endothelium in ischemia-reperfusion and circulatory shock, *Annu Rev Pharmacol Toxicol* 33:71, 1993.

Ludbrook J: Reflex control of blood pressure during exercise, *Annu Rev Physiol* 45:155, 1983.

Mitchell JH, Kaufman MP, Iwamoto GA: The exercise pressor reflex: its cardiovascular effects, afferent mechanisms, and central pathways, *Annu Rev Physiol* 45:229, 1983.

Rea RF, Eckberg DL, Fritsch JM, Goldstein DS: Relation of plasma norepinephrine and sympathetic traffic during hypotension in humans, *Am J Physiol* 258:R982, 1990.

Redl H, Gasser H, Schlag G, Marzi I: Involvement of oxygen radicals in shock related cell injury, *Br Med Bull* 49:556, 1993.

Reilly PM, Bulkley GB: Vasoactive mediators and splanchnic perfusion, *Crit Care Med* 21:S55, 1993.

Schadt JC, Gaddis RR: Renin-angiotensin system and opioids during acute hemorrhage in conscious rabbits, *Am J Physiol* 258:R543, 1990.

Share L: Role of vasopressin in cardiovascular regulation, *Physiol Rev* 68:1248, 1988.

Shen Y-T, Knight DR, Thomas JX Jr, Vatner SF: Relative roles of cardiac receptors and arterial baroreceptors during hemorrhage in conscious dogs, *Circ Res* 66:397, 1990.

Sheriff DD, Zhou XP, Scher AM, Rowell LB: Dependence of cardiac filling pressure on cardiac output during rest and dynamic exercise in dogs, *Am J Physiol* 265:H316, 1993.

Stoclet J-C, Fleming I, Gray G et al: Nitric oxide and endotoxemia, *Circulation* 87:V-77, 1993.

Szabo C: Alterations in nitric oxide production in various forms of circulatory shock, *New Horizons* 3:2, 1995.

Thiemermann C: Role of L-arginine: nitric oxide pathway in circulatory shock, *Adv Pharmacol* 28:45, 1994.

Triedman JK, Cohen RJ, Saul JP: Mild hypovolemic stress alters autonomic modulation of heart rate, *Hypertension* 21:236, 1993.

Vissing SF, Scherrer U, Victor RG: Stimulation of skin sympathetic nerve discharge by central command: differential control of sympathetic outflow to skin and skeletal muscle during static exercise, *Circ Res* 69:229, 1991.

Westerblad H, Lee JA, Lannergren J, Allen DG: Cellular mechanisms of fatigue in skeletal muscle, *Am J Physiol* 261:C195, 1991.

Books and monographs

Bond RF, Adams HR, Chaudry IH, associate editors: *Perspectives in shock research,* New York, 1988, Alan R Liss.

Brooks GA, Fahey TD: *Exercise physiology—human bioenergetics and its applications,* New York, 1984, John Wiley.

Janssen HF, Barnes CD, editors: *Circulatory shock: basic and clinical implications,* New York, 1985, Academic Press.

Lind AR: *Cardiovascular adjustments to isometric contractions: static effort.* In *Handbook of physiology,* Section 2: *The cardiovascular system—peripheral circulation and organ blood flow,* vol III, Bethesda, Md., 1983, American Physiological Society.

Mitchell JH, Schmidt RF: *Cardiovascular reflex control by afferent fibers from skeletal muscle receptors.* In *Handbook of physiology,* Section 2: *The cardiovascular system—peripheral circulation and organ blood flow,* vol III, Bethesda, Md., 1983, American Physiological Society.

Roth BL, Nielsen TB, McKee AE, editors: *Molecular and cellular mechanisms of septic shock.* In *Progress in clinical and biological research,* vol 286, New York, 1988, Alan R Liss.

Rowell LB: *Integration of body systems in exercise.* In Berne RM, Levy MN, editors: *Principles of physiology,* St Louis, 1990, Mosby–Year Book.

Rowell LB: *Human circulation: regulation during physical stress,* New York, 1986, Oxford University Press.

Answers to Self-Study Problems

■ CHAPTER 1: THE CIRCUITRY

1 The arterioles have a thick, smooth muscle layer and a small internal diameter. Hence, changes in the contractile state of the vascular smooth muscle in response to alterations in sympathetic nerve activity or to the concentration of vasoactive substances can affect blood pressure when the response is widespread, and can affect the distribution of blood flow when the response is regional.

2. The venous system has a greater compliance than does the arterial system. Therefore, it takes more blood to fill the venous system than it does to fill the arterial system at any given filling pressure.

3. The velocity of the systemic circulation is greatest in the aorta and slowest in the capillaries. This is so because the total cross-sectional area of the vasculature is smallest in the aorta and largest in the capillaries, and the entire cardiac output must flow through all segments of the vascular tree per unit of time.

4. Blood is pulsatile in the arterial system because of the intermittent ejection of blood by the left ventricle. Blood flow becomes non-pulsatile (steady flow) in the capillaries because (1) the pulsations are partially damped by the elastic arteries and (2) further damping is caused by frictional resistance in the arterioles and small arteries.

■ CHAPTER 2: ELECTRICAL ACTIVITY OF THE HEART

1. In a fast-response myocyte the resting transmembrane potential during phase 4 remains constant (at about -90 mV). Thus, no appreciable ion flux takes place. The membrane is most permeable to K^+ during phase 4, but the ratio of extracellular to intracellular K^+ concentration is close to the equilibrium value defined by the Nernst equation for this ion. Thus, the driving force that tends to move K^+ across the cell membrane is very small. When the cell is stimulated to depolarize, the steep upstroke (phase 1) of the action potential is associated with an abrupt opening of the fast Na^+ channels. Consequently, Na^+ rushes into the cell, and the charge on the cell membrane reverses very quickly; the interior of the cell is positive to the exterior. These channels inactivate very quickly, however, and Na^+ influx ceases. The transient outward K^+ channels are activated, and the outward flux of K^+ leads to early partial repolarization (phase 1). The

Ca^{++} channels are activated during the action potential upstroke, and Ca^{++} begins to enter the cell. The influx of Ca^{++} triggers the release of Ca^{++} from the sarcoplasmic reticulum, an important step in excitation-contraction coupling of cardiac cells. For about 100 to 300 ms the influx of charge carried by Ca^{++} is counterbalanced by the efflux of charge carried by K$^+$, and the inside of the cell remains at a fairly constant positive potential of about +10 to +20 mV; this is the plateau (phase 2). Near the end of the plateau, the efflux of charge carried by K$^+$ begins to exceed the influx of charge carried by Ca^{++} and repolarization (phase 3) begins. As repolarization proceeds, K$^+$ conductance increases, and the rate of repolarization accelerates until the cell is fully repolarized. This constitutes phase 4 again, and the cycle is completed.

2. An atrioventricular (AV) node cell is a slow-response fiber, whereas atrial and ventricular myocytes are fast-response fibers. In a myocyte the upstroke of the action potential is much steeper and the amplitude much greater than are the respective characteristics in an AV node cell. The steep upstroke in a myocyte reflects the rapid inrush of Na$^+$ through fast Na$^+$ channels. The rapid Na$^+$ flux at one point in the cell membrane of a myocyte allows a more rapid change in potential in an adjacent point in the membrane (i.e., it allows a more rapid propagation) than would prevail in the cell membrane of an AV node cell, in which the upstroke is achieved by the relatively slow influx of Ca^{++}. Furthermore, the greater amplitude of the action potential in a myocyte permits the electrotonic spread of potential to extend a greater distance down the fiber than is true for an AV node cell, which has a smaller-amplitude action potential. The greater electrotonic spread of excitation allows points at a greater distance from the reference point to be depolarized more

expeditiously. Thus, in a cell whose action potential has a greater amplitude, the cardiac impulse is propagated more rapidly than in a cell whose action potential has a smaller amplitude.

3. The cardiac impulse is ordinarily generated by automatic cells in the sinoatrial (SA) node. It then passes through the perinodal tissues and radiates through the atrial tissues. When the wave front reaches the AV node, it proceeds slowly through the node and then accelerates greatly when it reaches the bundle of His, in the interventricular septum. From this bundle, it spreads rapidly through the Purkinje fiber network in the endocardial region of both ventricles, and then spreads from endocardium to epicardium via ventricular myocardial fibers.

4. The electrophysiologic conditions that favor the occurrence of reentry are slow conduction and unidirectional block within the reentry loop. Furthermore, the refractory period of the reentered region must be less than the propagation time around the reentry loop. If conduction velocity is diminished in one region of the heart, an impulse that traverses this region will arrive relatively late at a more distal region. Hence, this distal region is more likely to have recovered its excitability, and therefore the tardy impulse may be able to reenter the original zone. Similarly, if one or more cardiac chambers are enlarged, the cardiac impulse has a longer path to traverse. Thus, the time required to traverse that path will be prolonged. If the path forms a loop, this longer time around the loop may allow sufficient time for the myocytes at the beginning of the loop to regain their excitability by the time the impulse completes the circuit. Reentrant rhythms do occur more commonly in enlarged ventricles or atria. Finally, unidirectional block in some region of the heart is an important factor in reentry. If two impulses

traveling in opposite directions invaded this region and both impulses could be conducted, they would collide and extinguish each other (each would arrive at a region that was absolutely refractory as a consequence of the passage of the other impulse). However, if only one of the impulses could traverse this region of unidirectional block, it might arrive at the opposite end and thus reenter that region, after the myocardial cells there had recovered their excitability.

5. First-degree AV block is characterized by an abnormally long P-R interval. In second-degree AV block, not every P wave is followed by an R wave; i.e., some atrial impulses are not conducted to the ventricles. In third-degree AV block, none of the atrial impulses reach the ventricles; the P waves and R waves are independent of each other.

■ CHAPTER 3: THE CARDIAC PUMP

1. Although not an anatomic syncytium, the heart behaves as if it were one, and an all or none response occurs with stimulation of the heart via the cardiac sympathetic nerves or by blood-borne catecholamines. Excitation spreads from cell to cell via gap junctions, and during the plateau of the action potential, some calcium enters the cells through the calcium channels and triggers the release of calcium from the sarcoplasmic reticulum. The calcium complexes with troponin C, and the Ca^{++}-troponin C complex interacts with tropomyosin to unblock active sites between actin and myosin; this interaction permits enhanced crossbridge cycling.

2. The preload is the degree of ventricular filling (distending pressure) by the end of diastole; the afterload is the aortic pressure during ventricular systole. Increases in preload increase developed pressure. Increases in afterload also increase developed pressure (until left ventricular pressure cannot open the aortic

valve) but decreases the velocity of contraction. Velocity is maximal at zero afterload.

3. Myocardial contractility can be gauged by (1) the slope of the upstroke of the ventricular pressure curve (change in pressure with time, dP/dt), (2) the initial velocity of the aortic flow curve, and (3) the ejection fraction (ratio of volume ejected per beat to the volume of blood in the ventricle at the end of diastole).

4. The pericardium restricts acute dilation of the heart but stretches with gradual enlargement of the heart or during the formation of pericardial effusion. Normally, the thin layer of fluid between the visceral and parietal layers of the pericardium serves as a lubricant for movement of the heart within the pericardial sac. In some disease states (e.g., tubercular pericarditis) the pericardium can become rigid and even calcified; such a condition can impair cardiac filling and thus reduce cardiac output.

5. In mitral stenosis the murmur is caused by the turbulence created during left ventricular filling, particularly during left atrial contraction when blood is forced through the stenotic mitral valve. Hence, the murmur just precedes the first heart sound. It is characteristically a rumbling crescendo murmur that ends with the first heart sound.

6.
$$\text{Cardiac output} = \frac{O_2 \text{ consumption/min}}{A - VO_2 \text{ difference}} = \frac{280}{0.19 - 0.12} = 4 \text{ L/min}$$

Myocardial O_2 consumption =
A − VO_2 difference × coronary blood flow =
$0.14 \times 150 = 21$ ml/min

■ CHAPTER 4: REGULATION OF THE HEARTBEAT

1. a. When the vagus nerves are stimulated the heart rate diminishes promptly to a new level, and then returns very quickly to the

control level when stimulation ceases. The response is so rapid because the acetylcholine (ACh) regulated K^+ channels that help mediate the response do not require a second messenger but are activated much more directly via a G protein. Also, the response decays so quickly after vagal activity ceases because acetylcholinesterase is abundant in the SA node, and it hydrolyzes the neurally released ACh very rapidly.

b. In response to sympathetic stimulation, the heart rate rises gradually to its steady-state value, and when stimulation ceases the heart rate decays very gradually to its control level. Two factors account for the gradual rise in heart rate in response to stimulation. First, a relatively slow second messenger system (the adenylyl cyclase system) is involved in the cascade of events that lead to the change in heart rate. Second, the cardiac sympathetic nerves release norepinephrine (NE) at a relatively slow rate. The response decays gradually after cessation of stimulation because the main processes (active neuronal reuptake and diffusion into the myocardial capillaries) that remove neurally released NE from the cardiac tissues are slow.

2. When the cardiac sympathetic and vagus nerves are stimulated simultaneously, the vagal effects on heart rate usually predominate. This is because the main neurotransmitters (NE and ACh) that mediate the cardiac response are both released simultaneously, and each inhibits the release of the other. However, the action of the ACh is much more rapid than the action of the NE. Therefore, very soon after the onset of stimulation, the vagally released ACh has markedly suppressed the release of NE from the sympathetic nerves. Therefore, the response to simultaneous stimulation is often equivalent to the response to vagal stimulation alone.

3. The rise in arterial blood pressure induced by a vasoconstrictor drug would stimulate the arterial baroreceptors in the carotid sinus and aortic arch. Consequently, the activity in the efferent sympathetic fibers to the heart and blood vessels would diminish, whereas the activity in the efferent vagal fibers to the heart would increase.

4. Rapid intravenous infusion of blood would first increase the venous return to the right ventricle. The consequent diastolic stretching of the right ventricle would increase its stroke volume by the Frank-Starling mechanism. The increase in right ventricular stroke volume would then increase the left ventricular end-diastolic volume, and the left ventricular stroke volume would then increase. The time delay between the increments in right and left ventricular stroke volume would be only the duration of two or three heartbeats.

5. Left atrial pressure usually exceeds right atrial pressure, for reasons explained in relation to Figure 4-20. If an opening were created in the interatrial septum, the left-to-right pressure differential would cause some blood to flow from the left to the right atrium through the interatrial septal defect. Hence, right atrial pressure would tend to rise and left atrial pressure would tend to fall. Consequently, right ventricular stroke volume would increase and left ventricular stroke volume would decrease. At equilibrium, right ventricular stroke volume would exceed left ventricular stroke volume by the amount of flow shunted from the left to the right atrium with each heartbeat.

6. The stroke volume ejected by the ventricles is markedly reduced during a premature ventricular beat; sometimes the premature contraction is so feeble that the peak intraventricular pressure does not exceed the prevailing arterial pressure, and no blood is ejected by the ventricle during that contrac-

tion. Conversely, the postextrasystolic contraction is much stronger than is the normal beat, and stroke volume may greatly exceed the normal stroke volume. Two major factors account for these changes in stroke volume. The first involves the Frank-Starling mechanism. With regard to the premature beat, the ventricles have insufficent time to fill adequately, and thus the subsequent contraction is weaker than normal. During the long pause between the premature and postextrasystolic beats, ventricular filling is greater than normal, and consequently the stroke volume is greater than normal. A second, less well understood mechanism also contributes to the changes in stroke volume, because substantial changes in ventricular contraction have been shown to occur in experimental isovolumic preparations, in which changes in ventricular filling are precluded (Figure 4-23). The weak premature contraction and the strong postextrasystolic contraction are believed to be produced in part by disparities in Ca^{++} release from the sarcoplasmic reticulum; such disparities are presumed to be associated with a substantial time delay in transfer of Ca^{++} from a putative uptake compartment to a putative release compartment of the sarcoplasmic reticulum.

■ CHAPTER 5: HEMODYNAMICS

1. The resistance to blood flow through one kidney equals the mean arterial pressure (100 mm Hg) divided by the blood flow (200 ml/min), or 0.5 mm Hg/ml/min; we shall assume that the renal venous pressure is approximately zero. The reciprocal of the resistance (R_t) to flow through both kidneys equals the sum of the reciprocals of the resistances (R_1 and R_r) of the left and right kidneys (the kidneys are aligned in parallel). That is, $1/R_t = 1/R_1 + 1/R_r$. Therefore, $R_t = 0.25$ mm Hg/ml/min. The hydraulic resistance of the two kidneys in parallel is less than the resistance of either kidney alone, because when both kidneys are being perfused, the blood has twice as many parallel channels through which the blood can flow than when only one of the kidneys is being perfused.

2. A murmur in the cardiovascular system denotes that flow is turbulent in some part of the cardiovascular system. Reynold's number denotes some of the factors that lead to turbulence; the tendency for flow to be turbulent increases directly with the velocity of flow and inversely with the fluid viscosity. In severe anemia the velocity of blood flow around the body is much greater than normal, and the viscosity of the blood is much less than normal.

3. The flow of blood in a blood vessel exerts a "viscous drag" on the endothelial lining of the blood vessels; it tends to pull the endothelium in the direction of the flowing blood. In a dissecting aneurysm of the aorta a tear exists in the endothelial lining; the tear tends to be oriented at right angles to the long axis of the vessel. If a small tear exists in the endothelial lining of the aorta, the flowing blood will tend to pull the distal lip of the tear caudally and may thereby extend the tear. This tendency will be more pronounced as the blood flow in the aorta increases. A dissecting aortic aneurysm is usually treated surgically, but before surgery the physician administers a drug (such as a β-adrenergic receptor antagonist) to lower the patient's arterial blood pressure and diminish the aortic flow (or cardiac output), in order to reduce the tendency for the tear in the aortic wall to be extended.

4. In the large arteries and veins the particles (such as red and white blood cells) are fairly evenly distributed over the cross section of the vessel. However, in blood vessels with cross-sectional areas that are only a few times greater than the average diameter of the

blood cells, the blood cells tend to be highly concentrated axially and the plasma is more concentrated near the vascular walls. However, the axial laminae of the bloodstream move much more rapidly than do the peripheral laminae. Because the more centrally located cells move more quickly than does the more peripherally located plasma, the ratio of cells to plasma (and therefore the hematocrit ratio) is less in the small blood vessels than in the large blood vessels.

■ CHAPTER 6: THE ARTERIAL SYSTEM

1. The arteries in patients with atherosclerosis are less compliant than in normal subjects, and hence less blood can be stored in the arteries during systole. Consequently, the heart must pump a greater flow during systole through the resistance vessels (small arteries and arterioles), and thus the heart must work harder than normal. The myocardium therefore needs a greater coronary blood flow to furnish more oxygen and nutrients than would be required in a subject with normal arteries.

2. Mean arterial pressure depends only on cardiac output and total peripheral resistance (TPR). Hence, mean arterial pressure would be the same in the two subjects. Because the cardiac outputs are the same in the two individuals, stroke volume must be much greater in the person with a heart rate of 45 beats/min than in the person with a heart rate of 75 beats/min. Therefore, the quantity of blood pumped into the aorta during the rapid ejection phase of systole would be expected to be much greater in the person with the slower heart rate. Consequently, the arterial pressure oscillation with each heartbeat about the mean arterial pressure level would be greater in the person with the greater stroke volume than in the other person; that is, the maximal arterial pressure (systolic pres-

sure) would be greater and the minimal pressure (diastolic pressure) would be less in the former than in the latter individual.

3. Because the 20- and 70-year old subjects had the same cardiac output, heart rate, and TPR under basal conditions, their mean arterial pressures must have been the same. Because the vasoconstrictor drug elicited the same (50%) increase in TPR in the two subjects, their mean arterial pressures must have increased by 50%. A rise in arterial pressure in general tends to decrease arterial compliance, but the reduction in compliance is ordinarily much more pronounced in older than in younger subjects. After the drug had elevated the arterial pressure, therefore, a given stroke volume ejected into the less compliant aorta of the older subject would produce a greater pressure oscillation (from the diastolic to the systolic pressure level) in the older than in the younger subject. Consequently, the systolic pressure would be higher and the diastolic pressure lower in the older subject.

4. The mean arterial pressures would be identical in the normal person and in the patient with aortic valve insufficiency, because mean arterial pressure depends only on cardiac output and TPR. However, the "volume increment" (i.e., the volume of blood ejected by the left ventricle during the rapid ejection phase of systole, minus the volume of blood that leaves the arteries through the resistance vessels during this same phase of systole) would be much greater in the patient than in the normal individual. The volume increment would be much greater in the patient because blood leaks back into the ventricle during diastole. Consequently, the greater diastolic filling leads to an augmented stroke volume (Frank-Starling mechanism). Hence, the patient's systolic pressure would be substantially greater and the diastolic pressure would be less than in the normal person.

■ CHAPTER 7: THE MICROCIRCULATION AND LYMPHATICS

1. Capillary blood flow is influenced by mean arterial pressure, precapillary resistance, and postcapillary resistance. When the cognate arterioles dilate, as occurs with section of sympathetic nerves to the vessels, or in response to local vasodilator metabolites, greater pressure is applied to blood in the capillaries, and the velocity of flow increases; arteriolar constriction has the opposite effect. An increase in venous pressure, as may occur in heart failure, is transmitted back to the capillaries and reduces the velocity of flow. An increase in blood viscosity, as occurs in polycythemia, also slows the velocity of blood flow in the capillaries. No active changes in capillary diameter occur because capillaries cannot independently constrict or dilate.

2. The reason the capillaries in the feet do not rupture when a person stands is explained in terms of the law of Laplace: $T = Pr$, where $T =$ wall tension, $P =$ transmural pressure, and $r =$ capillary radius. Although the pressure within the capillaries may reach very high levels, the small diameter of the capillaries "compensates" for the high pressure, and the increase in wall tension is very small relative to that of a large artery, like the aorta, at a similar transmural pressure.

3. The capillary will absorb fluid because the forces moving fluid from the interstitial space into the capillary lumen (plasma oncotic pressure plus tissue hydrostatic pressure) exceed the forces favoring filtration (capillary hydrostatic pressure plus tissue oncotic pressure) by 7 mm Hg.

4. Flow-limited transport means that lipid-insoluble, small solute molecules that pass through the capillary pores can move from capillary lumen to interstitial space faster than they are transported to the capillary by the flowing blood. Diffusion-limited transport means that the lipid-insoluble molecules are large enough to be partially or completely prevented from passing through the capillary pores, regardless of the rate at which they are brought to the capillaries by the flowing blood.

5. Lipid-insoluble solutes of small molecular size (e.g., NaCl, glucose) pass through capillary pores that are about 4 Å in diameter, whereas lipid-soluble molecules (e.g., CO_2 and O_2) pass directly through the endothelial cells as well as through the pores. Large lipid-insoluble molecules that cannot get through the capillary pores may be transported across the capillary endothelial cells by pinocytosis.

6. Albumin that has entered the interstitial space cannot be taken up directly by the capillaries because of the opposing concentration gradient and the endothelial barrier. Albumin enters the lymph capillaries, whose openings are facilitated by fine filaments that pull the lymphatic endothelial cells apart when the tissue moves, as in muscle contraction and relaxation. The albumin, along with interstitial fluid, travels through the lymphatic system. Its passage is aided by contraction of the lymphatic vessels, which have valves that prevent backflow, and by muscle contraction (squeezing of the vessels in the tissue). The lymph fluid moves through vessels of increasing size and finally enters the circulating blood at the junction of the subclavian and internal jugular veins.

■ CHAPTER 8: THE PERIPHERAL CIRCULATION AND ITS CONTROL

1. Autoregulation of blood flow describes the constancy of blood flow to an organ during alteration in perfusion pressure (blood pressure). When the metabolic activity of an organ is constant, an abrupt increase in perfusion pressure produces an immediate increase in blood flow. However, if the perfusion pressure is held at the new elevated level, blood flow

gradually returns to or toward the control level within a minute. With abrupt decreases in perfusion pressure, blood flow initially decreases but then increases to or toward the control level. Studies on isolated arterioles suggest that a myogenic mechanism is responsible for autoregulation; that is, stretch of the vascular smooth muscle (increased transmural pressure) elicits contraction (increased resistance), whereas a decrease in transmural pressure elicits relaxation (decreased resistance).

2. The endothelium can synthesize vasoactive substances that act locally on the vascular smooth muscle of the resistance vessels. Known vasodilator substances that can be released by the endothelium are nitric oxide, prostacyclin, and adenosine. The endothelium is also the source of endothelin, a powerful vasoconstrictor.

3. Vascular tone refers to the partially contracted state of vascular smooth muscle in the resistance vessels. It is in part attributable to tonic activity of the sympathetic nerves that innervate the arterioles and small arteries, and also to an intrinsic factor in the vascular smooth muscle that becomes evident after interruption of the vessel innervation. The intrinsic factor causes a partial contraction that is called basal tone; its cause has not been elucidated.

4. In resting skeletal muscle, blood flow is low and largely under sympathetic neural control. The low blood flow is commensurate with the low metabolic activity of the resting muscle. With muscle contractions, the increased metabolic activity engenders the local release of vasodilator metabolites. These metabolites dilate the resistance vessels and thereby produce an increase in blood flow in the active muscle (active hyperemia). This local mechanism can override the vasoconstriction produced by activation of the sympathetic nerves to the blood vessels.

5. When pressure within the carotid sinuses decreases, as may occur with blood loss, the number of impulses traveling up the sinus nerve and glossopharyngeal nerve to the medulla decreases. The vasomotor (vasoconstrictor) center becomes less inhibited, and the resulting increase in sympathetic activity causes arteriolar constriction and an increase in peripheral resistance. Heart rate and myocardial contractility are also increased. These factors operate to return blood pressure to the normal level. An increase in pressure in the carotid sinuses has the opposite effect.

■ CHAPTER 9: CONTROL OF CARDIAC OUTPUT: COUPLING OF HEART AND BLOOD VESSELS

1. The answer to both questions is "Yes." The preload is the filling pressure for the ventricles, and the extent of filling is an important determinant of the mechanical performance of the ventricles. As the myocardial cells are progressively stretched, calcium sensitivity of the myofilaments is augmented, and cardiac performance is enhanced. This association (the cardiac function curve) indicates that cardiac output is directly related to the preload. It is equally true, however, that the inverse relationship is also applicable. As cardiac performance is enhanced, the attendant increase in cardiac output will tend to increase the volume of blood contained in the arterial side of the vascular system. If total blood volume remains constant, any increment in arterial blood volume will be associated with an equivalent decrement in the venous blood volume. Hence, central venous pressure (preload) will diminish. This association (the vascular function curve) indicates that preload is inversely related to cardiac output.

2. Arterial blood pressure is not precisely equivalent to the ventricular afterload (because ventricular geometry is also a factor), but arterial blood pressure is the predominant determinant of the afterload. Arterial blood pressure is the main counterforce that opposes the ejection of blood by the contracting ventricle. This counterforce to any specific ventricular contraction has been built up as a result of the preceding ventricular contractions. Thus, the counterforce to ventricular ejection has been generated by the ventricle itself. This process is analogous to the compression of a coiled spring: as a person gradually compresses the spring, it exerts a greater and greater counterforce to further compression.

3. Isoproterenol would enhance myocardial contractility by increasing the Ca^{++} conductance of the myocyte cell membranes, and thereby augmenting the influx of Ca^{++}. Consequently, the ventricle would pump a greater cardiac output from any given filling pressure (preload). As cardiac output increases, more of the blood volume would tend to be sequestered on the arterial side of the circuit, and therefore less of the blood volume would tend to be located on the venous side of the circuit. Consequently, central venous pressure would tend to diminish, but cardiac output would be elevated.

4. The infused blood would be distributed to the arterial and venous segments of the vascular system. The increased venous volume would result in a greater ventricular filling pressure, and this would tend to increase cardiac output. The increased arterial blood volume would tend to increase afterload, but in general the inverse effect of afterload on cardiac output tends to be much less pronounced than the direct effects of preload on cardiac output. The net result of the blood transfusion tends to be an increase in cardiac output, central venous pressure, and mean arterial pressure.

5. Cardiac output equals stroke volume (SV) times heart rate (HR). When HR is only 35 beats/min, SV usually cannot increase sufficiently (mainly because of the limitation to filling associated with the pericardium and the compliance characteristics of the ventricles). Therefore, when HR is very low, cardiac output is subnormal. A low cardiac output causes a redistribution of blood volume from the arterial to the venous segments of the vascular system, and therefore central venous pressure tends to be elevated.

6. When a person on a tilt table is rotated to the upright position, gravity causes the pressure to rise in the vessels in the dependent regions of the body. Consequently, the pressure rises considerably in the veins of the legs and feet, and a substantial volume of blood is sequestered in the veins in this region. The hemodynamic results are similar to those that would be seen if an equivalent volume of blood were lost from the body (hemorrhage). Therefore, cardiac output, mean arterial pressure, and central venous pressures would all be diminished.

■ CHAPTER 10: CORONARY CIRCULATION

1. Stimulation of the cardiac sympathetic nerves has several effects on the heart. Heart rate, contractility, and the speed of impulse conduction in the heart are all increased. The primary effect on the coronary resistance vessels is vasoconstriction. However, the increase in metabolic activity releases vasodilator substances from the myocardium. The arteriolar dilation that ensues overrides the neural-mediated vasoconstriction, and the net effect is an increase in coronary blood flow. The same effects on coronary blood flow occur in the

perfused fibrillating heart, in which the extravascular compression factor is eliminated.

2. Metabolic regulation of coronary blood flow means that the flow is adjusted to the metabolic (oxygen) needs of the myocardium. When the heart works harder, coronary blood flow increases even though there is no increase in coronary perfusion pressure (blood pressure). In other words, the ratio of oxygen supply to oxygen need is important in the regulation of coronary blood flow. A decrease in this ratio, caused by either a decrease in supply (e.g., hypoxemia or partial coronary occlusion) or an increase in need (e.g., exercise), elicits the release of a vasodilator substance (e.g., adenosine) that dilates the resistance vessels and tends to restore the balance between oxygen supply and demand.

3. The net effect of tachycardia on coronary blood flow is an increase in flow secondary to the enhanced metabolism of the myocardium. Opposing the "metabolic vasodilation" is the extravascular compression of the coronary vessels by the contracting cardiac muscle. In tachycardia the heart spends more time per minute in systole (when the vessels are compressed in the left ventricular muscle) than it does at normal heart rates. However, the increase in this extravascular compression (or extravascular resistance) is small relative to the metabolic vasodilation. In bradycardia, the reverse occurs. Oxygen needs are reduced, and although extravascular compression is less, the net effect is an increase in coronary resistance and a decrease in coronary blood flow.

4. If reductions in coronary blood flow are sufficiently severe and prolonged, cardiac dysfunction will be caused mainly by the necrosis (death) of myocardial cells. However, if the reduction of coronary flow is neither prolonged nor severe, the cardiac contractility may be depressed only temporarily. A relatively brief period of severe ischemia, followed by reperfusion, may be associated with a pronounced mechanical dysfunction of the heart, which eventually will fully recover. This "myocardial stunning" is produced by Ca^{++} overload of the cardiac cells during the ischemic period, combined with the generation of free radicals during the period of reperfusion. During prolonged periods of moderate ischemia, "myocardial hibernation" may prevail. The impaired mechanical function of the heart is associated with a reduction in the metabolic activity of the myocardial cells. This biochemical response tends to preserve the viability of certain cells.

■ CHAPTER 11: SPECIAL CIRCULATIONS

1. In muscle at rest, blood flow is chiefly regulated by the sympathetic nerves to the muscle resistance vessels. In exercise, however, local (metabolic) factors supervene and blood flow increases, within limits, to meet the oxygen needs of the tissue. In skin, the major adjustments in blood flow help maintain a constant body temperature. Hence, skin blood flow (reflexly or directly) increases when there is a need to lose body heat, as in exercise or in a warm environment, and decreases when there is a need to conserve heat, as in a cold environment. Skin also serves as a blood reservoir. In hemorrhage or exhausting exercise, vasoconstriction occurs in the skin, thereby reducing the size of the total vascular bed and providing more blood to be pumped to essential organs such as the brain and heart.

2. Cerebral blood flow is remarkably constant, and because the brain is in a rigid structure, blood flow is affected by extravascular pressure, as well as by intravascular pressure. The autonomic nervous system exerts a minimal effect on cerebrovascular resistance. The pri-

mary regulatory factor is the metabolic activity of the brain tissue. An increase in brain metabolic rate (e.g., seizures) or a decrease in oxygen supply (e.g., hypoxia) causes an increase in cerebral blood flow by the release of a vasodilator substance (e.g., adenosine).

3. The pulmonary vascular resistance is low, and therefore pressures in the system are not very high. Hence, gravitational effects may affect the spatial distribution of blood flow substantially. When a person stands, the pressures in the lung apex are appreciably lower than in the lung base. Because the lung vessels are also very compliant, transmural pressures affect vascular calibers and thus affect vascular resistances. The higher pressures in the lung bases cause the vascular resistances there to be considerably less than the resistances in the lung apices. Consequently, the flow per unit weight of tissue tends to be greater in the lung bases than in the apices. In a recumbent person the gravitational effects do not differ appreciably in the bases and apices.

4. In association with the ultrafiltration of about 20% of the blood that enters the glomerular circulation, the kidneys are endowed with a very large blood flow per unit mass of kidney; renal blood flow is about 20% of cardiac output. Hence, the kidneys are relatively resistant to modest reductions in blood flow. The blood flow per unit mass of renal medulla is only about one tenth as great as that per unit mass of renal cortex, and therefore the renal medulla is much less resistant to blood flow reductions than is the renal cortex.

5. Normally, the renal blood flow and glomerular filtration rate (GFR) are well autoregulated; that is, the levels tend to be maintained over a substantial range of perfusion pressures. Hence, in the normal kidney, reduction of renal arterial pressure from 150 to 100 mm Hg would not affect renal blood flow or GFR sub-

stantially. Because renal vascular resistance is the ratio of renal arterial pressure to renal blood flow, the combination of a reduction in pressure and a constant flow indicates that renal vascular resistance must have diminished in proportion to the reduction in arterial pressure. The parallel responses of renal blood flow and of GFR indicate that the main resistance change involved the afferent rather than the efferent arterioles in the kidney.

6. The portal vein delivers about three fourths of the blood flow to the liver but only about one fourth of the oxygen supply; the hepatic artery delivers about one fourth of the blood flow but three fourths of the oxygen supply. The reason for the disproportionate delivery of oxygen by the hepatic artery is that hepatic artery blood is normally fully saturated with oxygen, whereas much of the oxygen in the portal venous blood had already been extracted as it flowed through the tissues of the gastrointestinal tract.

7. Chronic inflammation of the liver (hepatic cirrhosis) encroaches upon the blood vessels and sinusoids in the liver and elevates hepatic vascular resistance. The resulting elevation in portal venous pressure leads to extensive fluid transudation (ascites) from the splanchnic capillaries into the abdominal cavity and to esophageal varices. A portacaval shunt is often created surgically to alleviate these serious problems associated with a substantial elevation of portal venous pressure.

8. In the fetus, most of the right ventricular output passes through the ductus arteriosus and thus bypasses the lungs. When the lungs become filled with air, the resistance to blood flow through the lung vessels falls sharply. This decrease in lung vascular resistance in the newborn, in conjunction with closure of the ductus arteriosus by the higher oxygen pressure in the blood, directs right ventricular output through the pulmonary vessels.

■ **CHAPTER 12: INTERPLAY OF CENTRAL AND PERIPHERAL FACTORS IN THE CONTROL OF THE CIRCULATION**

1. The primary cardiovascular change in exercise is the increase in heart rate, which facilitates the increase in cardiac output in a sedentary person; only a small increase in stroke volume occurs. In the trained individual, heart rate also increases to the same maximal level, but stroke volume is greater at rest and increases further (before heart rate reaches a maximum) during exercise. Hence, the trained athlete can achieve a greater cardiac output. Vascular resistance in the active muscle decreases, producing a decrease in total peripheral resistance (TPR). However, despite this decrease in TPR, blood pressure increases a little because of the large increase in cardiac output. Oxygen extraction from blood perfusing the active muscles is increased, which results in an increase in the arteriovenous oxygen difference.

2. The limiting factor in the performance of whole body exercise is the pumping ability of the heart. Neither the ability of the active muscles to consume oxygen nor the oxygen-carrying capacity of the blood are limiting. Therefore, the supply of oxygen is a function of the amount of blood brought to the active muscles. Thus, with the vessels in the active muscles maximally dilated, the only way to transport more oxygen to the muscles is to increase cardiac output.

3. The arterial baroreceptor reflex is a very important mechanism for protecting the body from the effects of blood loss. When the baroreceptors signal a decline in arterial blood pressure, the reflex response is generalized arteriolar vasoconstriction, increased cardiac contractility, and increased heart rate, all of which attenuate the change in blood pressure evoked by the loss of blood. Other important mechanisms are the release of endogenous vasoconstrictors (vasopressin, angiotensin II, catecholamines), renal conservation of water and electrolytes, and the transfer of fluid from the interstitial and intracellular fluid compartments to the intravascular compartment.

4. Many factors act to aggravate the hypotension induced by blood loss. For example, the decreased arterial blood pressure tends to diminish coronary blood flow, which in turn tends to impair myocardial contractility. Diminished blood flow to the tissues generally leads to metabolic acidosis, and this in turn depresses myocardial contractility. Diminished cerebral blood flow tends to impair cerebral function, and thereby to depress the various reflex compensatory mechanisms. Aberrations of blood coagulation may lead initially to increased coagulability, which may lead to disseminated intravascular clotting, which in turn will then impair the circulation to the peripheral tissues. Subsequent impairment of coagulability may lead to internal hemorrhage, aggravating the effects of the initiating hemorrhage. Depression of the reticuloendothelial system may allow endotoxins to invade the cardiovascular system. The subsequent induction of nitric oxide synthase in the vessels may lead to generalized vasodilation and profound hypotension.

Review Examination

1. The mean systemic arterial pressure exceeds the mean pulmonary artery pressure because
   A. the blood flow through the systemic circulation exceeds the blood flow through the pulmonary circulation.
   B. the number of systemic capillaries exceeds the number of pulmonary capillaries.
   C. the low oxygen tension in the pulmonary arterial blood causes the pulmonary resistance vessels to dilate.
   D. the compliance is greater in the systemic than in the pulmonary arteries.
   E. the resistance to blood flow is much greater in the systemic than in the pulmonary vascular bed.

2. An increase in left ventricular end-diastolic volume increases the stroke volume because
   A. the increased preload diminishes the ventricular compliance.
   B. the increased preload diminishes the ventricular afterload.
   C. the increased ventricular volume diminishes the stiffness of the series elastic elements.

   D. the increased myocardial fiber length enhances the responsiveness of the contractile proteins to calcium.
   E. the increased preload increases the conductance of the I_{K1} potassium channels.

3. In a typical capillary
   A. the pressure at the venous end exceeds that at the arterial end.
   B. the radius exceeds that of a typical arteriole.
   C. the tension in the wall increases as the hydrostatic pressure rises.
   D. the radius is more than three times as great as the radius of a red blood cell.
   E. the tension in the wall is proportional to the fourth power of the radius.

4. If the red blood cells in a blood vessel move at a mean velocity of 100 cm/s and the blood flow through the vessel is 200 ml/s, the cross-sectional area of that vessel is
   A. 2.0 cm^2.
   B. 5.0 cm^2.
   C. 20.0 cm^2.
   D. 0.20 cm^2.
   E. 0.50 cm^2.

$$V = \frac{Q}{A}$$

5. In a normal person, most of the circulating blood is located in the
   A. systemic capillaries.
   B. systemic veins.
   C. pulmonary capillaries.
   D. pulmonary veins.
   E. systemic arteries and arterioles.

6. The colloid osmotic pressure of the plasma is determined mainly by the plasma concentration of
   A. vitamin K.
   B. albumin.
   C. globulin.
   D. sodium.
   E. collagen.

7. During the resting phase of a ventricular myocardial cell, the transmembrane potential depends mostly on the conductance of the cell membrane to
   A. calcium.
   B. acetylcholine.
   C. sodium.
   D. potassium.
   E. norepinephrine.

8. During moderate physical exercise,
   A. stroke volume increases in proportion to the cardiac output.
   B. renal blood flow increases in proportion to the cardiac output.
   C. blood flow to the exercising muscle increases in proportion to the cardiac output.
   D. heart rate increases in proportion to the cardiac output.
   E. splanchnic blood flow increases in proportion to the cardiac output.

9. Arteriovenous anastomoses in the skin
   A. show basal tone and autoregulation.
   B. are responsive to metabolic activity of the skin.
   C. are insensitive to circulating epinephrine.
   D. show reactive hyperemia.
   E. close in response to sympathetic nerve activity.

10. If a drug is given that acts specifically to increase myocardial contractility,
    A. mean arterial pressure will decrease.
    B. arterial pulse pressure will decrease.
    C. capillary blood flow will decrease.
    D. stroke volume will decrease.
    E. central venous pressure will decrease.

11. Neural regulation of vascular resistance in skeletal muscle is mediated by
    A. sympathetic nerves alone.
    B. parasympathetic nerves alone.
    C. motor nerves.
    D. combined action of sympathetic and parasympathetic nerves.
    E. sympathetic cholinergic nerves.

12. The cardiac fibers that normally display the property of post-repolarization refractoriness are
    A. atrial myocardial fibers.
    B. ventricular myocardial fibers.
    C. AV nodal fibers.
    D. His bundle fibers.
    E. Purkinje fibers.

13. Velocity of shortening of myocardial fibers is greatest when
    A. preload is moderate and afterload is zero.
    B. preload is zero and afterload is moderate.
    C. preload is high and afterload is high.
    D. preload is zero and afterload is high.
    E. preload is high and afterload is moderate.

14. The ultrafiltration of fluid from the capillaries into the interstitial spaces increases as the
    A. tissue hydrostatic pressure decreases.
    B. oncotic pressure of the interstitial fluid decreases.
    C. hydrostatic pressure in the capillaries decreases.
    D. radius of the upstream arteriole decreases.
    E. molecular weight of the plasma proteins decreases.

15. The most important cause of increased blood flow through a working skeletal muscle during exercise is
    A. increased cardiac output.
    B. stimulation of sympathetic vasodilator nerves to the muscle.
    C. release of epinephrine from the adrenal medulla.
    D. vasoconstriction in the viscera.
    E. products of local metabolism.

16. The contribution of atrial contraction to ventricular filling is greatest
    A. when vagal activity is pronounced.
    B. at rapid heart rates.
    C. when atria and ventricles contract simultaneously.
    D. during atrial flutter.
    E. during third-degree AV block.

17. An increase in ventricular contractility is indicated by
    A. an increase in cardiac output accompanied by an increase in ventricular end-diastolic volume.
    B. an increase in the amplitude of the QRS complex of the electrocardiogram.
    C. an increase in cardiac output accompanied by a decrease in mean arterial pressure.
    D. a decrease in cardiac output accompanied by an increase in ventricular end-diastolic volume.
    E. an increase in cardiac output accompanied by a decrease in ventricular end-diastolic volume.

18. The medullary vasomotor center is stimulated most effectively by
    A. decreased arterial blood oxygen tension.
    B. decreased arterial blood hydrogen ion concentration.
    C. increased arterial blood adenosine concentration.
    D. increased arterial blood carbon dioxide tension.
    E. increased arterial blood potassium ion concentration.

19. In response to a substantial hemorrhage
    A. the neural activity in the efferent vagus nerve fibers to the heart decreases.
    B. the neural activity in the carotid sinus baroreceptor nerve fibers increases.
    C. the neural activity in the efferent sympathetic nerve fibers to the heart decreases.
    D. the release of vasopressin from the posterior pituitary gland decreases.
    E. the release of renin from the kidney decreases.

20. During the cardiac catheterization of a person who was found to be normal, the blood withdrawn through the catheter had an oxygen saturation of 60%, and the recorded pressure oscillated each heartbeat between 14 and 26 mm Hg. Most likely, the catheter tip was located in the
    A. azygos vein.
    B. pulmonary artery.
    C. right atrium.
    D. foramen ovale.
    E. coronary sinus.

21. For a given patient, the results of laboratory and experimental studies are as follows:

Hematocrit	55%
Oxygen consumption	250 ml/min
Arterial-to-mixed venous blood oxygen difference	25 ml/L blood
Arterial oxygen saturation	70%

    The output of the left ventricle, L/min, is
    A. 1.25
    B. 5.0.
    C. 7.5.
    D. 10.0.
    E. 15.0.

22. In a physically trained person,
    A. heart rate can reach higher levels than in an untrained person.
    B. stroke volume is greater than in an untrained person.
    C. vagal tone is lower than in an untrained person.
    D. vascular resistance is higher than in an untrained person.
    E. left ventricular end-diastolic volume is less than in an untrained person.

23. A reduction in mean arterial pressure from 120 to 70 mm Hg causes a reflex
    A. decrease in myocardial contractility.
    B. increase in duration of the cardiac cycle.
    C. decrease in impulse conduction velocity through the AV node.
    D. increase in total peripheral vascular resistance.
    E. decrease in calcium conductance of myocytes during the action potential plateau.

24. If a person's resting heart rate, stroke volume, and total peripheral resistance did not change appreciably as he or she advanced from 20 to 70 years of age, but the arterial compliance did diminish substantially as the person grew older,
    A. pulmonary blood flow would decrease substantially with age.
    B. myocardial energy requirements would diminish with age.
    C. mean arterial pressure would not change appreciably with age.
    D. systemic capillary blood flow would become less pulsatile with age.
    E. arterial pulse pressure would diminish with age.

25. In a normal resting person, the organ with the greatest oxygen consumption (per gram of tissue) and highest venous oxygen content is the
    A. brain.
    B. heart.
    C. liver.
    D. kidney.
    E. skeletal muscle.

26. A sudden hemorrhage will cause
    A. a decrease in stroke volume and a decrease in central venous pressure.
    B. a decrease in arterial pressure but a rise in central venous pressure.
    C. an increase in stroke volume but a decrease in central venous pressure.
    D. a decrease in stroke volume but a rise in central venous pressure.
    E. an increase in stroke volume and a rise in central venous pressure.

27. The laminar flow of a newtonian fluid through a cylindric tube varies
    A. inversely with the difference in pressure at the two ends of the tube.
    B. directly with the viscosity of the fluid.
    C. inversely with the length of the tube.
    D. inversely with the fourth power of the radius.
    E. directly with the hydraulic resistance to flow.

28. If both the radius and the length of a cylindric tube are doubled, the resistance to the laminar flow of a newtonian fluid will
    A. increase twofold.
    B. remain unchanged.
    C. decrease to half its previous value.
    D. decrease to one fourth its previous value.
    E. decrease to one eighth its previous value.

29. Velocity of blood flow is greatest in the
    A. capillaries.
    B. venules.
    C. venae cavae.
    D. aorta.
    E. arterioles.

30. During the plateau of the action potential in a ventricular myocardial cell,
    A. the cell is relatively refractory.
    B. the efflux of calcium from the cell exceeds the influx of calcium into the cell.
    C. the transmembrane potential is slightly positive.
    D. the potassium conductance exceeds the potassium conductance that prevails during phase 4.
    E. the influx of calcium into the sarcoplasmic reticulum exceeds the efflux of calcium from the sarcoplasmic reticulum.

31. Cerebral blood flow is
    A. insensitive to Po_2.
    B. reduced by high $Paco_2$.
    C. characterized by autoregulation.
    D. uniform throughout the brain.
    E. primarily under neural control.

32. If a drug is given that acts specifically to constrict the arterioles in the systemic circulation,
    A. cardiac output will decrease but central venous pressure will rise.
    B. cardiac output and mean arterial pressure will both decrease.
    C. cardiac output will increase but mean arterial pressure will not be affected.
    D. cardiac output and central venous pressure will both decrease.
    E. mean arterial pressure and central venous pressure will both rise.

33. An increase in carotid sinus pressure will
    A. increase heart rate.
    B. increase peripheral resistance.
    C. increase capillary pressure.
    D. increase myocardial contractility.
    E. increase systemic blood pressure.

34. In a person with a prominent respiratory sinus arrhythmia,
    A. efferent vagal activity decreases during inspiration.
    B. efferent cardiac sympathetic activity decreases during inspiration.
    C. the slope of the slow diastolic depolarization of the sinoatrial cells decreases during inspiration.
    D. the arrhythmia will become more pronounced in response to hemorrhage.
    E. propranolol will abolish the arrhythmia.

35. During isovolumic relaxation,
    A. the aortic valve is closed and the mitral valve is open.
    B. the aortic valve is open and the mitral valve is closed.
    C. the pulmonic valve is open and the tricuspid valve is closed.
    D. the pulmonic valve is closed and the tricuspid valve is open.
    E. all valves are closed.

36. The Frank-Starling relation is essentially a restatement of
    A. the force-velocity relation of cardiac muscle.
    B. Poiseuille's law of the heart.
    C. the length-tension diagram of cardiac muscle.
    D. Laplace's law of the heart.
    E. excitation-contraction coupling of cardiac muscle.

37. One half-hour after a brief but substantial hemorrhage,
    A. the hematocrit ratio of the blood has increased.
    B. the renal tubular reabsorption of sodium has decreased.
    C. the secretion of epinephrine from the adrenal medulla had decreased.
    D. the secretion of aldosterone from the adrenal cortex has increased.
    E. the blood level of angiotensin II has decreased.

38. The mean pressure in the left renal artery of a normal experimental animal is 100 mm Hg but is reduced suddenly to 80 mm Hg by means of a clamp and then held at that lower level for 5 minutes. At the end of this period,
    A. the blood flow to the right kidney will have increased by about 20%.
    B. the oxygen consumption of the left kidney will be diminished by about 30%.
    C. the blood flow to the left kidney will not be appreciably different from the control value.
    D. the glomerular filtration rate of the left kidney will be decreased by about 30%.
    E. the free water clearance of the left kidney will be decreased by about 50%.

39. When cardiac sympathetic activity suddenly ceases, the effects of that activity subside gradually because
    A. norepinephrine continues to be released from the nerve endings long after the neural activity has ceased.
    B. neuropeptides co-released with norepinephrine delay its degradation.
    C. the processes that remove neurally released norepinephrine from the cardiac tissues are slow.
    D. the calcium channels in the myocyte membranes are connected to the beta-adrenergic receptors by G proteins.
    E. the neurally released norepinephrine alters the viscoelastic characteristic of the cardiac tissues.

40. When a person lying on a tilt table is shifted from a horizontal to an upright position, the cardiac output decreases because
    A. arterial compliance decreases.
    B. central venous pressure decreases.
    C. heart rate decreases.
    D. the arteriovenous shunts in the splanchnic vessels dilate.
    E. sympathetic nervous activity to the heart decreases.

41. If the radius of a cylindric tube is tripled, the laminar flow of a newtonian fluid through the tube will
    A. not be affected.
    B. increase threefold.
    C. increase sixfold.
    D. increase ninefold.
    E. increase 81-fold.

42. The total peripheral resistance (TPR) of a tall, stocky adult who has normal arterial blood pressure is
    A. greater than the TPR of an average 10-year-old child.
    B. greater than the TPR of a hypertensive adult of the same weight.
    C. less during rest than during exercise.
    D. less than the TPR of a normal adult of average height and build.
    E. greater than the renal vascular resistance.

43. The pressure drop in the systemic circulation is greatest in the
    A. arterioles.
    B. capillaries.
    C. venules.
    D. aorta.
    E. venae cavae.

44. The cardiac impulse is conducted most slowly in
    A. atrial myocardial fibers.
    B. AV nodal fibers.
    C. His bundle fibers.
    D. Purkinje fibers.
    E. ventricular myocardial fibers.

45. In the fetus,
    A. pulmonary resistance is lower than in a 1-day-old baby.
    B. the left ventricle pumps more than does the right ventricle.
    C. the ductus arteriosus closes in response to an increase in Pa_{CO_2}.
    D. fetal hemoglobin has a greater affinity for O_2 than does adult hemoglobin.
    E. the foramen ovale shunts blood from the pulmonary artery to the aorta.

46. If the heart rate of a resting, normal person is increased from 60 to 90 beats/min by artificial atrial pacing,
    A. cardiac output will increase by at least 50%.
    B. stroke volume will not be affected appreciably.
    C. cardiac output will not be affected appreciably.
    D. arterial pulse pressure will increase.
    E. central venous pressure will increase.

47. Hypoxia, as occurs at high altitude,
    A. increases partial pressure of arterial blood CO_2 (Pa_{CO_2}).
    B. decreases blood pH.
    C. decreases peripheral resistance.
    D. increases the respiratory rate.
    E. decreases blood pressure.

48. When vagal activity suddenly ceases, the cardiac response to that activity disappears rapidly because the
    A. cardiac cells become tachyphylactic.
    B. nerve endings rapidly take up the released acetylcholine.
    C. myocytes rapidly take up the released acetylcholine.
    D. acetylcholine in the nerve endings is rapidly depleted.
    E. abundant acetylcholinesterase rapidly degrades the released acetylcholine.

49. When a person is standing, the capillaries in the feet do not rupture because the
    A. arterioles reflexly constrict and prevent exposure of the capillaries to high pressure.
    B. tissue pressure rises and opposes an increase in capillary pressure.
    C. total capillary cross section is large enough to distribute and thereby reduce intracapillary pressure.
    D. capillary diameter is so small that the wall tension is low.
    E. capillaries constrict by a myogenic mechanism.

50. With regard to the blood supply to the normal liver,
    A. more than half of the blood flow and more than half of the oxygen supply is delivered by the hepatic artery.
    B. less than half of the blood flow and less than half of the oxygen supply is delivered by the hepatic artery.
    C. more than half of the blood flow and more than half of the oxygen supply is delivered by the portal vein.
    D. less than half of the blood flow and less than half of the oxygen supply is delivered by the portal vein.
    E. less than half of the blood flow and more than half of the oxygen supply is delivered by the hepatic artery.

51. In a 60-year-old hypertensive person, the commonly observed increase in arterial pulse pressure is caused by
    A. increased stroke volume.
    B. increased myocardial contractility.
    C. decreased mean circulatory pressure.
    D. decreased arterial compliance.
    E. increased heart rate.

52. The principal determinants of mean arterial pressure are
    A. cardiac output and peripheral resistance.
    B. arterial and venous compliance.
    C. cardiac output and arterial compliance.
    D. peripheral resistance and arterial compliance
    E. cardiac output and venous compliance.

53. The force of cardiac contraction is enhanced by
    A. a reduction in preload.
    B. an increase in interstitial fluid Na^+.
    C. inhibition of the Na^+,K^+-ATPase.
    D. phosphorylation of phospholamban.
    E. administration of a beta blocker.

54. Cardiac Purkinje fibers
    A. are located in the epicardial layers of the ventricles.
    B. do not possess the property of automaticity.
    C. do not display a prominent notch (phase 1) in their action potentials.
    D. have a very brief plateau.
    E. conduct action potentials more rapidly than do atrial or ventricular myocytes.

55. In severe exercise,
    A. stroke volume increases proportionately more than does heart rate.
    B. pulse pressure decreases.
    C. capillary hydrostatic pressure decreases.
    D. arterial oxygen levels fall.
    E. arteriovenous oxygen difference increases.

56. The most important factor in the regulation of coronary blood flow is the
    A. coronary perfusion pressure.
    B. metabolic activity of the myocardium.
    C. extravascular compression of the coronary vessels.
    D. activity of the cardiac sympathetic nerves.
    E. activity of the vagus nerves to the heart.

57. In metabolic regulation of blood flow,
    A. basal vascular tone is unchanged when tissue metabolism is altered.
    B. blood flow is held constant during changes in tissue metabolism.
    C. blood flow and tissue metabolism are inversely related.
    D. blood flow and arterial pressure are inversely related.
    E. blood flow and tissue metabolism are directly related.

58. The less compliant arterial system in old people than in young people
    A. allows blood to flow through the capillaries at a more steady rate.
    B. requires the heart to expend more energy to pump a normal cardiac output.
    C. prevents the arterial systolic pressure from attaining excessively high values.
    D. increases the total blood volume.
    E. decreases the mean arterial blood pressure.

59. The ejection fraction is the
    A. ratio of the blood ejected per beat by the left ventricle to the volume of blood in the left ventricle at the end of systole.
    B. ratio of the blood ejected per beat by the left ventricle to the volume of blood in the left atrium in early diastole.
    C. fraction of the cardiac output ejected per heartbeat.
    D. stoke volume minus residual volume.
    E. ratio of the blood ejected per beat by the left ventricle to the volume of blood in the left ventricle at the end of diastole.

60. In the coronary circulation,
    A. venous oxygen content is one of the lowest in the body.
    B. coronary blood flow to the left ventricle is greatest during ventricular systole.
    C. autoregulation does not occur.
    D. the epicardium and endocardium are equally vulnerable to reductions in coronary perfusion pressure.
    E. parasympathetic effects predominate over sympathetic neural effects on the vessels.

ANSWERS

1. E	31. C
2. D	32. D
3. C	33. C
4. A	34. A
5. B	35. E
6. B	36. C
7. D	37. D
8. D	38. C
9. E	39. C
10. E	40. B
11. A	41. E
12. C	42. D
13. A	43. A
14. A	44. B
15. E	45. D
16. B	46. C
17. E	47. D
18. D	48. E
19. A	49. D
20. B	50. E
21. D	51. D
22. B	52. A
23. D	53. C
24. C	54. E
25. D	55. E
26. A	56. B
27. C	57. E
28. E	58. B
29. D	59. E
30. C	60. A

Index

A

A receptors, 187
Abdominal aneurysms, 156
Accessory AV pathways, 33
Acetoacetate, 235
Acetylcholine
  coronary circulation and, 228
  heartbeat and, 84-85, 87
  heart rate and, 91
  in hyperpolarization, 35
  norepinephrine and, 105
Acetylstrophanthidin, 40, 41
Acidosis
  calcium ion and, 109
  diabetic, 235
  in hemorrhage, 280
Actin, 55, 173, 174
Action potentials, 7-8; *see also* Electrical activity
  amplitude and rate of change, 23
  from cell in sinoatrial node, 27-28
  ionic basis of fast response
    early repolarization genesis, 16-17
    final repolarization genesis, 20-21
    plateau genesis, 17-20
    restoration of ionic concentrations, 21
    statistical characteristics of gate concept, 15-16
    upstroke genesis, 12-15
  ionic basis of resting potential, 9-12
  ionic basis of slow response, 22
  phases, 7-8, 49
  types, 9, 49-50
Activation gate, 13
Active hyperemia, 178
Acute coronary artery occlusion, 231
Acute heart failure, 207
Addisonian crisis, 107
Addison's disease, 107
Adenosine
  in cerebral blood flow regulation, 247

Adenosine—cont'd
  in coronary circulation regulation, 229
  in intestinal circulation regulation, 258-259
  in vasodilation, 178
Adenosine hypothesis, 229
Adenosine monophosphate, cyclic, 19, 63, 87
Adenosine triphosphate, 235
Adenylyl cyclase, 19, 102
Adrenergic blocking drugs, 66
α-Adrenergic effect, 182
β-Adrenergic effect, 182
β-Adrenergic receptors, 19, 86
  blocking agents, exercise and, 272
Adrenocortical hormones, 107
Adrenocortical insufficiency, 107
Adrenomedullary hormones, 106-107
Afferent arterioles, 253
Afterdepolarizations, 39-41
Afterload, 19, 65
  in cardiac output, 195
  in Frank-Starling mechanism, 96
  velocity and, 63
Afterloaded isotonic contraction, 64
Afterload reducing drugs, 19
Aging, arterial elasticity and, 139-140
A-H interval, 45
Albumin
  lymphatics and, 167
  in oncotic pressure, 164
Aldosterone
  cardiopulmonary receptors and, 188
  in congestive heart failure, 90
  in hemorrhage, 279
All-or-none response, 57
Alpha-adrenergic effect, 182
Altitude, peripheral chemoreceptors and, 188
Alveolar pressure, 251, 252
Amplitude of action potential, 12, 23
Anastomoses, arteriovenous, 239

Anatomy
    coronary vessels, 223-225
    glomeruli, 255
    hepatic circulation, 259-260
    microcirculation, 153
    pulmonary circulation, 248-249
    renal circulation, 253
Anemia
    blood viscosity in, 127
    functional cardiac murmurs in, 125
    sickle cell, 131
    spherocytic, 131
Aneurysms
    abdominal, 156
    aortic, syphilitic, 156
    dissecting, 126
Angina pectoris, 188
    in aortic stenosis, 116
    drug treatment, 233
Angioplasty, balloon, 231, 232
Angiotensin
    cardiopulmonary receptors and, 187-188
    in hemorrhage, 279
Angiotensin converting enzyme, 257
Angiotensin I, 257
Angiotensin II, 257
Angiotensinogen, 257, 279
Anomalous viscosity, 126
ANP, 90
AN region of AV node, 32, 33
Anterior division of left bundle branch, 36
Anterior interatrial myocardial band, 31
Anterior internodal pathway, 31
Antidiuretic hormone
    cardiopulmonary receptors and, 188
    in diuresis, 90
    in hemorrhage, 279
Aorta
    static pressure-volume relationship for, 137
    vessel wall tension in, 156
Aortic aneurysms, syphilitic, 156
Aortic arch baroreceptors, 183, 184-185
Aortic bodies, 188
Aortic compliance, 139, 140
Aortic insufficiency, 73
Aortic pressure, 65
    in coronary blood flow, 225
    response to blood loss, 277
Aortic regurgitation, 146
Aortic stenosis, 227
    murmurs produced by, 73
    pressure and volume work in, 234
    velocity and pressure in, 115-116
Apnea, 218
Apparent viscosity, 126
Arcuate arteries, 253
Arrhythmias
    altered sinoatrial rhythms, 44-45
    atrioventricular transmission blocks, 45
    ectopic pacemakers and, 27

Arrhythmias—cont'd
    ectopic tachycardias, 46-47
    fibrillation, 47-49
    impulse initiation disturbances, 44, 50
    impulse propagation disturbances, 44, 50-51
    premature depolarizations, 45-46
    reentry loops in, 39
    respiratory cardiac, 44-46
Arterial baroreceptors, 183-187
Arterial blood pressure; see also Blood pressure
    determinants, 140-147
    heart rate and, 88-89, 91
    in hemorrhage, 276
    in mild to moderate exercise, 273
    myogenic mechanism and, 175
Arterial compliance, 196
    pulse pressure and, 144, 146
Arterial pressure curves, peripheral, 147-149
Arterial system, 135-152
    blood pressure measurement in humans, 149-150
    determinants of arterial blood pressure, 140-147
    elasticity, 137, 139-140
    hydraulic filter, 135-137
    peripheral arterial pressure curves, 147-149
Arterial volume increment, 145-146
Arteries
    blood flow resistance in, 2
    coronary; see Coronary circulation
    in renal circulation, 253
Arteriolar tone, vascular function curve and, 203
Arterioles, 171
    afferent and efferent, 253
    in cutaneous circulation, 239
    diameter of, 156
    flow resistance in, 2, 120-121, 123-124
    functional anatomy, 153
    pulmonary, 248
    standing and, 177
    transmural pressure and, 154
    vasoconstriction, in hemorrhage, 277
    vasodilation, in hyperthyroidism, 2
Arterioluminal vessels, 225
Arteriosclerosis, 227
Arteriosinusoidal vessels, 225
Arteriovenous anastomoses, 239
Arteriovenous shunts, 154
Artificial respiration, 219
Ascites, 261
Asystole, 31
Atherosclerosis, 139, 140
    coronary, 230
    surgical treatment, 232
Athletes, well-trained, heart rates of, 146
ATP, 235
Atria, 66, 68
Atrial conduction, 31-32
Atrial depolarization, premature, 46
Atrial fibrillation, 47-49
Atrial flutter, 47
Atrial natriuretic peptide, 90

Atrial pacemaker complex, 27
Atrial receptors, 187
  heart rate and, 89-90
Atrial septal defects, congenital, 99
Atrial sound, 72, 73
Atrial systole, 75
Atrioventricular blocks, 33-35, 213
Atrioventricular conduction, 32-36
Atrioventricular node, 9
  parasympathetic influences, 84-85
  regions, 32-33
Atrioventricular node pacemaker cells, ionic basis of automaticity in, 30
Atrioventricular pathways, accessory, 33
Atrioventricular transmission blocks, 45
Atrioventricular valves, 68-71
Atropine, 84, 94, 96
Auscultatory method, 149
Automaticity, 26, 50
  ionic basis of, 29-30
Autonomic nervous system; see Nervous system
Autoregulation of blood flow
  cerebral, 248
  coronary, 225
  intestinal, 258-259
  microcirculation, 166
  peripheral, 175
  renal, 255-257
Auxiliary pump, respiratory muscles and venous valves as, 218
Auxiliary pumping mechanism, 218
AV; see Atrioventricular entries

B

B receptors, 187
Bachmann's bundle, 31
Bainbridge reflex
  atrial receptors and, 89-90
  respiratory sinus arrhythmia and, 91
Balloon angioplasty, 231, 232
Baroreceptor reflex, 88-89, 91, 95, 106, 216
  in hemorrhage, 276-278, 282
  in skeletal muscle circulation, 244, 274-275
Baroreceptors
  arterial, 183-187
  cardiopulmonary, 187-188
Basal tone, 179, 182, 239
Beta-adrenergic effect, 182
Beta-adrenergic receptors, 19, 86
  blocking agents, exercise and, 272
Beta-endorphin, 281
Birth, circulatory changes at, 263-264
Blanching, 241
Blocks
  atrioventricular, 33-35, 213
  atrioventricular transmission, 45
  bundle branch, 37
  unidirectional, 38-39

Blood
  loss; see Hemorrhage
  rheologic properties of, 126-131
  viscosity, 126-128, 129-130
Blood-brain barrier, 246
Blood clotting aberrations after hemorrhage, 282
Blood flow, 113; see also Circulation
  capillary, 135
  cerebral, estimation of, 245-246
  coronary
    diminished, 230-231
    measurement, 223-225
  laminar and turbulent, 124-125
  in microcirculation, 153-154
  pressure and, 113, 116-120
  pulmonary, 250-252
  pulsatile arterial, 2
  reactive hyperemia and, 179
  renal, 254-255
  resistance to, 2, 120-124
  velocity of, 4
Blood gases, in myocardial performance, 108-109
Blood pressure
  arterial, determinants of, 140-147
  arterial baroreceptors and, 184-187
  critical closing, 157
  flow and, 116-120, 154
  heart rate and, 88-89, 91
  in hemorrhage, 276
  hydrostatic-osmotic balance disturbances, 166-167
  measurement in humans, 149-150
  in mild to moderate exercise, 273
  myogenic mechanism and, 175
  transmural, 154
  velocity and, 114-116
Blood reservoirs, vascular function curve and, 202-203
Bloodstream velocity, 4, 113-114
Blood transfusions, 207
Blood vessels
  caliber of, 120
  coronary, functional anatomy, 223-225
  dimensions in 20-kg dog, 4
  of pulmonary circulation, 248-249
  series and parallel arrangement, 5
  walls, 1-2
Blood volume, 4
  arterial blood pressure and, 140
  cardiac output and, 207-208
  vascular function curve and, 201-202
Blushing, 241
Body temperature, in skin blood flow regulation, 241-242
Bowman's capsule, 253, 254
Bradycardia
  blood pressure and, 184, 188
  cardiac output and heart rate in, 213
  coronary blood flow and, 227
  fetal, 263
  sinus, 44
  after tracheal catheter disconnection, 94
Bradykinin, 182, 241

Brain
    cerebral blood flow and, 246
    in heart rate control, 87-88
    vascular control in, 190
Bronchial vasculature, 248-249
Bundle branch block, 37
Bundle branches, 36
Bundle of His, 32
    electrograms, 35, 45
Burns, 167
Bypass surgery
    coronary, 231
    right ventricle, 211

C

c wave, 74
Calcium (ion), 55
    in cardiac excitation and contraction, 61-63
    conductance during plateau, 18-19
    delayed afterdepolarizations and, 41
    in electrical activity of heart, 9-10, 17-22, 29-30
    in heartbeat regulation, 101-102, 104, 109
    increases in intracellular content of, 100-101
    in smooth muscle contraction, 173, 174
Calcium channel antagonists, 18
    effects and uses of, 19, 30, 33
Calcium channels, 173, 176
    L-type and C-type, 18
Caliber of vessel, 120
Calmodulin, 174
cAMP, 19, 63, 87
Capacitance vessels, 153
    sympathetic constrictor influence on, 181-182
Capillaries, 153-155
    density of, 153
    flow resistance in, 120
    flow velocity in, 2
    glomerular, 253-254
    injury, 167
    lymph, 167
    myocardial, 59
    peritubular, 253
    pulmonary, 248, 251-252
    recruitment, 166, 271
    in splanchnic circulation, 257
    transcapillary exchange, 158-160
        diffusion, 160-162
        filtration, 162-167, 176-177
        pinocytosis, 167
    vessel wall tension in, 156
Capillary blood flow, 135
Capillary filtration coefficient, 165-166
Carbohydrate, 235
Carbon dioxide
    in cerebral blood flow regulation, 246
    chemoreceptors and, 188, 190
    in metabolic vasodilation, 178
    movement, 161-162

Carbon dioxide—cont'd
    in myocardial performance, 108-109
Cardiac arrest, 196-198
Cardiac arrhythmias; see Arrhythmias
Cardiac chambers, 66, 68
Cardiac cycle
    ventricular diastole, 74-76
    ventricular systole, 73-74
Cardiac defects, congenital, 211
Cardiac efficiency, 234-235
Cardiac excitability, 24-26; see also Excitation of heart
Cardiac factors, 195
Cardiac failure; see Heart failure
Cardiac function curves, 195, 204-205
Cardiac output, 195-221
    ancillary factors affecting venous system and, 213-219
    arterial pressure and, 140, 141-144
    coupling between heart and vasculature, 204-208
    equation for, 83
    factors determining, 195
    heart rate and, 83, 140, 195, 211-213
    measurement
        Fick principle, 76-77
        indicator dilution techniques, 78-79
    in mild to moderate exercise, 272
    right ventricle function and, 208-211
    vascular function curve and, 195-203
    venous return and, 204
Cardiac pump, 55-82
    chambers, 66, 68
    contractility indices, 66
    cycle, 73-76
    myocardial cells, 55-66
    output measurement, 76-79
    pericardium, 71-73
    valves, 68-71
Cardiac valves, 68-71
Cardiopulmonary baroreceptors, 187-188
Cardiovascular system
    components, 1
    exercise effects on, 274
    model, 197, 209
Cardioversion, 213
Carotid bodies, 188
Carotid sinus baroreceptors, 183, 184-186
Carotid sinus pressure, cardiac autonomic nerves and, 88
Catecholamines, 74, 106
    cutaneous circulation and, 241
    effects of, 19, 63, 108
    in hemorrhage, 279
Catheters
    in cardiac output measurement, 76-77, 78
    pulmonary artery wedge pressure and, 250
Cells
    ischemic, 9
    membrane permeability, action potentials and, 9
    myocardial, 55-66
    pacemaker, 27-31
    in sinoatrial node, 27, 28
    smooth muscle, 171, 173

Central chemoreceptors, 190
Central command, 269
Central nervous system depression, in hemorrhage, 280-282
Central terminal, 44
Central venous pressure, 195
Cerebral circulation, 244-245, 265
    estimation of blood flow, 245
    regulation, 246-248
Cerebral cortex, in heart rate control, 87
Cerebral ischemia, 190, 278
Cerebrum, in vascular reflexes, 189
Cervical venous distension, 216
Chambers of heart, 66, 68
Chemical control of myocardial performance, 106-109
Chemoreceptor reflex, 92-94, 278
Chemoreceptors
    central, 190
    peripheral, 188
Cholecystokinin, 259
Cholinesterase, 84
Chordae tendinae, 70
Chord conductance equation, 12
Chronic heart failure, 97, 207
Circle of Willis, 244
Circuitry, 1-6
Circulation; see also specific circulations
    coronary, 223-237
    interplay of central and peripheral factors in, 269-285
    microcirculation and lymphatics, 153-170
    peripheral, 171-194
    pulmonary, 1, 4
    special circulations, 239-268
    systemic, 1, 4
Circulatory system, 1-6
Cirrhosis, 261
Claudication, intermittent, 180
Clotting aberrations after hemorrhage, 282
Coagulation aberrations after hemorrhage, 282
Cold exposure, cutaneous circulation and, 241-242
Colloid osmotic pressure, 163-164
Compensatory pause, 46
Complete AV heart block, 35, 213
Compliance
    aortic, 139, 140
    arterial, 196
        pulse pressure and, 144, 146
    venous, 196
Compression, extravascular, 225
Conditioning, 275
Conductance
    hydraulic, 122
    ionic, 16
        during plateau, 18-20
Conduction
    atrial, 31-32
    atrioventricular, 32-36
    in cardiac fibers, 22-24
    system, 32
    ventricular, 36-38
Congenital atrial septal defects, 99

Congenital cardiac defects, 211
Congestive heart failure, 216, 261
    arterial pulse pressure in, 146
    calcium channel antagonists in, 19
    hormones in, 90
    norepinephrine in, 96
Connexons, 57, 59
Contractile element, 64
Contractility, 65, 98
    in cardiac output, 195, 205-207
    drugs and, 66
    indices, 66
    myocardial contractile machinery and, 63-65
    norepinephrine and, 106-107
    residual volume and, 74
Contraction
    afterloaded isotonic, 64
    atrial, 75
    of heart, excitation-contraction coupling, 61-63
    isometric, 63-64
    isovolumic, 73
    of vascular smooth muscle, 171, 173, 175-176
Converting enzyme for angiotensin, 257
Coronary artery disease, action potentials in, 9, 24
Coronary artery occlusion, 227
    acute, 231
Coronary atherosclerosis, 230
Coronary bypass surgery, 231, 232
Coronary circulation, 223-237
    cardiac efficiency and, 234-235
    cardiac oxygen consumption and work, 233-234
    collateral circulation and vasodilators, 231-233
    effects of diminished flow, 230-231
    factors influencing
        metabolic, 228-230
        neural and neurohumoral, 227-228
        physical, 225-227
    functional anatomy of coronary vessels, 223-225
    substrate utilization and, 235-236
Coronary steal, 233
Coughing, intrathoracic pressure increased by, 218
Countercurrent, 242
Countercurrent exchange, 162, 258
Counterpulsation, 226
Coupled extrasystoles, 40-41, 45
Coupling factors, 195
Coupling interval, 45, 101
Coupling of heart and vascular system, 195
Crista dividens, 262
Critical closing pressure, 157
Current
    long lasting, 18
    transient, 16, 18, 41
Cushing's phenomenon, 246
Cutaneous circulation, 239, 264
    color of skin and, 242
    regulation, 239-242
Cycle length, action potential duration and, 26
Cyclic adenosine monophosphate, 19, 63, 87

D

Delayed afterdepolarizations (DADs), 39, 40-41
Delayed rectifier K+ channels, 20
Delayed rectifier K+ current, 21
Denervated hearts, 95-96
Denervation hypersensitivity, 241
Dependent variable
    in cardiac function curve, 205
    in vascular function curve, 196
Depolarizations, 7
    premature, 25, 27, 45-46
    slow diastolic, 30
Depressor area, 180
Diabetic acidosis, 235
Diastasis, 75
Diastole, 1
    ventricular, 74-76
Diastolic arterial pressure, 140, 145, 149
    total peripheral resistance and, 146-147
Diastolic depolarization, slow, 30
Diffusion, in transcapillary exchange, 160-162
Diffusion limited, 161
Digitalis, 66, 74
    electrogenic pump and, 11
    in heart failure, 63
Diltiazem, 18, 20, 34
Dipyridamole, 233
Discontinuous endothelium, 160
Disks, intercalated, 57
Dissecting aneurysm, 126
Distension of heart, Laplace's law and, 56
Diuretics, 63
Doppler ultrasonography, in coronary blood flow measurement, 223-224
Dorsal motor nucleus of vagus, 84
Driving force, 20
Drugs
    afterload reducing, 19
    in angina pectoris, 233
    contractility and, 66
    in hypertension, 216
Ductus arteriosus, 263, 264
Ductus venosus, 261

E

Early afterdepolarizations (EADs), 39-40
Early repolarization, genesis of, 16-17
Echocardiogram of mitral valve leaflet movement, 70
Echocardiography, 70
    in coronary blood flow measurement, 224-225
Ectopic foci/pacemakers, 27
Ectopic tachycardias, 46-47
Edema, 166-167, 168, 211
    arteriolar resistance and, 177
    pulmonary, 165, 209
EDRF, 157-158, 177
Effective refractory period, 15, 25

Efferent arterioles, 253
Efficiency of heart, 234-235
Einthoven triangle, 42
Ejection, 73-74
Ejection fraction, 66
E_K, 10
Elastic characteristics, 140
Elastic element, 64
Elasticity of arteries, 137, 139-140
Elastic modulus, 140
Electrical activity, 7-53
    arrhythmias, 44-49, 50-51
    cardiac excitability, 24-38, 50
    conduction in cardiac fibers, 22-24
    electrocardiography, 41-44, 51
    historical perspective, 7
    reentry, 38-39
    transmembrane potentials, 7-22, 49-50
    triggered activity, 39-41
Electric shock, for fibrillation, 49
Electrocardiograms, 51
    deflections and intervals in, 34
    scalar, 41
    in Wolff-Parkinson-White syndrome, 33
Electrocardiography
    benefits, 41
    scalar, 41
        configuration, 41-42
        standard limb leads for, 42-44
Electrogenic pump, 11
Electrograms, His bundle, 35, 45
Electrolytes, in hemorrhage, 279
Electrolyte solutions, 22
Electromechanical coupling, 173
Electron micrographs
    of interalveolar septum, 249
    of myocardium, 57-61
Embolism, pulmonary, 250
Emphysema, 250
E_{Na}, 11
End-diastolic myocardial fiber length, 97
End-diastolic volume, 56, 65
Endocrine system, 1
Endothelial cells of capillaries, 154-155
Endothelin, 158
Endothelium
    discontinuous, 160
    passive role of, 158-167
    vasoactive role of, 157-158
Endothelium-derived relaxing factor, 157-158, 177
Endothelium-mediated regulation of peripheral circulation, 177
Endotoxins, 282
Endurance training, 275
Enkephalins, 281
Enlargement of heart, 44, 71
Epicardial fibers, early repolarization and, 17
Epinephrine
    contractility and, 66
    cutaneous circulation and, 241

Epinephrine—cont'd
  excessive doses of, 66
  in hemorrhage, 279
  peripheral circulation and, 182-183
  skeletal muscle circulation and, 244
Equilibrium point, 205
Erythrocytes, deformability of, 130, 131
Esophageal varices, 261
Essential hypertension, 207
Excitability, cardiac, 24-26
Excitation-contraction coupling, 19, 61-63
Excitation of heart, natural, 26-27, 50
  atrial conduction, 31-32
  atrioventricular conduction, 32-36
  ionic basis of automaticity, 29-30
  overdrive suppression, 30-31
  sinoatrial node, 27-29
  ventricular conduction, 36-38
Exercise, 269-270, 283
  cardiac output during, 213
  mild to moderate, 270-273
  performance limits, 274-275
  physical training and conditioning, 275
  recovery, 274
  severe, 273-274
  vascular control in, 190-191
Extracoronary resistance, 225
Extrasystoles (coupled), 40-41, 45
Extravascular compression, 225

F

f waves, 47
Fast channels, 12
Fast response, 9
  cardiac excitability and, 25
  conduction of, 23-24
  ionic basis of, 12-21
Fatty acids, 235
Febrile infectious diseases, 28
Fenestrations, capillary, 160
Fetal circulation, 261-263, 265
  changes at birth, 263-264
  schematic diagram, 262
Fetal hemoglobin, 263
Fibers
  cardiac
    conduction in, 22-24
    parasympathetic, 84
    sympathetic, 86
  early repolarization and, 17
  length and force, 56
  length and volume, 97
  Purkinje, 9, 23-24, 26, 27, 36-38
Fibrillation, 25, 47-49
  as random reentry, 38
  ventricular, 218
Fick equation, 245

Fick principle, 76-77, 245
Fick's law, 160
Filtration
  hydraulic, 135-137
  in transcapillary exchange, 158, 162-167
Final repolarization, genesis of, 20-21
First-degree AV block, 33, 35
Flow; see also Blood flow
  nutritional and nonnutritional, 154
  pressure and
    in coronary circulation, 225
    in hydraulic systems, 138
  steady, 117
  streamlined, 124, 125
  turbulent, 124-125, 126
  volume flow, 113
Flow limited, 161, 230
Fluids
  blood pressure and, 187
  capillaries and, 162-167, 177
  in hemorrhage, 278-279
  laminar and turbulent flow of, 124-125
  lymphatics and, 167
  in mild to moderate exercise, 272
  viscosity of, 118-119, 120, 126-128
Flutter, atrial, 47
Foramen ovale, 262
Force, contraction and, 63
Frank-Starling mechanism
  exercise and, 272, 273
  intact preparations and, 97-99
  isolated hearts and, 96-97
  premature contractions and, 101
Frank-Starling relationship, 56, 195
Functional cardiac murmurs, 125
Functional hyperemia, in intestinal circulation, 259

G

Gain, of positive feedback mechanism, 280
Gallop rhythms, 73
Galvanometer connections, 43, 44
Gap junctions, 57, 59
Gastrin, 259
Gate concept statistical characteristics, 15-16
Gates for sodium channel, 13-15
Gibbs-Donnan effect, 164
Glomerular capillaries, 253-254
Glomerular filtration rate, 257
Glomeruli, 253, 255
Glucagon, 108
Glucose, 235
Glycocalyx, 62
Glycogen, 263
Graves disease, 2
Gravity, in cardiac output, 214-216

H

h gates, 13, 14, 15, 23
Heart; *see also* Cardiac *entries*
    chambers, 66, 68
    coupling of vascular system and, 195
    denervated, 95-96
    distension, Laplace's law and, 56
    efficiency, 234-235
    electrical activity, 7-53
    enlargement, 44, 71
    excitation, 26-32, 50
    extrinsic and intrinsic vascular control in, 190
    hyperdynamic, 66
    hypodynamic, 66
    oxygen consumption by, work and, 233-234
    substrate utilization by, 235-236
    valves, 68-71
Heartbeat, 83-112
    extrinsic regulation of myocardial performance, 102-109
    intrinsic regulation of myocardial performance, 95-102
    nervous control of heart rate, 83-95
Heart block, complete, 35
Heart failure, 207
    acute, 207
    chronic, 97, 207
    congestive, 216, 261
        arterial pulse pressure in, 146
        calcium channel antagonists in, 19
        hormones in, 90
        norepinephrine in, 26
    contractility in, 98
    digitalis and diuretics in, 63
    in hemorrhage, 280
    left, 250
    residual volume in, 74
    right, 211
Heart pump; *see* Cardiac pump
Heart rate
    cardiac output and, 83, 140, 195, 211-213
    intrinsic, 84
    nervous control, 83-84
        Bainbridge reflex and atrial receptors, 89-90
        baroreceptor reflex, 88-89
        chemoreceptor reflex, 92-94
        control by higher centers, 87-88
        parasympathetic pathways, 84-86
        respiratory cardiac arrhythmia and, 90-92
        sympathetic pathways, 86-87
        ventricular receptor reflexes, 94-95
    in training, 275
Heart sounds, 71-73
Hematocrit ratio, 126-129
Hemodynamics, 113-133
    flow resistance, 120-124
    hepatic, 260-261
    laminar and turbulent flow, 124-125
    pressure-flow relationship, 116-120
    pulmonary, 250-252
    renal, 253-255

Hemodynamics—cont'd
    rheologic properties of blood, 126-131
    shear stress on vessel wall, 126
    velocity of bloodstream, 113-114
    velocity-pressure relationship, 114-116
Hemoglobin, fetal, 263
Hemorrhage, 166, 190, 204
    arterial pulse pressure in, 146
    compensatory mechanisms, 276-279
    course of arterial blood pressure changes in, 276
    decompensatory mechanisms, 280-282
    effects of, 276, 283
    interactions of positive and negative feedback mechanisms in, 282-283
Hemorrhage curve, 202
Hemorrhagic shock, 182, 276
Hepatic artery, 259, 261
Hepatic circulation, 265
    anatomy, 259-260
    hemodynamics, 260-261
    regulation, 261
Hepatic cirrhosis, 261
His bundle, 32
    branches, 36
    electrograms, 35, 45
Hormones, 90; *see also specific hormones*
    adrenocortical, 107
    adrenomedullary, 106-107
    gastrointestinal, 259
    thyroid, 107-108
Humoral factors, peripheral circulation and, 182-183
H-V interval, 45
Hydraulic conductance, 122
Hydraulic filter, 135-137
Hydraulic resistance equation, 120
Hydraulic resistance in series and in parallel, 121-124
Hydraulic systems, pressure-flow relationships in, 138
Hydrocortisone, 107
Hydrogen ions, in metabolic vasodilation, 178
Hydrostatic forces, 162
Hydrostatic-osmotic balance disturbances, 168-169
Hydrostatic pressure
    arteriolar resistance and, 177
    in capillary filtration, 162-163, 164-165
Hypercapnia, hypoxia with, 188
Hyperdynamic heart, 66
Hyperemia
    active, 178
    functional, in intestinal circulation, 259
    reactive, 179, 229, 241, 248
Hyperpolarization, 29, 30, 31, 35-36
Hypersensitivity, denervation, 24
Hypertension
    baroreceptor sensitivity in, 186
    chronic, 147
    drugs treating, 216
    epinephrine and, 66
    essential, 207
    heart sounds in, 72
    peripheral resistance in, 127

Hypertension—cont'd
  viscous drag in, 126
Hyperthyroidism, 2, 108
Hypertrophy, ventricular, 44
Hyperventilation, 94
Hypervolemia, 201-202
Hypodynamic heart, 66
Hypotension, 227
  arterial, 182
  carotid sinus and, 186
  during exercise, 273
  hemorrhagic, 278, 280, 282
  orthostatic, 216
Hypothalamus
  in heart rate control, 87
  in vascular reflexes, 188-189
Hypothyroidism, 108
Hypovolemia, 188, 201
Hypovolemic shock, 251
Hypoxia
  effects on heart, 108
  fetal circulation and, 263
  hypercapnia with, 188
  pulmonary vascular resistance and, 252-253
  substrate utilization in, 235

I

Idioventricular pacemakers, 27
Impulse propagation or initiation disturbances, 44, 50-51
Inactivation gate, 13
Inactivation of ion channel, 15
Incisura, 74, 148
Independent variable
  in cardiac function curve, 205
  in vascular function curve, 196
Indicator dilution techniques, 78-79
Infectious diseases, febrile, 28
Inositol trisphosphate, 174
Insulin, 108
Intercalated disks, 57
Interlobar arteries, 253
Interlobular branches, 253
Intermittent claudication, 180
Internodal pathways, 31
Interstitial fluids, resorption, in hemorrhage, 278-279
Intestinal circulation, 258-259, 265
Intrathoracic pressure, 218
Intravenous infusions, heart rate and, 89
Intrinsic heart rate, 84
Inwardly rectified K^+ current, 21
Inwardly rectifying K^+ current, 10
Inward Na^+ current, 13
Ion channels, 9, 15
Ionic conductance, 16
Ions; *see also* Calcium; Potassium; Sodium
  automaticity and, 29-30
  fast response and, 12-21
  resting potential and, 9-12

Ions—cont'd
  slow response and, 22
Ischemia
  in angina pectoris, 233
  cerebral, 190, 278
  hemorrhage and, 278
  lactic acid in, 235
  myocardial, 230, 233
Ischemic cells, 9
Ischemic heart disease, 207
Isoelectric line, 42
Isometric contraction, 63-64
Isoproterenol, 19, 86, 104, 258
Isotonic contraction, 64
Isovolumic contraction, 73
Isovolumic relaxation, 74

J

Juxtaglomerular apparatus, 257
Juxtamedullary glomeruli, 253

K

K^+; *see* Potassium
Ketone bodies, 235
Kidney; *see* Renal *entries*
Korotkoff sounds, 149

L

Lactate, 235
Lactic acid, in metabolic vasodilation, 178
Laminar flow, 117, 124, 125
Laplace's law, 56, 155-156
Lateral pressure, 114, 115
Law of Laplace, 56, 155-156
Leads for electrocardiography, 42-44
Leaflets of cardiac valves, 68-71
Left anterior hemiblock, 37
Left bundle branch, 36
  blocks, 37
Left coronary artery, 223
  phasic coronary flow curve, 225, 226
Left heart failure, 250
Left posterior hemiblock, 37
Left ventricle
  exercise effects on, 275
  failure, 165, 209
  pressure-volume relationship, 75-76
Legs
  pain in, from intermittent claudication, 180
  venous pressure in, 216-217
Limb leads for electrocardiography, 42-44
Linear velocity, 113-114
Lipid solubility, 161
Liver; *see* Hepatic *entries*

Long lasting current, 18
Lower extremities
   pain in, from intermittent claudication, 180
   venous pressure in, 216-217
L-type Ca^{++} channels, 18
Lungs; *see also* Pulmonary *entries*
   capillary hydrostatic pressure in, 165
Lymphatics, 167-168

M

m gate, 13, 14, 15
Macrophages, 282
Macula densa of juxtaglomerular apparatus, 257
Mayer waves, 181
Mean arterial pressure, 140, 141-144
Mean circulatory pressure, 198
Mean electrical axis, 43-44
Mechanical restitution curve, 101
Medications
   afterload reducing, 19
   in angina pectoris, 233
   contractility and, 66
   in hypertension, 216
Medulla
   adrenal, 106
   peripheral chemoreceptor stimulation and, 92, 93
   respiratory sinus arrhythmia and, 91-92
   vascular reflexes and, 183
Mesenteric arteries, 258
Mesenteric circulation, 258-259
Metabolic factors affecting coronary circulation, 228-229
Metabolic regulation of peripheral circulation, 177-180
Metarterioles, 153, 154
Microcirculation, 153-157
   passive role of endothelium in, 158-167
   vasoactive role of endothelium in, 157-158
Middle internodal pathway, 31
Mitochondria
   calcium ion and, 63
   in cardiac and skeletal muscle, 59
Mitral insufficiency, 73
Mitral valve, 68
   leaflet movements, 70-71
   stenosis, 73, 165
Monokines, 282
Müller's maneuver, 218
Murmurs, 73
   aneurysms and, 156
   functional cardiac, 125
   turbulence and, 125
Muscarinic receptors, 87
Muscle
   activity, venous valves and, 216-217
   cardiac, 55-66
      conduction in fibers, 22-24
      electrical behavior of, 7-8
   papillary, 64, 68

Muscle—cont'd
   skeletal
      circulation, 242-244, 265
      myocardial vs., 55, 57, 59
      performance, oxygen and, 274-275
      vascular control in, 190-191
   vascular smooth, 171-179
      tone of, 171, 179, 181
Myocardial cells, 55-61
   contractility and, 63-66, 74
   electrical activity and, 9-10; *see also* Action potentials
   excitation-contraction coupling, 61-63
Myocardial contractility, in cardiac output, 195, 205-207
Myocardial hibernation, 231
Myocardial infarction, 201
Myocardial ischemia, 230, 233
Myocardial metabolic activity, coronary circulation and, 228-229
Myocardial performance
   extrinsic regulation, 102
      chemical control, 106-109
      nervous control, 102-106
   intrinsic regulation, 95-96
      Frank-Starling mechanism, 96-99
      rate-induced, 99-102
Myocardial stunning, 230
Myoendothelial junctions, 171
Myogenic mechanism, 175-177
   of renal autoregulation, 257
Myosin, 55, 173, 174

N

N region of AV node, 32, 33
Na^+; *see* Sodium
Na^+,K^+-ATPase, 11, 24, 31
Naloxone, 282
Natural pacemaker, 27
Neck, venous distension in, 216
Necrosis, 230
   coronary collateral vessels in, 231-232
Negative feedback mechanisms, in hemorrhage, 276-279, 282-283
Nernst equation, 10, 11, 12
Nervous system, 1; *see also* Parasympathetic nervous system; Sympathetic nervous system
   in circulation regulation
      cerebral blood flow, 246
      coronary, 227-228
      cutaneous, 239, 241
      hepatic, 261
      intestinal, 258
      peripheral, 182
      pulmonary, 252
      renal, 257
      skeletal muscle blood flow, 243-244
   in heart rate control, 83-84
      Bainbridge reflex and atrial receptors, 89-90

Nervous system—cont'd
  in heart rate control—cont'd
    baroreceptor reflex, 88-89
    chemoreceptor reflex, 92-94
    control by higher centers, 87-88
    parasympathetic pathways, 84-86
    respiratory cardiac arrhythmia and, 90-92
    sympathetic pathways, 86-87
    ventricular receptor reflexes, 94-95
  in myocardial performance control
    baroreceptor reflex, 106
    parasympathetic influences, 105-106
    sympathetic influences, 102-105
  vascular reflexes and, 183-190
  in vasoconstriction, 180-182
Neurohumoral factors affecting coronary circulation, 227-228
Neuropeptide Y, 106
Newtonian fluids, 117, 119, 126
Nexi, 57, 59
NH region of AV node, 32, 33
Nifedipine, 18, 31
Nitrates, in angina pectoris, 233
Nitric oxide, 157-158, 177
Nitrites, in angina pectoris, 233
Nitroprusside, 158
Nitrous oxide method of cerebral blood flow measurement, 245
Nonnewtonian fluids, 119, 126
Nonnutritional flow, 154
Norepinephrine, 19
  AV node and, 36
  in congestive heart failure, 96
  contractility and, 66, 106, 107
  cutaneous circulation and, 241
  in exercise, 273
  in heartbeat regulation, 86, 87, 91
  in hemorrhage, 279
  peripheral circulation and, 180, 181, 182-183, 186
  in skeletal muscle circulation, 244
  ventricular function curve and, 97-98
Normovolemia, 201
NPY, 106
Nucleus ambiguus, 84
Nucleus of tractus solitarius, 183
Nutritional flow, 154

O

Occlusion, coronary artery, 227, 231
Ohm's law, 252
Oncotic pressure, 163-164
Opioids, 281-282
Ordered reentry, 38
Orthostatic hypotension, 216
Osmolarity, in vasodilation, 178
Osmotic forces, 163-165
Osmotic-hydrostatic balance disturbances, 168-169
Output; *see* Cardiac output

Outward K^+ current, 11
Overdrive suppression, 30-31
Overshoot of cardiac action potential, 15
Oxygen
  cardiac consumption of
    efficiency and, 234-235
    work and, 233-234
  circulation and
    coronary, 229
    fetal, 261, 263, 264
    hepatic, 259, 261
    intestinal, 258
    peripheral, 177-178
    pulmonary, 252-253
    renal, 255
  consumption, 76, 77
  exercise and, 271, 274-275
  in Fick principle, 76-77
  movement, 161-162
  in myocardial performance, 108
Oxygen tension
  arteriolar diameter and, 178
  central chemoreceptors and, 190
  of fetal blood, 263
  myocardial performance and, 108

P

P wave, 32
  in AV blocks, 35
  in premature depolarizations, 46
Pacemaker cells, 27-31
Pacemaker potential, 28
Pacemakers
  in AV blocks, 35
  ectopic, 27
  idioventricular, 27
  natural (SA node), 27
Pacemaker shift, 29
Pa_{CO_2}
  in cerebral blood flow regulation, 246
  chemoreceptors and, 188, 190
  myocardial performance and, 108-109
Palpatory method, 149
Pa_{O_2}
  chemoreceptors and, 188
  myocardial performance and, 108
Papillary muscle, 64, 68
Parasympathetic nervous system
  in heart rate control, 83-86
  in myocardial performance, 105-106
  peripheral circulation and, 182
Parasystole, 45
Paroxysmal supraventricular tachycardia, 47
Paroxysmal tachycardias, 27, 47
Paroxysmal ventricular tachycardia, 47
Patch-clamping technique, 15
Peptides, 90, 257; *see also* Hormones

Perfusion pressure, myogenic mechanism and, 175
Pericardium, 71, 97
Peripheral arterial pressure curves, 147-149
Peripheral chemoreceptors, 188
Peripheral circulation, 171-194
   balance between intrinsic and extrinsic factors in regula-
      tion of, 190-191
   extrinsic control, 180
      humoral factors, 182-183
      neural sympathetic vasoconstriction, 180-181
      parasympathetic neural influence, 182
      sympathetic constrictor influence on resistance and ca-
        pacitance vessels, 181-182
      vascular reflexes, 183-190
   intrinsic or local control
      autoregulation and myogenic regulation, 175-177
      endothelium-mediated regulation, 177
      metabolic regulation, 177-180
   vascular smooth muscle and, 171-175
Peripheral resistance, 196
   arterial pressure and, 140, 143, 144
   cardiac function curve and, 208
   in mild to moderate exercise, 270-271
   total
      arterial diastolic pressure and, 146-147
      in hypertension, 147
      vascular function curve and, 199, 203, 208
Peripheral runoff, 141, 196
Peritubular capillaries, 253
pH
   calcium ion and, 109
   central chemoreceptors and, 190
   in cerebral blood flow regulation, 246, 247
Pharmacomechanical coupling, 173
Phonocardiogram, 71, 72
Phosphate, in vasodilation, 178
Phospholamban, 63, 104
Phospholamban gene, 65
Phospholipase C, 173-174
Physical training, 275
Physiologic shunting of blood flow, 154
Pinocytosis, 167
Pitot tubes, 114
Plasma
   osmotic and oncotic pressure, 163-164, 165
   proteins, 167
Plateau of transmembrane potentials, 7
   genesis of, 17-20
Po$_2$, vascular smooth muscle and, 178
Poise, 120
Poiseuille's law, 117, 165, 214
   full statement of, 120
Polycythemia, 127
Pores, capillary, 158, 161
Portacaval shunt, 261
Portal vein, 259, 261
Positive feedback mechanisms, in hemorrhage, 280-283
Positive inotropic effect, 66
Posterior division of left bundle branch, 36
Posterior internodal pathway, 31

Postextrasystolic potentiation, 101
Post-repolarization refractoriness, 25
Potassium (ion)
   in cardiac excitation and contraction, 61
   in cerebral blood flow regulation, 246-247
   conductance during plateau, 19-20
   current
      delayed rectifier, 21
      inwardly rectified, 21
      inwardly rectifying, 10
      outward, 11
   in electrical activity of heart, 9-12, 16-21, 23-24, 30
   in vasodilation, 178
Potassium (ion) channels, 10
   delayed rectifier, 21
Potassium equilibrium potential, 10
P-P interval, 44
Precordial leads, 44
Preload, 65
   in cardiac output, 195
   in Frank-Starling mechanism, 96
Preloaded (isometric) contraction, 63-64
Premature atrial depolarization, 46
Premature depolarizations, 25, 27, 45-46
Premature ventricular depolarization, 46, 101-102
Pressoreceptors, 183-187
Pressor region, 180
Pressure; *see also* Blood pressure
   aortic, 65, 225, 277
   arterial
      diastolic, 140, 145, 146-147, 149
      mean, 140, 141-144
      in mild to moderate exercise, 273
      peripheral arterial pressure curves, 147-149
      systolic, 65, 140, 145, 149
   carotid sinus, cardiac autonomic nerves and, 88
   central venous, 195
   colloid osmotic (oncotic), 163-164
   critical closing, 157
   flow and, 116-120, 154
      in coronary circulation, 225
      in hydraulic systems, 138
   in Frank-Starling relationship, 56
   hydrostatic, 162-163, 177
   hydrostatic-osmotic balance disturbances, 166-167
   intrathoracic, 218
   lateral, 114, 115
   mean circulatory (static), 198
   perfusion, myogenic mechanism and, 175
   in pulmonary circulation, 250-252
   pulse, 144-147
   total, 114, 115
   transmural, 154, 175-176, 252
   velocity and, 114-116
   venous, 166, 196-201
Pressure-volume relationship for aorta, 137, 139-140
Pressure-volume relationship/loop, left ventricular, 75-76
Presystolic gallop, 73
P-R interval, 42
Procainamide, 28

Propranolol, 84, 86, 96
Prostacyclin, 157
Prostaglandins, in vasodilation, 178
Proteins, 167-168
Protodiastolic gallop, 73
Pulmonary artery, 248
Pulmonary artery wedge pressure, 250
Pulmonary circulation, 1, 4, 248, 265
    functional anatomy, 248-249
    hemodynamics, 250-252
    regulation, 252-253
Pulmonary edema, 165, 209
Pulmonary embolism, 250
Pulmonary hyperventilation, 94
Pulmonary reflexes, 189
Pulmonary vascular resistance in newborn, 264
Pulmonary vasculature, 248
Pulsatile arterial blood flow, 2
Pulse pressure, 144-147
Pump
    auxiliary, respiratory muscles and venous valves as, 218
    electrogenic, 11
    heart as, 196; *see also* Cardiac pump
Purkinje fibers, 9, 27
    cycle length changes and, 26
    external K⁺ concentration changes and, 23-24
    refractory period of, 38
    in ventricular conduction, 36-38

Q

QRS complex, 32, 42, 43-44
    in AV blocks, 35
    in premature depolarizations, 46
Q-T interval, 42
Quinidine, 28

R

Random reentry, 38
Rapid ejection, 73
Rapid filling phase, 747
Rate-induced regulation, 99-102
Rate of change of action potentials, 23
Raynaud's disease, 241
Reactive hyperemia, 179, 229, 241, 248
Recovery of ion channels from inactivation, 15
Red blood cells, deformability of, 130, 131
Reduced ejection, 73
Reentry, 38-39
Reflection coefficient, 161, 164
Reflex(es)
    Bainbridge, 89-90, 91
    baroreceptor, 88-89, 91, 95, 106, 216
        in hemorrhage, 276-278, 282
        in skeletal muscle circulation, 244, 274-275
    chemoreceptor, 92-94, 278
    exercise and, 269-270

Reflex(es)—cont'd
    pulmonary, 189
    vascular, 183-190
    ventricular receptor, 94-95
Refractory period
    effective, 15, 25
    of Purkinje fibers, 38
    relative, 25
Regenerative process, 13
Regulation
    of heartbeat, 83-112
    of peripheral circulation, 175-191
    of special circulations; *see specific circulations*
Relative refractory period, 25
Relaxation, isovolumic, 74
Renal artery, 253
Renal circulation, 265
    anatomy, 253
    hemodynamics, 253-255
    regulation, 255-257
Renal conservation of salt and water, in hemorrhage, 279
Renal vasoconstriction, in hemorrhage, 277-278
Renin, 188, 257, 279
Renin-angiotensin system, 257
Repolarization, 7
    early, genesis of, 16-17
    final, genesis of, 20-21
RES, in hemorrhage, 282
Reserpine, 96
Residual volume, 74
Resistance
    coronary vascular, 229-230
    extracoronary, 225
    peripheral, 196
        arterial pressure and, 140, 142, 144
        cardiac function curve and, 208
        in mild to moderate exercise, 270-271
        total, 146-147
        vascular function curve and, 199, 203, 208
    in peripheral vascular beds, 186
    pulmonary vascular, in newborn, 264
    segmental, in renal circulation, 253-254
Resistance vessels, 153, 171; *see also* Arterioles
    in cutaneous circulation, 239
    diameter of, 156
    functional anatomy, 153
    in skeletal muscle circulation, 243
    sympathetic constrictor influence on, 181-182
Respiration, artificial, 219
Respiratory activity, in cardiac output, 217-218
Respiratory cardiac arrhythmia, 44-46
Resting membrane potential, 9
    conduction velocity and, 23
    ionic basis of, 9-12
Resultant cardiac vector, 42
Reticuloendothelial system, in hemorrhage, 282
Reynold's number, 125
Rheologic properties of blood, 126-131
Rhythm
    disturbances; *see* Arrhythmias

Rhythm—cont'd
    gallop, 73
Rhythmicity, 26
Right bundle branch, 36
    blocks, 37
Right coronary artery, 223
    phasic coronary flow curve, 226
Right heart failure, 211
Right ventricle, function of, 208-211

S

SA; *see* Sinoatrial *entries*
Salt, renal conservation of, in hemorrhage, 279
Sarcolemma, excitation-contraction coupling and, 61, 62, 63
Sarcomeres, 55, 56
Sarcoplasmic reticulum, 61, 63
Sarcosomes, 59
Scalar electrocardiography, 41-44
Scalar quantities, 41
Second-degree AV block, 35
Segmental resistance, in renal circulation, 253-254
Semilunar valves, 69, 71
Shear rate, 119, 120
    blood viscosity and, 129-130
Shear stress, 119
    on vessel wall, 126
Shear thinning, 130, 131
Shock
    hemorrhagic, 182, 276
    hypovolemic, 251
Shunt flow, 154
Shunts
    arteriovenous, 154
    portacaval, 261
Sickle cell anemia, 131
Sick sinus syndrome, 31, 213
Sinoatrial node, 9, 27-29
    ionic basis of automaticity in, 29-30
    parasympathetic influences, 84-85
Sinoatrial node pacemaker cells, ionic basis of automaticity
        in, 29-30
Sinoatrial rhythms, altered, 44-45
Sinus bradycardia, 44
Sinuses of Valsalva, 71
Sinus node recovery time, 31
Sinus tachycardia, 44
Skeletal muscle
    circulation, 242-243, 265
        regulation, 243-244
    myocardial vs., 55, 57, 59
    performance, oxygen and, 274-275
    vascular control in, 190-191
Skin
    color, 242
    vascular control in, 190
    in vascular reflexes, 189
Skin circulation, 239, 264
    regulation, 239-242

Slow diastolic depolarization, 30
Slow response, 9
    cardiac excitability and, 25-26
    conduction of, 24
    ionic basis of, 22
Smooth muscle, vascular, 171-179
    tone of, 171, 179, 181
Sodium (ion)
    in cardiac excitation and contraction, 61, 63
    in electrical activity of heart, 9-17, 21-24, 29, 31
    in hemorrhage, 279
    inward Na$^+$ current, 13
Sodium equilibrium potential, 11
Sounds produced by heart, 71-73
Spherocytic anemias, 131
Sphygmomanometer, 149, 150
Splanchnic circulation, 257-261, 265
Splanchnic vasoconstriction, in hemorrhage, 278
Split sound, 73
Staircase phenomenon, 99
Standard limb leads for electrocardiography, 42-44
Standing
    blood pressure and, 176-177
    cardiac output and, 214, 215-216
    venous valves and, 216-217
Starling hypothesis, 164-165
Starling's law of the heart, 96, 204; *see also* Frank-Starling
        mechanism
Static pressure, 114, 198
Static pressure-volume relationship, 137
Steady flow, 117
Stenosis
    aortic, 73, 115-116, 227, 234
    mitral valve, 73, 165
Steroids, 107
ST interval, 42
Stokes-Adams attacks, 35
Streamlined flow, 124, 125
Strength exercises, 275
Stretch of elastic element, 64-65
Stroke volume, 66, 97
    atrial pacing and, 212
    cardiac output and, 83, 140
    pulse pressure and, 144-146
Stroke work, 233
Substrate utilization, 235-236
Superior mesenteric artery, 258
Supraventricular tachycardia, 33, 213
    paroxysmal, 47
Sweat glands, 241
Sympathetic nerves, section of, 181
Sympathetic nervous system, 175
    in circulation regulation
        cerebral blood flow, 246
        coronary, 227-228
        hepatic, 261
        intestinal, 258
        renal, 257
        skeletal muscle blood flow, 243-244
    in heart rate control, 83, 86-87

Sympathetic nervous system—cont'd
  in myocardial performance, 102-105
  in vasoconstriction, 180-182
Syncope, 75
  third-degree block and, 35
  vasovagal, 28, 95
Syncytium, cardiac muscle functioning as, 57
Syphilitic aortic aneurysm, 156
Systemic circulation, 1, 4
Systole, 1
  atrial, 75
  ventricular, 73-74
Systolic arterial pressure, 140, 145
  afterload and, 65
  Korotkoff sounds and, 149

T

T waves, 42
Tachycardia
  atrial contraction in, 75
  contractility and, 66
  coronary blood flow and, 227
  ectopic, 46-47
  experimental induction of, 87
  fetal, 263
  hypothalamus and, 188
  paroxysmal, 27, 47
  sinus, 44
  supraventricular, 33, 213
  ventricular, 213
Temperature, in skin blood flow regulation, 241-242
Tetanus, 15
Tetrodotoxin, 9, 12, 22, 33
Thebesian vessels, 225
Thermodilution, 78-79, 223
Third-degree AV block, 35
Thoracic duct, 168
Threshold for action potentials, 12
Thrombi, 125, 282
Thromboangiitis obliterans, 180
Thromboxane A_2, 282
Thyroid dysfunction, 108
Thyroid hormones, 107-108
Tissue fluids, resorption, in hemorrhage, 278-279
Tissue pressure, capillary filtration and, 163
Tone
  arteriolar, vascular function curve and, 203
  of vascular smooth muscle, 171
    basal, 179, 182, 239
    section of sympathetic nerves and, 181
  venomotor, vascular function curve and, 202
Total peripheral resistance, 123
  arterial diastolic pressure and, 146-147
  in hypertension, 127, 147
Total pressure, 114, 115
Tractus solitarius, 183
Training, physical, 275

Transcapillary exchange, 158-160
  diffusion, 160-162
  filtration, 162-167
  pinocytosis, 167
Transfusion curve, 202
Transfusions, 207
Transient current, 18
Transient inward current, 41
Transient outward current, 16
Transmembrane potentials; see Action potentials
Transmural pressure, 154, 175-176, 252
Transverse-tubular system, 59-61
Traube-Hering waves, 180
Treppe phenomenon, 99
Tricuspid valve, 68
Trigger Ca^{++}, 62
Triggered activity, 39-41
Troponin C, 62, 63
T-tubular system, 59-61
T-type Ca^{++} channels, 18
Tubuloglomerular feedback, in renal autoregulation, 257
Turbulent flow, 124-125, 126

U

U tubes, 214-216
Ultrasonography, in coronary blood flow measurement, 223-224
Umbilical vessels, 263-264
Unidirectional block, 38-39
Upstroke, genesis of, 12-15
Urine volume, increased by atrial receptor stimulation, 89-90

V

Vagal activity
  coronary circulation and, 228
  in heartbeat regulation, 105-106
  in heart rate control, 84-85
  increased, 28
Vagus nerves, 84, 85, 105
Valsalva sinuses, 71
Valsalva's maneuver, 218
Valves
  cardiac, 68-71
  semilunar, 65, 71
  venous, muscular activity and, 216-217
Varices, esophageal, 261
Varicose veins, 217, 243
Vasa recta, 253
Vascular function curve, 195-200
  blood reservoirs and, 202-203
  blood volume and, 201-202
  definition, 195
  mathematical analysis, 199-200
  peripheral resistance and, 203
  venomotor tone and, 202

Vascular function curve—cont'd
  venous pressure dependence on cardiac output and, 200-201
Vascular reflexes, 183-190
Vascular resistance, in training, 275
Vascular system, coupling of heart and, 195
Vasoconstriction
  in cerebral ischemia, 190
  from cold exposure, 241, 242
  in hemorrhage, 277-278
  in kidney, 188
  neural sympathetic, 180-182
  in severe exercise, 273
  in skeletal muscle circulation, 244
Vasoconstrictors, endogenous, in hemorrhage, 279
Vasodilation
  arterial and arteriolar, coordination of, 179-180
  bradykinin in, 182
  by calcium channel antagonists, 19
  cold exposure and, 242
  from endothelium-derived relaxing factor, 177
  metabolic, 177-180
  in skeletal muscle circulation, 244
Vasodilators, coronary collateral circulation and, 231-233
Vasomotion, 153-154
Vasopressin
  cardiopulmonary receptors and, 188
  in diuresis, 90
  in hemorrhage, 279
Vasovagal syncope, 28, 95
Veins, varicose, 217, 243
Velocity
  of bloodstream, 4, 113-114
    pressure and, 114-116
  conduction, 23
  contraction and, 63
Vena caval flow, 4, 219
Venoconstriction, 202
Venomotor tone, vascular function curve and, 202
Venous compliance, 196
Venous pooling, 215
Venous pressure
  cardiac output and, 196-201
  increases, 166
Venous return, in mild to moderate exercise, 272-273
Venous valves, muscular activity and, 216-217
Ventilation-perfusion ratio, 252
Ventricles, 68
Ventricular conduction, 36-38
Ventricular depolarization, premature, 46
Ventricular diastole, 74-76
Ventricular ejection, 73-74
Ventricular fibrillation, 47-49, 218
Ventricular function, 209-211
Ventricular function curves, 97-98, 281
Ventricular hypertrophy, 44

Ventricular pressure curves, 66
Ventricular receptor reflexes, 94-95
Ventricular systole, 73-74
Ventricular tachycardia, 47, 213
Ventricular volume, end-diastolic, in Frank-Starling relationship, 56
Ventricular walls in newborn, 264
Verapamil, 18
Videodensitometry, in coronary blood flow measurement, 224
Viscera, in vascular reflexes, 189
Viscosity, 118-119, 120
  anomalous and apparent, 126
  hematocrit ratio and, 126-128
  shear rate and, 129-130
Viscous drag, 126
V_m, 11-15, 18-21, 23-24
Voltage clamping, 10
Voltage-dependent phenomenon, 13
Volume
  blood, 4
    arterial blood pressure and, 140
    cardiac output and, 207-208
    vascular function curve and, 201-202
  end-diastolic, 56, 65
  pressure and, left ventricular, 75
  residual, 74
  stroke, 66, 97
    atrial pacing and, 212
    cardiac output and, 83, 140
    pulse pressure and, 144-146
Volume flow, 113
Volume-pressure relationship for aorta, 137, 139-140
Volume-pressure relationship/loop, left ventricular, 75-76
$\dot{V}O_{2max}$, 274, 275
Vulnerable period, 47

W

Wall tension, 155-156
Water
  capillaries and, 162-167
  renal conservation of, in hemorrhage, 279
Waterfall effect, 252
Willis circle, 244
Windkessels, 135
Wolff-Parkinson-White syndrome, 33
Work; see also Exercise
  cardiac oxygen consumption and, 233-234

Z

Z line, 55, 61